Physical Activity, Physical Fitness, and Exercise Interventions for Preserving Human Health and Preventing and Treating Chronic Conditions across the Lifespan

Physical Activity, Physical Fitness, and Exercise Interventions for Preserving Human Health and Preventing and Treating Chronic Conditions across the Lifespan

Editor

Alberto Soriano-Maldonado

MDPI • Basel • Beijing • Wuhan • Barcelona • Belgrade • Manchester • Tokyo • Cluj • Tianjin

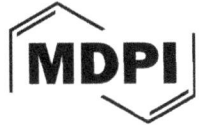

Editor
Alberto Soriano-Maldonado
University of Almería
Spain

Editorial Office
MDPI
St. Alban-Anlage 66
4052 Basel, Switzerland

This is a reprint of articles from the Special Issue published online in the open access journal *International Journal of Environmental Research and Public Health* (ISSN 1660-4601) (available at: https://www.mdpi.com/journal/ijerph/special_issues/physical_activity_fitness).

For citation purposes, cite each article independently as indicated on the article page online and as indicated below:

LastName, A.A.; LastName, B.B.; LastName, C.C. Article Title. *Journal Name* **Year**, *Volume Number*, Page Range.

ISBN 978-3-0365-2500-6 (Hbk)
ISBN 978-3-0365-2501-3 (PDF)

© 2021 by the authors. Articles in this book are Open Access and distributed under the Creative Commons Attribution (CC BY) license, which allows users to download, copy and build upon published articles, as long as the author and publisher are properly credited, which ensures maximum dissemination and a wider impact of our publications.

The book as a whole is distributed by MDPI under the terms and conditions of the Creative Commons license CC BY-NC-ND.

Contents

About the Editor vii

Preface to "Physical Activity, Physical Fitness, and Exercise Interventions for Preserving Human Health and Preventing and Treating Chronic Conditions across the Lifespan" ix

Jonas Verbrugghe, Dominique Hansen, Christophe Demoulin, Jeanine Verbunt, Nathalie Anne Roussel and Annick Timmermans
High Intensity Training Is an Effective Modality to Improve Long-Term Disability and Exercise Capacity in Chronic Nonspecific Low Back Pain: A Randomized Controlled Trial
Reprinted from: *Int. J. Environ. Res. Public Health* **2021**, *18*, 10779, doi:10.3390/ijerph182010779 . 1

Osama Abdelkarim, Julian Fritsch, Darko Jekauc and Klaus Bös
Examination of Construct Validity and Criterion-Related Validity of the German Motor Test in Egyptian Schoolchildren
Reprinted from: *Int. J. Environ. Res. Public Health* **2021**, *18*, 8341, doi:10.3390/ijerph18168341 . . . 13

Sergio Sola-Rodríguez, José Antonio Vargas-Hitos, Blanca Gavilán-Carrera, Antonio Rosales-Castillo, José Mario Sabio, Alba Hernández-Martínez, Elena Martínez-Rosales, Norberto Ortego-Centeno and Alberto Soriano-Maldonado
Relative Handgrip Strength as Marker of Cardiometabolic Risk in Women with Systemic Lupus Erythematosus
Reprinted from: *Int. J. Environ. Res. Public Health* **2021**, *18*, 4630, doi:10.3390/ijerph18094630 . . . 23

Lin Chi, Chiao-Ling Hung, Chi-Yen Lin, Tai-Fen Song, Chien-Heng Chu, Yu-Kai Chang and Chenglin Zhou
The Combined Effects of Obesity and Cardiorespiratory Fitness Are Associated with Response Inhibition: An ERP Study
Reprinted from: *Int. J. Environ. Res. Public Health* **2021**, *18*, 3429, doi:10.3390/ijerph18073429 . . . 35

Dauda Salihu, Eliza M. L. Wong and Rick Y. C. Kwan
Effects of an African Circle Dance Programme on Internally Displaced Persons with Depressive Symptoms: A Quasi-Experimental Study
Reprinted from: *Int. J. Environ. Res. Public Health* **2021**, *18*, 843, doi:10.3390/ijerph18020843 . . . 49

Elena Martínez-Rosales, Sergio Sola-Rodríguez, José Antonio Vargas-Hitos, Blanca Gavilán-Carrera, Antonio Rosales-Castillo, Alba Hernández-Martínez, Enrique G. Artero, José Mario Sabio and Alberto Soriano-Maldonado
Heart Rate Variability in Women with Systemic Lupus Erythematosus: Association with Health-Related Parameters and Effects of Aerobic Exercise
Reprinted from: *Int. J. Environ. Res. Public Health* **2020**, *17*, 9501, doi:10.3390/ijerph17249501 . . . 67

Jiangang Chen, Yuan Zhou, Xinliang Pan, Xiaolong Li, Jiamin Long, Hui Zhang and Jing Zhang
Associations between Health-Related Physical Fitness and Cardiovascular Disease Risk Factors in Overweight and Obese University Staff
Reprinted from: *Int. J. Environ. Res. Public Health* **2020**, *17*, 9031, doi:10.3390/ijerph17239031 . . . 81

Ahmad Salman and Patrick Doherty
Is Weight Gain Inevitable for Patients Trying to Quit Smoking as Part of Cardiac Rehabilitation?
Reprinted from: *Int. J. Environ. Res. Public Health* **2020**, *17*, 8565, doi:10.3390/ijerph17228565 . . . 91

Eduardo Vásquez-Araneda, Rodrigo Ignacio Solís-Vivanco, Sandra Mahecha-Matsudo, Rafael Zapata-Lamana and Igor Cigarroa
Characteristics of Physical Exercise Programs for Older Adults in Latin America: A Systematic Review of Randomized Controlled Trials
Reprinted from: *Int. J. Environ. Res. Public Health* **2021**, *18*, 2812, doi:10.3390/ijerph18062812 . . . **103**

Waleska Reyes-Ferrada, Luis Chirosa-Rios, Angela Rodriguez-Perea, Daniel Jerez-Mayorga and Ignacio Chirosa-Rios
Isokinetic Trunk Strength in Acute Low Back Pain Patients Compared to Healthy Subjects: A Systematic Review
Reprinted from: *Int. J. Environ. Res. Public Health* **2021**, *18*, 2576, doi:10.3390/ijerph18052576 . . . **131**

Daniel Sur, Shanthi Sabarimurugan and Shailesh Advani
The Effects of Martial Arts on Cancer-Related Fatigue and Quality of Life in Cancer Patients: An Up-to-Date Systematic Review and Meta-Analysis of Randomized Controlled Clinical Trials
Reprinted from: *Int. J. Environ. Res. Public Health* **2021**, *18*, 6116, doi:10.3390/ijerph18116116 . . . **145**

About the Editor

Alberto Soriano-Maldonado, PhD, Associate Professor at the University of Almería, Spain. The research activities of Dr. Soriano-Maldonado are focused on understanding the role of physical fitness and exercise interventions on the health status of individuals with several chronic conditions including rheumatological and cardiovascular diseases, obesity and cancer. He has published over 95 articles in international journals indexed in the Journal of Citation Reports. Dr. Soriano-Maldonado has participated in over 20 research projects and has been the principal investigator of two funded projects in Spain. He currently is the director of the SPORT Research Group (CTS-1024) at the University of Almería.

Preface to "Physical Activity, Physical Fitness, and Exercise Interventions for Preserving Human Health and Preventing and Treating Chronic Conditions across the Lifespan"

Increasing global physical activity levels is one of the most important public health goals of the 21st century. Physically active individuals present better sleep patterns, increased wellbeing and quality of life, as well as better physical function and fitness levels. In addition, physical activity might stimulate brain function and improve both cognition and mental health. The risk of many chronic diseases is also reduced in physically active individuals, and physical activity might counteract the detrimental metabolic effects of long sedentary periods.

Physical fitness is not only a key marker of health in healthy individuals, but in people with chronic conditions. Compelling evidence indicates that low levels of both cardiorespiratory fitness and muscular strength are associated with an increased risk of morbidity and premature mortality for a variety of causes, including cardiovascular diseases and cancer. Consequently, preserving fitness levels throughout life is a major clinical and public health interest.

Exercise interventions represent the most efficient form of physical activity to enhance physical fitness and improve health outcomes at all ages and chronic statuses. However, exercise prescription in many populations is underdeveloped and further insights are needed for practitioners and the research community to understand how exercise should be administered, depending on the health and clinical status of different populations.

This Special Issue focuses on the influence of fitness and physical activity and the effects of exercise interventions on human health- and disease-related outcomes. This includes, but is not restricted to, the following article types:

- Observational studies assessing the association of physical fitness (alone or in combination with other risks/protective factors) with health- and disease-related outcomes.

- Observational studies assessing the association of physical activity (alone or in combination with other lifestyle behaviors) with health- and disease-related outcomes. *This includes studies assessing physical activity through either objective or subjective means.*

- Experimental studies assessing the effects of exercise interventions (alone or in combination with other interventions) on health- and disease-related outcomes across the lifespan.

- Systematic reviews and meta-analyses on the above-mentioned topics are also welcome.

Alberto Soriano-Maldonado
Editor

Article

High Intensity Training Is an Effective Modality to Improve Long-Term Disability and Exercise Capacity in Chronic Nonspecific Low Back Pain: A Randomized Controlled Trial

Jonas Verbrugghe [1,*], Dominique Hansen [1,2], Christophe Demoulin [3], Jeanine Verbunt [4,5], Nathalie Anne Roussel [6] and Annick Timmermans [1]

1. REVAL—Rehabilitation Research Center, Faculty of Rehabilitation Sciences, Hasselt University, 3590 Diepenbeek, Belgium; dominique.hansen@uhasselt.be (D.H.); Annick.Timmermans@uhasselt.be (A.T.)
2. Heart Centre Hasselt, Jessa Hospital, 3500 Hasselt, Belgium
3. Department of Sport and Rehabilitation Sciences, University of Liege, 4000 Liege, Belgium; christophe.demoulin@uliege.be
4. Adelante Centre of Expertise in Rehabilitation and Audiology, 6432CC Hoensbroek, The Netherlands; jeanine.verbunt@maastrichtuniversity.nl
5. Department of Rehabilitation Medicine, Maastricht University, 6211LK Maastricht, The Netherlands
6. Faculty of Medicine and Health Sciences, University of Antwerp, 2000 Antwerp, Belgium; nathalie.roussel@uantwerpen.be
* Correspondence: jonas.verbrugghe@uhasselt.be; Tel.: +32-11269224

Abstract: Previous research indicates that high intensity training (HIT) is a more effective exercise modality, as opposed to moderate intensity training (MIT), to improve disability and physical performance in persons with chronic nonspecific low back pain (CNSLBP). However, it is unclear how well benefits are maintained after intervention cessation. This study aimed to evaluate the long-term effectiveness of HIT on disability, pain intensity, patient-specific functioning, exercise capacity, and trunk muscle strength, and to compare the long-term effectiveness of HIT with MIT in persons with CNSLBP. Persons with CNSLBP ($n = 35$) who participated in a randomized controlled trial comparing effects of an HIT versus MIT intervention (24 sessions/12 weeks) were included for evaluation at baseline (PRE), directly after (POST), and six months after program finalization (FU) on disability, pain intensity, exercise capacity, patient-specific functioning, and trunk muscle strength. A general linear model was used to evaluate PRE-FU and POST-FU deltas of these outcome measures in each group (time effects) and differences between HIT and MIT (interaction effects). Ultimately, twenty-nine participants (mean age = 44.1 year) were analysed (HIT:16; MIT:13). Six participants were lost to follow-up. At FU, pain intensity, disability, and patient-specific functioning were maintained at the level of POST (which was significant from PRE, $p < 0.05$) in both groups. However, HIT led to a greater conservation of lowered disability and improved exercise capacity when compared with MIT ($p < 0.05$). HIT leads to a greater maintenance of lowered disability and improved exercise capacity when compared to MIT six months after cessation of a 12-week supervised exercise therapy intervention, in persons with CNSLBP.

Keywords: chronic low back pain; exercise therapy; high intensity training

1. Introduction

Chronic nonspecific low back pain (CNSLBP) is a common musculoskeletal disorder affecting many individuals worldwide [1]. It is characterized by fluctuating pain and high levels of functional disability, and consequently has a major impact on activities of daily living, work, and social interactions [2]. As it is thought to have a multi-factorial origin at its base [3], guidelines for CNSLBP highlight the need for a multimodal therapy design [4]. Exercise therapy (ET) is hereby consistently advocated as an important component in management [5,6]. However, while it is presented as the best-evidenced approach, treatment effect sizes in CNSLBP remain only modest [7].

In this regard, a novel ET method, i.e., high intensity training (HIT), has recently been proven to be a feasible and more effective therapy modality than training protocols at moderate intensity in CNSLBP [8,9]. It produces notably greater decreases in functional disability and improves exercise capacity more in the short term [9]. Also, different HIT protocol modalities have been shown to be equally effective to each other in CNSLBP [10]. Indeed, HIT might be better adapted on a physiological level to increase the physical fitness levels in this population [5,11]. Furthermore, these outcomes are in line with studies in other musculoskeletal disorders such as spondyloarthritis or chronic neck pain using various HIT protocols to improve disease specific outcomes such as pain intensity and physical functioning [12,13].

However, CNSLBP by nature often fluctuates over longer periods [14]. As such, recurrences of gradual pain or episodes with increased pain are very common [15,16]. It is thus necessary to obtain a better insight into how exercise-induced benefits directly measured at the cessation of an intervention are retained [17]. While minimal to moderate improvements are observed consistently upon completion of various exercise interventions, these improvements are typically lost over time [18]. Considering this, the ability to maintain the long-term impact of exercise interventions for CNSLBP remains a challenge [18].

The long-term effectiveness of HIT on specific outcomes has been studied in other musculoskeletal populations, such as improving walking speed in persons with knee osteoarthritis and aerobic fitness and functional ability in rheumatoid arthritis [19,20]. However, currently, no data are available on retention effects of HIT on therapy outcomes in rehabilitation of persons with CNSLBP. Because of the better short-term results by HIT on disability and exercise capacity versus MIT, it is expected that HIT leads to a better retaining of these benefits after cessation of intervention in the long-term, when compared with MIT.

Therefore, the aim of this study is (1) to evaluate long-term effectiveness of HIT on disability, pain intensity, patient-specific functioning, exercise capacity, and trunk muscle strength, and (2) to compare long-term effectiveness of HIT with MIT in persons with CNSLBP.

2. Materials and Methods

2.1. Trial Design

This exploratory study is part of a larger trial that evaluated the effects of training intensity and training mode in CNSLBP rehabilitation through a prospectively registered, five-arm, RCT organized at REVAL (Hasselt University, Diepenbeek, Belgium). The current article evaluates the effectiveness of HIT in comparison to MIT at six months of follow-up. A comprehensive research design flowchart is displayed in Figure 1. This project was approved by the Medical Ethics Committee of Jessa Hospital (Hasselt, Belgium) and registered at clinicaltrials.gov as NCT02911987.

2.2. Participants and Recruitment

Participants were recruited through local study advertisements in Limburg (Belgium). To be eligible, persons had to speak Dutch, be 25–60 years old, and have medically diagnosed CNSLBP [21,22]. Persons were excluded when they had a history of spinal fusion, had a musculoskeletal disorder aside from CNSLBP that could affect the execution of the therapy program, had co-morbidities (e.g., paresis and/or sensory disturbances by neurological causes), were pregnant, had ongoing compensation claims and/or a work disability >six months, had followed an exercise intervention for low back pain in the past three months, or were not able to attend regular therapy appointments. Interested persons received a patient information letter and were invited for an intake session. During that session, the information letter was reviewed, study inclusion and exclusion criteria were evaluated, the informed consent was signed, and a study specific screening form concerning red flags for low back pain rehabilitation was filled out.

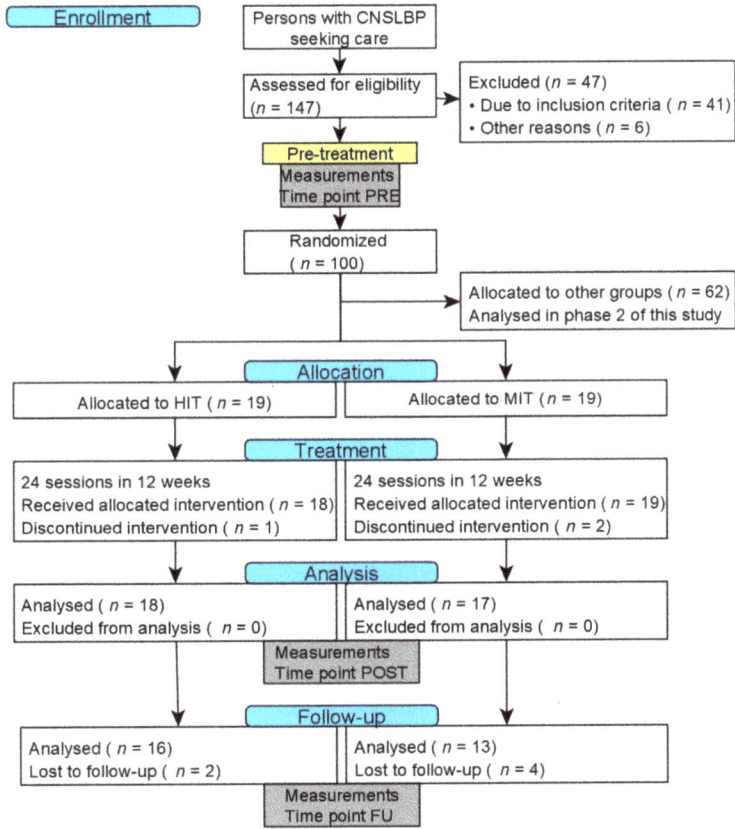

Figure 1. CONSORT flowchart of the research design. Abbreviations: CNSLBP: chronic nonspecific low back pain; HIT: High intensity training; MIT: moderate intensity training.

2.3. Randomization and Blinding

Participants were randomly assigned to an experimental group ('HIT') performing a high intensity training program, or a control group ('MIT') performing the same training program at moderate intensity. To ensure concealment of allocation, a research assistant not involved in the study picked a sealed, opaque envelope containing the allocated group for each participant. Given the nature of the exercise intervention it was not possible to blind the participants and physiotherapists for group assignment. To limit the performance bias of the participants, the study was described to the participants as 'a comparison between different modes of exercise therapy treatment'.

2.4. Interventions

Participants of both groups were enrolled in a 12-week exercise therapy program consisting of 24 supervised individual therapy sessions (2 × 1.5 h/week). The training protocols have been published more extensively previously [9].

Experimental group ('HIT'): This group performed a protocol consisting of cardiorespiratory training, general resistance training, and core muscle training, all at high intensity (see also Table 1).

Cardiorespiratory training consisted of an interval protocol on a cycle ergometer containing five high intensity one-minute bouts (110 revolutions per minute (RPM) at 100% of the VO_2 max workload achieved during the maximal cardiopulmonary exercise test, separated by one minute of active recovery (75 RPM at 50% of the same VO_2 max workload). High intensity bouts increased every two sessions by 10". Recovery time between bouts remained stable. This protocol was repeated from session 13 to 24 with an updated workload, based on the results from a complementary cardiopulmonary exercise test.

General resistance training consisted of three upper and three lower body exercises executed on fitness devices. A one repetition maximum (1 RM) testing [23] was performed for each exercise. One set of a maximum of twelve repetitions was performed at 80% 1 RM for each exercise. Researchers progressively increased the exercise weight when the participant was able to perform more than 10 repetitions on two consecutive training sessions.

Core strength training consisted of six static core exercises. Exercises were chosen as a function of their ability to load the core muscles at an intensity of at least 40–60% of the maximum voluntary contraction [24]. Participants performed one set of ten repetitions of a ten second static hold. Participants were encouraged to hold the last repetition as long as possible. Exercises were made more difficult by increasing the static hold time and progressing to a more demanding posture when they were executed with a stable core posture for the indicated time by the participant on two consecutive training sessions.

Control group ('MIT'): This group performed a protocol consisting of cardiorespiratory training, general resistance training, and core muscle training, all at moderate intensity (see also Table 1).

Cardiorespiratory training consisted of a continuous training protocol on a cycle ergometer containing 14 min of cycling (90 RPM at 60% VO_2 max workload). Duration increased every two sessions with 1 min 40 s up to 22 min 40 s. This protocol was repeated from sessions 13 to 24 with an updated workload, extracted from a complementary cardiopulmonary exercise test.

General resistance training was identical to the HIT protocol with the exception of the exercise intensity. One set of 15 repetitions was performed at 60% of 1 RM.

Core training was identical to the HIT protocol with the exception of the exercise intensity. Participants performed one set of 10 repetitions of a 10 s static hold. Exercises were made more difficult when they were executed with a stable core posture for the indicated time by increasing the time of the static hold each six sessions.

Table 1. Overview of the content of the intervention program for the experimental (HIT) and control (MIT) group.

Training Modalities	HIT	MIT
Cardiorespiratory protocol	Interval cycling protocol at 100% VO_2 max	Continuous cycling protocol at 50–60% VO_2 max
General resistance protocol	Three upper and three lower body exercises at 80% 1 RM	Three upper and three lower body exercises at 60% 1 RM
Core strength protocol	Six static core exercises at an intensity of at least 40–60% MVC until failure	Six static core exercises at an intensity of up to 40% MVC

Abbreviations: VO_2 max: maximal oxygen uptake; 1 RM: one repetition maximum; MVC: maximum voluntary contraction.

2.5. Testing Procedure and Outcomes

The following baseline participant characteristics were collected: gender, age (years), weight (kg), and height (cm), to calculate BMI, time of onset of CNSLBP (years, months), fear of movement (Tampa Scale for Kinesiophobia), and physical activity (Physical Activity Scale for Individuals with Physical Disabilities) [25,26]. Outcome measures are described below and were collected at baseline ('PRE'), at the end of the intervention program ('POST'), and six months after cessation of the intervention program ('FU'). At POST, participants were only advised to stay active and were not assisted or tracked in any way. They were not aware they would be invited for a test six months later.

Disability level—The Modified Oswestry Disability Index (MODI) evaluates CNSLBP-related disability and consists of 10 items scored on a five-point scale [27]. Total score is expressed in percentage of disability (higher is more) and displays a degree of functional limitation.

Pain intensity—The Numeric Pain Rating Score (NPRS) evaluates average pain intensity in the previous six-week period by choosing a number of the 0–10 scale (0 means no pain and 10 means worst pain imaginable) [28].

Patient-specific functioning—The Patient-Specific Functioning Scale (PSFS) evaluates individual-specific functioning [29]. Participants state three to five of the most relevant activities compromised due to physical disability and rate them on a 0–10 numeric rating scale (0 means unable to perform and 10 means able to perform at preinjury level). An overall mean percentage is calculated.

Exercise capacity—A maximal cardiopulmonary exercise test (75 RPM) on an electronically braked cycle ergometer (eBike Basic, General Electric GmbH, Frankfurt am Main, Germany) evaluates exercise capacity through maximal oxygen uptake (VO_2 max) and maximal workload through cycling time (min.) [30]. Participants started at a low workload that gradually increased each minute (♂: 30 W + 15 W/min, ♀: 20 W + 10 W/min). Supplementary, respiratory exchange ratio (RER) and heart rate were determined through breath-by-breath gas exchange analysis (MetaMax 3B, Cortex Medical, Leipzig, Germany) and heartrate monitoring (Polar, Kempele, Finland).

Trunk muscle strength—A maximal isometric muscle strength test of the trunk flexors and extensors using an isokinetic dynamometer (System 3, Biodex, Enraf-Nonius [31]) evaluates peak torque of trunk flexors and extensors during three maximal repetitions of isometric trunk flexion and trunk extension [32]. Peak torque was expressed in Newton meter (Nm) and normalized to bodyweight (Nm/kg).

2.6. Data Analysis

JMP Pro (12.0, SAS Institute Inc., Cary, NC, USA) was used for data analysis. A sample size calculation was performed to detect differences in the primary outcome measure (disability measured by the MODI) between the groups at POST in the primary analysis [9], resulting in a total needed amount of $n = 34$ ($n = 17$ per group). A post-hoc observed power analysis was performed to confirm the specific power for each evaluated outcome measure in the current analysis. Descriptive statistics were used to display baseline group characteristics. Normality and homoscedasticity of each primary outcome were checked by fitting a general linear model of the PRE-FU and POST-FU deltas and plotting the residuals to look for equal variance, symmetry, and identify possible outliers. A general linear model (MANOVA) was used to evaluate the PRE-FU and POST-FU deltas of each outcome measure in each group and the differences between the HIT and MIT group (interaction effect). An alpha level of 0.05 (two-tailed) was used. Percentage improvement of PRE-FU deltas was calculated to evaluate minimal clinically important differences [33]. Regarding the drop-outs, no imputation of data was performed, under the assumption that data were missing at random. However, to check for selective drop-out, differences between participants completing the trial and drop-outs were examined (independent *t*-tests, Mann-Whitney U tests, X^2 tests).

3. Results

3.1. Recruitment and Baseline Data

Thirty-eight participants were included in the initial PRE-POST analysis (HIT: $n = 19$, MIT: $n = 19$). Significantly more women (69%) were included. Mean age was 44.1 years (SD = 9.8) and mean pain onset was 11.7 years (SD = 7.7). Both study groups had similar demographics, clinical characteristics, and outcome measures at baseline ($p > 0.05$), except for trunk extensor strength (higher in the HIT group). Nonetheless, all treatment effects were adjusted for these baseline estimates. An overview of the patient characteristics at baseline is displayed in Table 2.

Table 2. Demographic and clinical characteristics of participants at baseline ($n = 38$).

Variables	HIT ($n = 19$)	MIT ($n = 19$)	p-Value
Gender (m/f)	6/13	6/13	1.000
Age (y)	44.3 (8.8)	44.0 (11.0)	0.769
Symptom duration (y)	11.8 (8.4)	10.3 (7.1)	0.268
BMI (kg/m^2)	25.6 (4.0)	25.9 (3.6)	0.609
PASIPD, 0–199	16.5 (10.6)	14.9 (11.7)	0.637
TSK, 17–68	32.0 (6.0)	34.7 (7.2)	0.218

Categorical variables are expressed as number, continuous variables are expressed as mean (SD). Abbreviations: m/f: male/female; y: years; kg: kilograms; m: meters; PASIPD: The Physical Activity Scale for Individuals with Physical Disabilities; TSK: Tampa Scale for Kinesiophobia.

3.2. Intervention and Follow-Up Drop-Outs

During the intervention phase, three drop-outs were noted (HIT: $n = 1$, MIT: $n = 2.8\%$ of all participants from PRE to POST). During the six-month follow-up phase, another six drop-outs (HIT: $n = 2$, MIT: $n = 4.17\%$ of all participants from POST to FU) were noted. Of these, three participants reported practical issues and three participants did not report any reason for drop-out. No differences in baseline characteristics were found between drop-outs with or without reasons, or drop-outs and other participants. Finally, 29 participants were included in the FU analysis (corresponding to a 24% drop-out in total). No adverse events were noted during this study.

3.3. Outcomes at the 6-Month Follow-Up Assessment

An overview of the results is presented in Table 3.

MODI outcomes remained significantly lower compared to PRE in both groups (−13.0 points, 62% improvement in HIT; −5.8 points, 36% improvement in MIT). No significant difference was found from POST to FU in either group. A significant difference of 3.6 points was found in the deltas of PRE to FU between groups.

NPRS outcomes remained significantly lower compared to PRE in both groups (−3.3 points, 59% improvement in HIT; −2.7 points, 54% improvement in MIT). A significant decrease was also found from POST to FU in MIT, but not in HIT. No significant difference was found in the deltas of PRE to FU between groups.

PSFS outcomes remained significantly higher compared to PRE in both groups (+26%, +57% improvement in HIT; +36%, +90% improvement in MIT). No significant difference was found from POST to FU in either group nor in the deltas of PRE to FU between groups.

VO$_2$ max remained significantly higher compared to PRE in HIT (3.1 mL/kg/min, 10% improvement), but not in MIT (no improvement at FU). No significant difference was found from POST to FU in either group. A significant difference of 3.2 mL/kg/min was found in the deltas of PRE to FU between groups.

Abdominal muscle strength did not improve compared to PRE in both groups (0.05 Nm/kg, 4% improvement in HIT; 0.03 Nm/kg, 2% improvement in MIT). Back muscle strength remained significantly better compared to PRE in in MIT (0.34 Nm/kg, 13% improvement), but not in HIT (0.19 Nm/kg, 6% improvement). No significant difference was found from POST to FU in either group nor in the deltas of PRE to FU between groups in both outcomes.

Table 3. Results of the outcome measures collected from participants at PRE, POST, and FU together with between group differences and post hoc power calculations at FU).

n = 29	HIT (n = 16)			MIT (n = 13)			Interaction at FU (T0-FU)	
Outcome Measures	PRE	POST	FU	PRE	POST	FU	DOD	Power
Primary								
Disability								
MODI, %	20.9 (8.7)	7.5 (5.4) *	7.9 (8.4) *	16.2 (8.2)	10.6 (3.0) *	10.4 (9.6) *	3.6 **	0.52
Pain intensity								
NPRS, 0–10	5.6 (1.5)	2.6 (1.3) *	2.3 (2.1) *	5.0 (1.7)	3.5 (1.7) *	2.3 (1.1) *,†	0.5	0.09
Secondary								
Function								
PSFS, %	46 (18)	71 (15) *	72 (13) *	40 (14)	67 (17) *	76 (15) *	10	0.22
Exercise capacity								
VO$_2$ max, mL/kg/min	30.6 (6.8)	35.7 (6.8) *	33.7 (6.5) *	31.6 (7.6)	32.5 (6.3)	31.6 (7.2)	3.2 **	0.61
Relative Muscle strength								
Abdominal, Nm/kg	1.38 (0.28)	1.43 (0.31)	1.43 (0.24)	1.26 (0.37)	1.29 (0.33)	1.29 (0.37)	0.02	0.06
Back, Nm/kg	3.28 (0.82)	3.53 (0.86) *	3.47 (0.84)	2.58 (0.61)	2.87 (0.76) *	2.92 (0.91) *	0.15	0.11

Values in HIT and MIT are reported as mean (standard deviation) and represent results of the Numeric Pain Rating Scale (NPRS), Modified Oswestry Disability Index (MODI), Patient-Specific Functioning Scale (PSFS), a cardiopulmonary exercise capacity test, and a maximum isometric muscle strength test of the abdominals and back, before (PRE) and after (POST) 24 sessions of high intensity training (HIT, 100% VO$_2$ max interval cardio training + >80% 1 RM general resistance training + >60% MVC core strength training) or moderate intensity training (MIT, 50–60% VO$_2$ max cardio training + 60% 1 RM general resistance training + 20–40% MVC core strength training). Delta displays the post-pre difference. Abbreviations: DOD: difference of deltas of PRE to FU in HIT compared to MIT; CI: 95% confidence interval. * $p < 0,05$ compared to PRE. † $p < 0.05$ compared to POST. ** $p < 0.05$ HIT compared to MIT.

4. Discussion

This study was the first to evaluate the long-term effects of HIT in CNSLBP. Results show that initial positive therapy effects at the finalization of the therapy program were retained for all outcomes until at least six months later, as no differences could be found between POST and FU results. Furthermore, improvements since baseline on disability level and exercise capacity remained clinically relevant and remained significantly larger in the HIT than in the MIT group at FU [27,34]. These results corroborate the effectiveness of HIT as a working therapeutic modality in the rehabilitation of CNSLBP.

The evaluation of long-term effects of ET studies in CNSLBP has been incorporated in systematic review analyses [5,7]. However, there is still a paucity of pooled data due to heterogeneous ET protocols. Furthermore, FITT-VP principles of exercise prescription (i.e., frequency, intensity, time, and type—volume and progression [35]) are often insufficiently defined, making it even more difficult to evaluate the impact of these program methodology characteristics on therapy success [5]. Only three other studies were found with a clear description of training intensity and a comparison between ET protocols in CNSLBP. Firstly, Michaelson et al. (2016) depicted no differences between a high and low load training program at 12 or 24 months follow-up [36]. However, in this article, the magnitude of the load was actually based on an analysis of volume rather than intensity. Besides, an indirect estimation of intensity was made, and no clear objective test was performed to show the actual percentage (e.g., 1 RM testing). Secondly, both Harts et al. (2004) and Helmhout et al. (2008) evaluated the difference between a high and low intensity lumbar extensor program [37,38]. Neither found differences between exercise intensities in the short nor the long term. However, these studies reflected on the use of a very specific strength training mode focused solely on the rationale of restoring back muscle function. Also, training volume was significantly lower, and the high intensity protocols that were used (ranging from 35% 1 RM to max. 70% 1 RM in the HIT group) did not meet the standards used in the present analysis (80% 1 RM strength training).

In the current study, significant differences were noted between PRE and FU in both the experimental HIT and the control MIT group, indicating the effective longevity of ET as a therapy modality. However, no additional improvements from POST to FU were found in either group. This result supports the outcomes of previous research showing that patients who present with low back pain often improve markedly in the first six weeks of rehabilitation therapy. After that, improvement often slows down [18]. This process can even be magnified after cessation of the therapy program. Low to moderate levels of pain and disability are frequently still present at one year after cessation of therapy, especially in the cohorts with persistent pain [39]. It should be noted that the sample in our study already showed low pain intensity (HIT: 2.6/10; MIT: 3.5/10) and disability level (HIT: 7.5/100; MIT: 10.6/100) at POST, which would make further significant improvements very hard to achieve. The only significant difference found from POST to FU was a pain intensity decrease in MIT (3.5/10 to 2.3/10), but not in HIT (2.6/10 to 2.3/10). Thus, while at first glance this might look like an important outcome to support the long-term application of MIT, this difference was actually due to the faster decrease in HIT already achieved at POST (i.e., during the therapy phase). As such, HIT seems to be able to lower pain intensity more quickly. As this was only evaluated with a subjective measure in this study, future research could try to incorporate more objective measures to improve our understanding of pain and pain processing such as pain pressure thresholds through quantitative sensory testing [40,41].

As participants did still display residual pain at FU, adaptations to further optimize the HIT modality should also be investigated. Following current clinical guidelines [6], the authors believe HIT should be incorporated in a multimodal therapy design, as this might stimulate the impact on other factors related to CNSLBP [6]. As such, HIT can be coupled with other important therapy modalities such as delivery of (pain) education and evaluation of and adaptation of therapy to individual therapy goals [42,43]. In addition, further research towards the predictors for therapy success is needed.

4.1. Limitations

Limitations of the initial RCT methodology have been discussed previously [9]. Nonetheless, some limitations specifically related to this follow-up analysis should be mentioned. Firstly, because the follow-up analysis was a secondary analysis, study group sample sizes were not initially designed for long-term follow-up. However, even with low power (as measured in a post-hoc analysis), significant results were found in this study, supporting its outcomes. Furthermore, the depicted MODI and VO_2 max outcomes were still in line with the results from the short-term analysis (that were fully powered). As such, we believe these outcomes to give a fair representation of the expected outcomes in a fully powered sample. Secondly, a follow-up of only six months was performed, which might be low for evaluating the effects of an intervention on long term health behavior. Other research has shown that, up to two years, the same outcomes might be expected but later a regression might occur if behaviors are not changed [44]. However, as this was the first study to evaluate HIT at follow-up, we chose a measurement point at which we expected loss to follow-up would still be manageable (to ensure proper statistical analysis). It is not yet clear whether continuing to perform HIT protocols after a rehabilitation program is needed to retain results beyond six months. Thirdly, physical activity might be a confounder in the maintaining of results during the period between POST and FU. The absence of any longitudinal data related to physical activity performed by the participants might therefore have caused a performance bias when comparing between participants. Indeed, keeping up regular physical activity and adhering to specific exercise programs after the rehabilitation phase have been noted to support therapy success and prevent reoccurrence of chronic low back pain in the long term [45,46]. Besides, multiple psychosocial factors such as perceived stress, self-efficacy, and patients' perceptions about back pain have also been found to predict development and chronification of low back pain [47,48]. As such, future research should emphasize more on incorporating these factors and evaluating their mediating effects. Fourthly, nine participants dropped out during the course of the protocol from PRE to FU. Results of these persons might have been less favorable. However, no significant differences in baseline characteristics were found between these drop-outs and the included patients. Moreover, no claims with regard to a CNSLBP-related cause to abort the protocol were made by any participant.

4.2. Future Recommendations

To be able to provide guidelines, better insights on the working mechanism of this therapy modality are needed. It is still unclear whether HIT improves outcomes due to its increased physical demands and the accompanied physiological factors such as improved muscle characteristics and anti-inflammatory factors, or other non-physiological factors such as increased self-efficacy or fear of movement [49,50].

5. Conclusions

High intensity training is an effective therapy modality to decrease disease-specific and physical performance related outcomes in the long term in CNSLBP. Moreover, at six months after cessation, HIT shows greater improvements in disability and exercise capacity than an equal exercise therapy program performed at moderate intensity. Future research is needed to evaluate the exact working mechanisms of this therapy modality and optimize therapy protocols.

Author Contributions: A.T., D.H. and J.V. (Jonas Verbrugghe) were involved in both the design of the follow-up study and the protocols for the assessments. J.V. (Jonas Verbrugghe) supervised the communication with the patients and performed the practical planning and execution of the assessments, as well as the data processing and statistical analysis. A.T., D.H., C.D., N.A.R., J.V. (Jeanine Verbunt) and J.V. (Jonas Verbrugghe) were involved in the interpretation of the results. J.V. (Jonas Verbrugghe) wrote the manuscript with substantial contributions to the conception, the design and the drafting of the manuscript of all authors via substantive feedback and textual corrections. All authors have read and agreed to the published version of the manuscript.

Funding: This project was funded by the UHasselt research fund BOF New initiatives (project number R-5211).

Institutional Review Board Statement: The study was conducted according to the guidelines of the Declaration of Helsinki, and approved by the Medical Ethics Committee of Jessa Hospital (Hasselt, Belgium) (protocol code: 15.142/REVA15.14).

Informed Consent Statement: Informed consent was obtained from all subjects involved in the study.

Data Availability Statement: The data that support the findings of this study are available on request from the corresponding author [JoV]. The data are not publicly available due to restrictions i.e., their containing information that could compromise the privacy of research participants.

Acknowledgments: The authors would like to express their gratitude to F. Vandenabeele, A. Agten, and Sjoerd Stevens from the Faculty of Rehabilitation Sciences of UHasselt, for their contribution to the conceptualisation of, and/or data-collection within the original RCT study [9,10]. The authors would like to thank all the persons with CNSLBP that participated in this study.

Conflicts of Interest: The authors declare no conflict of interest. The funders had no role in the design of the study; in the collection, analyses, or interpretation of data; in the writing of the manuscript, or in the decision to publish the results.

References

1. Manchikanti, L.; Singh, V.; Falco, F.J.E.; Benyamin, R.M.; Hirsch, J.A. Epidemiology of Low Back Pain in Adults. *Neuromodulation* **2014**, *17*, 3–10. [CrossRef] [PubMed]
2. Hartvigsen, J.; Hancock, M.; Kongsted, A.; Louw, Q.; Ferreira, M.L.; Genevay, S.; Hoy, D.; Karppinen, J.; Pransky, G.; Sieper, J.; et al. What low back pain is and why we need to pay attention. *Lancet* **2018**, *391*, 2356–2367. [CrossRef]
3. Maher, C.; Underwood, M.; Buchbinder, R. Non-specific low back pain. *Lancet* **2017**, *389*, 736–747. [CrossRef]
4. Vlaeyen, J.W.S.; Maher, C.G.; Wiech, K.; van Zundert, J.; Meloto, C.B.; Diatchenko, L.; Battié, M.C.; Goosens, M.; Koes, B.; Linton, S.J. Low back pain. *Nat. Rev. Dis. Primers* **2018**, *4*, 52. [CrossRef] [PubMed]
5. Searle, A.; Spink, M.; Ho, A.; Chuter, V. Exercise interventions for the treatment of chronic low back pain: A systematic review and meta-analysis of randomised controlled trials. *Clin. Rehabil.* **2015**, *29*, 1155–1167. [CrossRef]
6. Oliveira, C.B.; Maher, C.G.; Pinto, R.Z.; Traeger, A.C.; Lin, C.-W.C.; Chenot, J.-F.; van Tulder, M.; Koes, B.W. Clinical practice guidelines for the management of non-specific low back pain in primary care: An updated overview. *Eur. Spine J.* **2018**, *27*, 2791–2803. [CrossRef] [PubMed]

7. van Middelkoop, M.; Rubinstein, S.M.; Verhagen, A.P.; Ostelo, R.; Koes, B.; van Tulder, M.W. Exercise therapy for chronic nonspecific low-back pain. *Best Pract. Res. Clin. Rheumatol.* **2010**, *24*, 193–204. [CrossRef] [PubMed]
8. Verbrugghe, J.; Agten, A.; Eijnde, B.O.; Olivieri, E.; Huybrechts, X.; Seelen, H.; Vandenabeele, F.; Timmermans, A. Feasibility of high intensity training in nonspecific chronic low back pain: A clinical trial. *J. Back Musculoskelet. Rehabil.* **2018**, *31*, 657–666. [CrossRef]
9. Verbrugghe, J.; Agten, A.; Stevens, S.; Hansen, D.; Demoulin, C.; Eijnde, B.O.; Vandenabeele, F.; Timmermans, A. Exercise Intensity Matters in Chronic Nonspecific Low Back Pain Rehabilitation. *Med. Sci. Sports Exerc.* **2019**, *51*, 2434–2442. [CrossRef]
10. Verbrugghe, J.; Agten, A.; Stevens, S.; Hansen, D.; Demoulin, C.; Eijnde, B.O.; Vandenabeele, F.; Timmermans, A. High Intensity Training to Treat Chronic Nonspecific Low Back Pain: Effectiveness of Various Exercise Modes. *J. Clin. Med.* **2020**, *9*, 2401. [CrossRef]
11. Meng, X.-G.; Yue, S.-W. Efficacy of aerobic exercise for treatment of chronic Low back pain: A meta-analysis. *Am. J. Phys. Med. Rehabil.* **2015**, *94*, 358–365. [CrossRef]
12. Sveaas, S.H.; Bilberg, A.; Berg, I.J.; Provan, S.A.; Rollefstad, S.; Semb, A.G.; Hagen, K.B.; Johansen, M.W.; Pedersen, E.; Dagfinrud, H. High intensity exercise for 3 months reduces disease activity in axial spondyloarthritis (axSpA): A multicentre randomised trial of 100 patients. *Br. J. Sports Med.* **2020**, *54*, 292–297. [CrossRef]
13. Zebis, M.K.; Andersen, L.L.; Pedersen, M.T.; Mortensen, P.; Andersen, C.H.; Pedersen, M.M.; Boysen, M.; Roessler, K.K.; Hannerz, H.; Mortensen, O.S.; et al. Implementation of neck/shoulder exercises for pain relief among industrial workers: A randomized controlled trial. *BMC Musculoskelet. Disord.* **2011**, *12*, 205. [CrossRef]
14. Lemeunier, N.; Leboeuf-Yde, C.; Gagey, O. The natural course of low back pain: A systematic critical literature review. *Chiropr. Man. Ther.* **2012**, *20*, 33. [CrossRef]
15. Macedo, L.G.; Maher, C.G.; Latimer, J.; McAuley, J.H.; Hodges, P.W.; Rogers, W.T. Nature and Determinants of the Course of Chronic Low Back Pain Over a 12-Month Period: A Cluster Analysis. *Phys. Ther.* **2014**, *94*, 210–221. [CrossRef]
16. Verkerk, K.; Luijsterburg, P.A.J.; Heymans, M.; Ronchetti, I.; Pool-Goudzwaard, A.L.; Miedema, H.S.; Koes, B.W. Prognosis and Course of Disability in Patients with Chronic Nonspecific Low Back Pain: A 5- and 12-Month Follow-up Cohort Study. *Phys. Ther.* **2013**, *93*, 1603–1614. [CrossRef]
17. Glette, M.; Stiles, T.C.; Borchgrevink, P.C.; Landmark, T. The Natural Course of Chronic Pain in a General Population: Stability and Change in an Eight-Wave Longitudinal Study Over Four Years (the HUNT Pain Study). *J. Pain* **2020**, *21*, 689–699. [CrossRef] [PubMed]
18. Beattie, P.F.; Silfies, S. Improving Long-Term Outcomes for Chronic Low Back Pain: Time for a New Paradigm? *J. Orthop. Sports Phys. Ther.* **2015**, *45*, 236–239. [CrossRef] [PubMed]
19. Waller, B.; Munukka, M.; Rantalainen, T.; Lammentausta, E.; Nieminen, M.; Kiviranta, I.; Kautiainen, H.; Häkkinen, A.; Kujala, U.; Heinonen, A. Effects of high intensity resistance aquatic training on body composition and walking speed in women with mild knee osteoarthritis: A 4-month RCT with 12-month follow-up. *Osteoarthr. Cartil.* **2017**, *25*, 1238–1246. [CrossRef] [PubMed]
20. De Jong, Z.; Munneke, M.; Kroon, H.M.; Van Schaardenburg, D.; Dijkmans, B.A.C.; Hazes, J.M.W.; Vlieland, T.V. Long-term follow-up of a high-intensity exercise program in patients with rheumatoid arthritis. *Clin. Rheumatol.* **2009**, *28*, 663–671. [CrossRef] [PubMed]
21. Balagué, F.; Mannion, A.F.; Pellise, F.; Cedraschi, C. Non-specific low back pain. *Lancet* **2012**, *379*, 482–491. [CrossRef]
22. Airaksinen, O.; Brox, J.I.; Cedraschi, C.; Hildebrandt, J.; Klaber-Moffett, J.; Kovacs, F.; Mannion, A.F.; Reis, S.; Staal, B.; Ursin, H.; et al. Chapter 4 European guidelines for the management of chronic nonspecific low back pain. *Eur. Spine J.* **2006**, *15*, s192–s300. [CrossRef] [PubMed]
23. Pescatello, L.S.; Riebe, D.; Thompson, P.D. *ACSM's Guidelines for Exercise Testing and Prescription*; Lippincott Williams & Wilkins: Philadelphia, PA, USA, 2014.
24. DiGiovine, N.M.; Jobe, F.W.; Pink, M.; Perry, J. An electromyographic analysis of the upper extremity in pitching. *J. Shoulder Elb. Surg.* **1992**, *1*, 15–25. [CrossRef]
25. Swinkels-Meewisse, E.J.C.M.; Swinkels, R.A.H.M.; Verbeek, A.L.M.; Vlaeyen, J.W.S.; Oostendorp, R.A.B. Psychometric properties of the Tampa Scale for kinesiophobia and the fear-avoidance beliefs questionnaire in acute low back pain. *Man. Ther.* **2003**, *8*, 29–36. [CrossRef] [PubMed]
26. Washburn, R.A.; Zhu, W.; McAuley, E.; Frogley, M.; Figoni, S.F. The physical activity scale for individuals with physical disabilities: Development and evaluation. *Arch. Phys. Med. Rehabil.* **2002**, *83*, 193–200. [CrossRef] [PubMed]
27. Fairbank, J.C.T.; Pynsent, P.B. The Oswestry Disability Index. *Spine* **2000**, *25*, 2940–2953. [CrossRef] [PubMed]
28. Hawker, G.A.; Mian, S.; Kendzerska, T.; French, M.R. Measures of adult pain: Visual Analog Scale for Pain (VAS Pain), Numeric Rating Scale for Pain (NRS Pain), McGill Pain Questionnaire (MPQ), Short-Form McGill Pain Questionnaire (SF-MPQ), Chronic Pain Grade Scale (CPGS), Short Form-36 Bodily Pain Scale (SF-36 BPS), and Measure of Intermittent and Constant Osteoarthritis Pain (ICOAP). *Arthritis Care Res.* **2011**, *63*, S240–S252. [CrossRef]
29. Horn, K.K.; Jennings, S.; Richardson, G.; Van Vliet, D.; Hefford, C.; Abbott, J.H. The Patient-Specific Functional Scale: Psychometrics, Clinimetrics, and Application as a Clinical Outcome Measure. *J. Orthop. Sports Phys. Ther.* **2012**, *42*, 30–42. [CrossRef] [PubMed]
30. Medicine ACoS. *ACSM's Guidelines for Exercise Testing and Prescription*; Lippincott Williams & Wilkins: Philadelphia, PA, USA, 2013.

31. Biodex Medical Systems, Inc. *Dual Position Back Ex/Flex Attachment Operation Manual*; Biodex Medical Systems, Inc: Shirley, NY, USA.
32. Verbrugghe, J.; Agten, A.; Eijnde, B.O.; Vandenabeele, F.; De Baets, L.; Huybrechts, X.; Timmermans, A. Reliability and agreement of isometric functional trunk and isolated lumbar strength assessment in healthy persons and persons with chronic nonspecific low back pain. *Phys. Ther. Sport* **2019**, *38*, 1–7. [CrossRef]
33. Ostelo, R.W.; Deyo, R.A.; Stratford, P.; Waddell, G.; Croft, P.; Von Korff, M.; Bouter, L.M.; de Vet Henrica, C. Interpreting change scores for pain and functional status in low back pain: Towards international consensus regarding minimal important change. *Spine* **2008**, *33*, 90–94. [CrossRef]
34. Myers, J.; Prakash, M.; Froelicher, V.; Do, D.; Partington, S.; Atwood, J.E. Exercise Capacity and Mortality among Men Referred for Exercise Testing. *N. Engl. J. Med.* **2002**, *346*, 793–801. [CrossRef] [PubMed]
35. Riebe, D.; Franklin, B.A.; Thompson, P.D.; Garber, C.E.; Whitfield, G.P.; Magal, M.; Pescatello, L.S. Updating ACSM's Recommendations for Exercise Preparticipation Health Screening. *Med. Sci. Sports Exerc.* **2015**, *47*, 2473–2479. [CrossRef] [PubMed]
36. Michaelson, P.; Holmberg, D.; Aasa, B.; Aasa, U. High load lifting exercise and low load motor control exercises as interventions for patients with mechanical low back pain: A randomized controlled trial with 24-month follow-up. *J. Rehabil. Med.* **2016**, *48*, 456–463. [CrossRef] [PubMed]
37. Helmhout, P.H.; Harts, C.C.; Staal, J.B.; Candel, M.J.J.M.; De Bie, R.A. Comparison of a high-intensity and a low-intensity lumbar extensor training program as minimal intervention treatment in low back pain: A randomized trial. *Eur. Spine J.* **2004**, *13*, 537–547. [CrossRef] [PubMed]
38. Harts, C.C.; Helmhout, P.H.; De Bie, R.A.; Staal, J.B. A high-intensity lumbar extensor strengthening program is little better than a low-intensity program or a waiting list control group for chronic low back pain: A randomised clinical trial. *Aust. J. Physiother.* **2008**, *54*, 23–31. [CrossRef]
39. Costa, L.D.C.M.; Maher, C.G.; Hancock, M.; McAuley, J.; Herbert, R.; Costa, L. The prognosis of acute and persistent low-back pain: A meta-analysis. *Can. Med. Assoc. J.* **2012**, *184*, E613–E624. [CrossRef]
40. Treede, R.-D. The role of quantitative sensory testing in the prediction of chronic pain. *Pain* **2019**, *160*, S66–S69. [CrossRef]
41. Uddin, Z.; MacDermid, J.C. Quantitative Sensory Testing in Chronic Musculoskeletal Pain. *Pain Med.* **2016**, *17*, 1694–1703. [CrossRef]
42. Malfliet, A.; Ickmans, K.; Huysmans, E.; Coppieters, I.; Willaert, W.; Van Bogaert, W.; Rheel, E.; Bilterys, T.; Van Wilgen, P.; Nijs, J. Best Evidence Rehabilitation for Chronic Pain Part 3: Low Back Pain. *J. Clin. Med.* **2019**, *8*, 1063. [CrossRef]
43. Tegner, H.; Frederiksen, P.; Esbensen, B.A.; Juhl, C. Neurophysiological Pain Education for Patients with Chronic Low Back Pain. *Clin. J. Pain* **2018**, *34*, 778–786. [CrossRef]
44. Toobert, D.J.; Strycker, L.A.; Barrera, M.; Glasgow, R.E. Seven-year follow-up of a multiple-health-behavior diabetes intervention. *Am. J. Health Behav.* **2010**, *34*, 680–694. [CrossRef]
45. Cecchi, F.; Pasquini, G.; Paperini, A.; Boni, R.; Castagnoli, C.; Pistritto, S.; Macchi, C. Predictors of response to exercise therapy for chronic low back pain: Result of a prospective study with one year follow-up. *Eur. J. Phys. Rehabil. Med.* **2014**, *50*, 143–151. [PubMed]
46. Shiri, R.; Falah-Hassani, K. Does leisure time physical activity protect against low back pain? Systematic review and meta-analysis of 36 prospective cohort studies. *Br. J. Sports Med.* **2017**, *51*, 1410–1418. [CrossRef]
47. Puschmann, A.-K.; Drießlein, D.; Beck, H.; Arampatzis, A.; Catalá, M.M.; Schiltenwolf, M.; Mayer, F.; Wippert, P.-M. Stress and Self-Efficacy as Long-Term Predictors for Chronic Low Back Pain: A Prospective Longitudinal Study. *J. Pain Res.* **2020**, *13*, 613–621. [CrossRef]
48. Chen, Y.; Campbell, P.; Strauss, V.Y.; Foster, N.E.; Jordan, K.; Dunn, K.M. Trajectories and predictors of the long-term course of low back pain: Cohort study with 5-year follow-up. *Pain* **2018**, *159*, 252–260. [CrossRef] [PubMed]
49. Fernandes, I.M.D.C.; Pinto, R.; Ferreira, P.; Lira, F.S. Low back pain, obesity, and inflammatory markers: Exercise as potential treatment. *J. Exerc. Rehabil.* **2018**, *14*, 168–174. [CrossRef] [PubMed]
50. Poon, E.T.-C.; Sheridan, S.; Chung, A.P.-W.; Wong, S.H.-S. Age-specific affective responses and self-efficacy to acute high-intensity interval training and continuous exercise in insufficiently active young and middle-aged men. *J. Exerc. Sci. Fit.* **2018**, *16*, 106–111. [CrossRef] [PubMed]

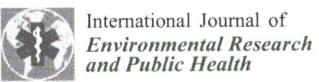

Article

Examination of Construct Validity and Criterion-Related Validity of the German Motor Test in Egyptian Schoolchildren

Osama Abdelkarim [1,2,*], Julian Fritsch [1], Darko Jekauc [1] and Klaus Bös [1]

1. Institute of Sports and Sports Science, Karlsruhe Institute of Technology, 76131 Karlsruhe, Germany; julian.fritsch@kit.edu (J.F.); darko.jekauc@kit.edu (D.J.); klaus.boes@kit.edu (K.B.)
2. Faculty of Physical Education, Assiut University, Assiut 71515, Egypt
* Correspondence: osama.abdelkarim@kit.edu

Citation: Abdelkarim, O.; Fritsch, J.; Jekauc, D.; Bös, K. Examination of Construct Validity and Criterion-Related Validity of the German Motor Test in Egyptian Schoolchildren. *Int. J. Environ. Res. Public Health* **2021**, *18*, 8341. https://doi.org/10.3390/ijerph18168341

Academic Editor: Alberto Soriano-Maldonado

Received: 9 May 2021
Accepted: 22 July 2021
Published: 6 August 2021

Publisher's Note: MDPI stays neutral with regard to jurisdictional claims in published maps and institutional affiliations.

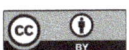

Copyright: © 2021 by the authors. Licensee MDPI, Basel, Switzerland. This article is an open access article distributed under the terms and conditions of the Creative Commons Attribution (CC BY) license (https://creativecommons.org/licenses/by/4.0/).

Abstract: Physical fitness is an indicator for children's public health status. Therefore, the aim of this study was to examine the construct validity and the criterion-related validity of the German motor test (GMT) in Egyptian schoolchildren. A cross-sectional study was conducted with a total of 931 children aged 6 to 11 years (age: 9.1 ± 1.7 years) with 484 (52%) males and 447 (48%) females in grades one to five in Assiut city. The children's physical fitness data were collected using GMT. GMT is designed to measure five health-related physical fitness components including speed, strength, coordination, endurance, and flexibility of children aged 6 to 18 years. The anthropometric data were collected based on three indicators: body height, body weight, and BMI. A confirmatory factor analysis was conducted with IBM SPSS AMOS 26.0 using full-information maximum likelihood. The results indicated an adequate fit (χ^2 = 112.3, df = 20; p < 0.01; CFI = 0.956; RMSEA = 0.07). The χ^2-statistic showed significant results, and the values for CFI and RMSEA showed a good fit. All loadings of the manifest variables on the first-order latent factors as well as loadings of the first-order latent factors on the second-order superordinate factor were significant. The results also showed strong construct validity in the components of conditioning abilities and moderate construct validity in the components of coordinative abilities. GMT proved to be a valid method and could be widely used on large-scale studies for health-related fitness monitoring in the Egyptian population.

Keywords: physical fitness; construct validity; schoolchildren

1. Introduction

Physical fitness (PF) is classified as a public health indicator affecting physical, mental, and psychological aspects [1–5]. In addition, PF is also suggested to play a vital role in brain functions and learning performance [6–8]. Thus, to effectively combat numerous public health problems, especially childhood obesity, there is a critical need for increasing PF levels among children [9]. In this context, PF should be ideally promoted at a young age in order to avoid long-lasting health problems and possibly improve cognitive functions and mental health [10].

A low level of PF and insufficient physical activity are associated with greater somatic and psychological problems [1,2]. Therefore, increased levels of PF, specifically muscular strength, could have significant benefits for the psychological health of overweight/obese children [11]. In addition, high PF levels are associated with less unfavorable body composition among children with elevated school stress [12]. Moreover, PF is also related to social health, such that the school environment is more conducive to the development of PF for promoting the students' social health [5].

Indeed, PF is usually determined in school-aged children using health-related PF batteries (e.g., field tests) [13]. Therefore, having good criteria for collecting PF data among children and youths is useful for identifying problems or optimizing performances in order to provide intervention programs that develop children's status [14–16]. Indeed, the assessment of PF became a necessary topic in epidemiological studies, since a reduction in

PF is directly associated with the incidence of obesity, coronary heart diseases, diabetes, and hypertension in adults [17–19].

Motor Performance Abilities (MPA)

There is a large body of historical work on the differentiation of motor abilities [20–27]. All approaches are based on the idea that the motor system is a complex, multidimensional construct that cannot be adequately described by one single characteristic. Differentiations of motor abilities are mostly based on the assumption of so-called basic qualities [28] or major forms of physical performance [29] and allow for a sufficiently accurate initial diagnosis and orientation for controlling the exercise load in physical education in the basic training of competitive sports but also in health and rehabilitation sports. However, differentiations according to ability categories are not sufficiently precise for performance explanations and prognoses, for training control at a high performance level, for sport-specific description models, or for disease-specific questions in rehabilitation. Here, diagnoses require a more process- and function-oriented approach with the help of sports-medicine or biomechanical measurement methods.

According to Bös and Mechling [30], MPA is on a first level differentiated according to the poles of energy and information into physical (energetic) and coordinative (information-oriented) abilities. On a second level, there is a breakdown into the much-cited "basic motor qualities" of endurance, strength, speed, coordination, and flexibility. The assignment of endurance and strength abilities to the energetically determined functional processes results from the distinction between the cardiovascular system and the skeletal muscles as central systems of energy production and energy transport in the human organism. The extent, the mass, and the structure of skeletal muscle are considered prerequisites for strength performance. The performance of the cardiovascular system represents determining and limiting variables for endurance performance.

In this context, the German motor test (GMT) [31] was developed as an objective tool to measure a complete fitness profile involving speed, endurance, strength, coordination under precision demands, coordination under time pressure, and flexibility [32,33]. The test battery was designed to be easily used in sports gym for physical examination. The content-related validity of all test items was consistently rated as good in terms of significance and feasibility based on expert ratings.

In Egypt, the health-related fitness components of schoolchildren were not sufficiently studied in recent decades, which negatively affects any intervention strategies, plans, or programs. Currently, it is useful for educational settings, parents, clinicians, and sports organizations to have valid and reliable health-related fitness data about children. In this context, this test could be used in Egypt as a data-collection tool for identifying problems or excellent performance in the field of public health, talent identification, exercise pediatric, and epidemiological studies [9,11,14–16].

Indeed, providing a valid and reliable tool for measuring health-related fitness components is very helpful for long-term and sustainable development of sport and health ecosystems in Egypt. Therefore, the aim of this study was to examine the construct validity and the criterion-related validity of the German motor test in Egyptian children aged 6 to 11 years.

2. Materials and Methods

2.1. Study Design and Sampling

A cross-sectional study was conducted between 2014 and 2017 at 13 public primary schools in the city of Assiut, which is the largest town in upper Egypt and is located about 234 miles south of Cairo. The size of the primary-school student population aged 6 to 11 years in Assiut is about 76,334 students. The total number of public schools is 69, distributed in 7 districts. The final sample was randomly selected from the chosen schools and consisted of 931 children aged 6 to 11 years (age: 9.1 ± 1.7 years) with 484 (52%) males and 447 (48%) females in grades 1 to 5 of primary schools in Assiut.

Precisely, the test development was based on an international expert survey involving 40 selected fitness experts in 25 European countries who were asked about the relevance of the test contents and requirements in sport-motor tests with respect to MPA documentation [34]. Subsequently, 13 experts evaluated the significance and the practicality of the study exercises on a scale of 1 (very good) to 5 (very bad). The evaluations in both regions were found to be within a good range ($M_{Significance}$ = 1.9; $M_{Practicality}$ = 1.7). To determine test–retest reliability, the motor tests were performed twice within 4 days on the same children using the same test situation and the same study investigator. All in all, there were good test–retest reliability coefficients (R_{min} = 0.74 to R_{max} = 0.96).

2.2. Data Collection

2.2.1. Anthropometric Characteristics Data

Assessment of the anthropometric characteristics of the children was based on three indicators: body height, body weight, and BMI. The instruments were calibrated according to the standard preparation prior to measurement. Measurements were taken with schoolchildren wearing light clothing and no shoes. Body weight was measured with a beam balance to the nearest 0.1 kg. Body height was measured with a stadiometer to the nearest 0.5 cm. BMI was defined as the ratio of body weight to body height squared, expressed in kg/m. Subjects were classified as underweight, normal weight, and overweight (i.e., overweight and obese) according to the published standards by the International Obesity Task Force based on age and sex difference characteristics [35].

2.2.2. Physical Fitness Data

The German motor test (GMT) was used to measure five health related-physical fitness components of children aged 6 to 18 years [36]. To determine test–retest reliability in the Egyptian sample, the test was performed twice within 7 days with the same children using the same test situation and the same study investigator. Good test–retest reliability coefficients were obtained (R-values between 0.68 and 0.94). The test items were described and performed according to Lämmle et al. [37] and Abdelkarim et al. [38] as the following:

Speed: The 20 m sprint test is used to measure speed ability. The child must cover a distance of 20 m in as short a time as possible in two trials; the best trial is evaluated. The time required for the sprint is measured to the nearest tenth of a second using a stopwatch (the start is from a standing position).

Coordination: Balancing backwards (BB) is used to measure coordination under precision demands. The child must walk backwards over three beams of approximately the same length (300 cm) but different widths (6 cm, 4.5 cm, and 3 cm) in two valid trials while maintaining balance. The goal is to stay on each of the beams, i.e., not miss, during the course of two valid trials. A total of six successful trials are evaluated. The number of steps taken while walking backwards is counted. The variable used for the analysis is the sum of the steps taken during all six trials while walking backwards. Side jumping (JS) is used to measure whole-body coordination under time pressure, speed, and muscular endurance of the lower extremities. The child must jump sideways across the center line of the carpet mat with both legs at the same time as fast as possible without exceeding the given field size (50–100 cm). Two trials of 15 s each are performed. The recovery time between the trials is 1 min. The number of jumps made during the two trials is evaluated, and the average of the two trials is analyzed.

Strength: Push-ups (PU) and sit-ups (SU) are used to measure dynamic muscular endurance of the upper extremities and the abdominal muscles, respectively. The child is asked to perform as many push-ups or sit-ups as possible in two trials of 40 s each. The starting position of the push-ups is the lying position with hands clasped behind the back. The second position is the raised position of the standard push-up (i.e., with arms extended). In the third position, one hand touches the top of the hand of the supporting arm before returning to the starting position. The average of the two attempts is used. The standing long jump (SLJ) test is used to measure the jumping strength and the spring strength of the leg muscles. The test person jumps with both legs and tries to reach the greatest possible distance. The propulsion may only be increased by swinging the arms, but it is not allowed to reach back with one or both hands. The distance (in cm) from the starting line to the heel of the foot behind when landing is measured. The best of two jumps is used for analysis.

Endurance: A six-minute running test is used to measure aerobic endurance. The child is asked to run around a volleyball court as many times as possible within six minutes. The measurement for each child is the distance in meters covered within six minutes. The length of the path is the number of laps (1 lap = 54 m) plus the distance covered in the last lap.

Flexibility: The stand-and-reach (SR) test is used to measure trunk flexibility and the elasticity of back and leg muscles. The test person stands on a wooden box and slowly bends forward at the waist. The arms and the hands must reach down as far as possible with the legs extended. The better of two trials is noted in centimeters.

2.3. Statistical Analysis

A confirmatory factor analysis was conducted with IBM SPSS AMOS 26. (IBM Corp.: Armonk, NY, USA) [39] using full-information maximum likelihood, which has the advantage that, when models with missing values are computed, the estimates are less biased than when classical methods such as listwise deletion, pairwise deletion, or mean imputation are used to handle missing values [40]. A five-factor structure with a global factor of physical fitness was assessed. The assessment of global goodness-of-fit was based on several fit indices. First, a non-significant p-value in the χ^2-statistic indicates a good model fit [41]. However, this test depends on the sample size, and even minor differences between the implied model and the observed covariance matrix led to significant results [42].

Second, the comparative fit index (CFI) shows the relative fit improvement by comparing the proposed model with the baseline model. Cut-off values for CFI are desirable above 0.95 and adequate above 0.90 [43]. Third, the root mean square error of approximation (RMSEA) describes the error of approximation in the population. RMSEA values are adequate below 0.08 and desirable below 0.05 [44]. To examine criterion-related validity, the relationship between physical fitness and children's BMI was assessed using bivariate correlations. For that purpose, a dummy variable was created to compare children who are classified as overweight or obese with those not classified as such [35]. Separate models were estimated for each calculation of bivariate correlations between the dummy variable and the latent variables.

3. Results

3.1. Descriptive Statistics

Table 1 contains raw score means, standard deviations, and correlations between all test indicators. The correlation coefficient between test items was easily demonstrated. The highest correlation coefficient values were shown between the 20 m sprint test and the long jump test (R = −0.67). On the other hand, the lowest correlation coefficient was demonstrated between the 6 min run and flexibility (R = 0.08), which is classified as a passive system of energy transfer. However, significant correlations between the 6 min run test and the test items related to strength ability were shown (R_{pushup} = 0.30, R_{situp} = 0.42, and $R_{longjump}$ = 0.46). There was also a strong correlation between the test item for the 20 m sprint and the test items for push-ups (R = 0.39), sit-ups in 40 s (R = 0.50), and the long jump (R = −0.67), respectively. The test items measuring coordination ability (jumping sideways, balancing backwards) showed a moderate significant correlation with the test items measuring sprint and strength ability. High correlations were shown between the jumping sideways test item and the 20 m sprint (R = −0.51), the long jump (R = 0.47), the push-ups (R = 0.43), and the sit-ups in 40 s (R = 0.40).

Table 1. Descriptive statistics.

	M	SD	Run	Spr	Pup	Sit	Lgj	Jsw	Bbw	Fbt
Run	7840.19	1690.42	1							
Spr	40.66	00.63	−0.43 **	1						
Pup	90.77	40.64	0.30 **	−0.39 **	1					
Sit	140.54	70.44	0.42 **	−0.50 **	0.46 **	1				
Lgj	1110.12	260.06	0.46 **	−0.67 **	0.42 **	0.54 **	1			
Jsw	230.16	70.48	0.36 **	−0.51 **	0.43 **	0.40 **	0.47 **	1		
Bbw	260.66	110.04	0.26 **	−0.27 **	0.25 **	0.27 **	0.38 **	0.26 **	1	
Fbt	−20.90	60.76	0.08 *	−0.12 **	0.15 **	0.16 **	0.18 **	0.13 **	0.20 **	1

* $p < 0.05$; ** $p < 0.01$; M = mean; SD = standard deviation; run = 6-min run; spr = 20-m-sprint; pup = push-ups; sit = sit-ups in 40 s; lgj = long jump; jsw = jumping sideways; bbw = balancing backwards; fbt = forward bending.

3.2. Construct Validity

Bös and Mechling's model [30] was presented in (Figure 1) as a structural equation model. The dimensions of endurance, coordination under time pressure, coordination with precision demands, and flexibility were operationalized with one item each. The strength dimension included four indicators. The superordinate dimension was motor performance ability (see Figure 2). The results of the model indicated an adequate fit (χ^2 = 112.3, df = 20, $p < 0.01$; CFI = 0.956; RMSEA = 0.07). Although the χ^2-statistic showed significant results, the values of CFI and RMSEA showed a good fit. All loadings of the manifest variables on the first-order latent factors and the loadings of the first-order latent factors on the second-order superordinate factor were significant.

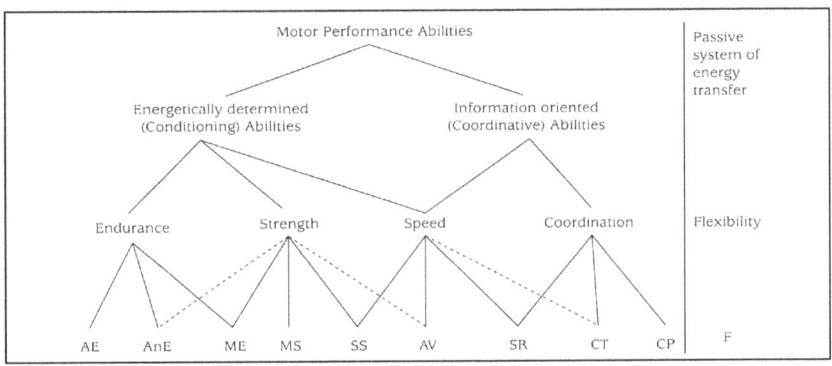

Figure 1. Motor performance abilities [30]. AE = aerobic endurance; AnE = anaerobic endurance; ME = muscular endurance; MS = maximum strength; SS = speed strength; AV = action velocity; SR = speed of response; CT = coordination under time pressure; CP = coordination with precision demands; F = flexibility.

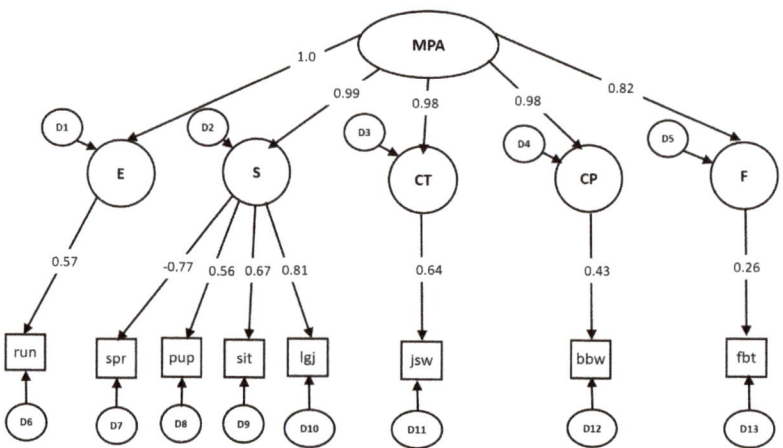

Figure 2. MPA = motor performance ability; E = endurance; S = strength; CT = coordination under time pressure; CP = coordination with precision demands; F = flexibility; run = 6 min run; spr = 20 m sprint; pup = push-ups; sit = sit-ups in 40 s; lgj = long jump; jsw = jumping sideways; M; fbt = forward bending of the trunk.

3.3. Criterion-Related Validity

Regarding BMI, we used a variable comparing children classified as overweight or obese with those not classified as such. This variable correlated significantly with endurance (R = −0.22, Z = −4.58, $p < 0.01$), coordination with precision demands (R = −0.40, Z = −5.98, $p < 0.01$), and overall motor performance ability (R = −0.16, Z = −4.66, $p < 0.01$) but not with flexibility (R = 0.04, Z = 0.34, $p = 0.73$) or strength (R = −0.04, Z = −1.51, $p = 0.13$). Interestingly, contrary to our expectations, the results showed that time pressure was positively correlated with BMI (R = 0.17, Z = 4.19, $p < 0.01$).

4. Discussion

Construct validity and criterion-related validity of the German motor test (GMT) were studied in Egyptian schoolchildren. The results of the confirmatory factorial analysis showed a good fit of Bös and Mechling's model [30] for the structure of motor performance abilities with good values for CFI and RMSEA. The criterion validity coefficient was acceptable for the majority of the test items. GMT showed strong construct validity in the components of energetically determined (conditioning) abilities including cardiorespiratory capacity (endurance), muscle strength, and speed. However, the test showed moderate construct validity in the components of information-oriented (coordinative) abilities including coordination with precision demands and coordination under time pressure.

The results showed a good construct validity with high significant values for the loading of the test items. The second-order factor was based on the five first-order factors of endurance, strength, coordination under time pressure, coordination with precision demands, and flexibility. The results suggested comparable results to other studies using the same test battery [36,45]. In addition, the current results confirmed the previous results of another test battery consisting of a combination of speed, endurance, strength, coordination, and flexibility that were shown to be valid, functional, and easy to administer for measuring children's physical fitness in different European populations in the same age groups [16,46].

The results also showed high loadings for the test items for strength, coordination with precision demands, and coordination under time pressure. These high loadings point to the potential of these test items as indicators of performance level [37]. In contrast, the loading of flexibility showed the lowest loading value. This confirmed the assumption that flexibility is a rather independent dimension (passive system of energy transfer). Moreover, flexibility shows a general deterioration in performance with age growing in both genders, especially in girls [47].

Indeed, the validity of the German motor test (GMT) in Egyptian children confirms the importance of measuring the levels of PF based on quantitative measurements such as anthropometric data and health-related fitness batteries [48,49]. These types of measurements are more practical, motivating, and provide an accurate overview of fitness levels, especially in the child population. In addition, the association between physical fitness and body mass index was shown to provide an indication of test validity, especially in prepubertal school children [38,50]. However, greater effort and logistical support are needed for data collection in large-scale studies [17,51,52].

This study provides an economical and objective data collection tool to increase the possibility of national representative studies for health-related physical fitness in Egypt. The tests included in the tool can help to provide an overview about Egyptian children's rate of involvement in physical activity. PF provides objective data which could predict the rate of participation in physical activity. Guthold et al. [53] point out that nationally representative data for physical activity using scientific measurements, such as accelerometers, are only available for high-income countries. Low-income countries, mainly in the Middle East and North Africa, had a very low proportion of available data with the estimated overall percentage of insufficient physical activity reaching 32%. Here, the WHO recommendation on physical activity and sedentary behavior should be strongly considered to achieve benefits in children and adolescents for improved physical fitness (cardiorespiratory and muscular fitness), cardiometabolic health (blood pressure, glucose, and insulin resistance), bone health, cognitive outcomes (academic performance, executive function), mental health (reduced symptoms of depression), and reduced obesity [54].

5. Conclusions

The German motor test (GMT) was shown to be a valid method for measuring PF in children in Egypt. This valid tool for data collection opens a large window for researchers to use in large-scale studies monitoring health-related fitness components in the fields of epidemiology, talent identification, and health-related educational studies. However, larger and representative samples are needed to establish reference standards in Egyptian children to correctly interpret the results of such tests by generating sex- and age-specific normative percentile values to be available for comparative studies and to establish a national database and fitness profile for the Egyptian population.

Author Contributions: Conceptualization, O.A. and K.B.; methodology, D.J.; software, J.F.; validation, O.A., D.J. and K.B.; formal analysis, J.F.; investigation, O.A.; resources, O.A.; data curation, D.J.; writing—original draft preparation, O.A.; writing—review and editing, J.F.; visualization, D.J.; supervision, K.B.; project administration, O.A.; funding acquisition, K.B. All authors have read and agreed to the published version of the manuscript.

Funding: This research received no external funding.

Institutional Review Board Statement: The study was conducted according to the guidelines of the Declaration of Helsinki, and approved from the Institutional Review Board of Assiut University as a part from (DAAD project ID: 57078220 in 2014).

Informed Consent Statement: Informed consent was obtained from all subjects involved in the study.

Data Availability Statement: The data presented in this study are available on request from the corresponding author. The data are not publicly available due to technical issue.

Conflicts of Interest: The authors declare no conflict of interest.

References

1. Poitras, V.J.; Gray, C.E.; Borghese, M.M.; Carson, V.; Chaput, J.; Janssen, I.; Katzmarzyk, P.T.; Pate, R.R.; Gorber, S.C.; Kho, M.E.; et al. Systematic review of the relationships between objectively measured physical activity and health indicators in school-aged children and youth. *Appl. Physiol. Nutr. Metab.* **2016**, *41*, 197–239. [CrossRef] [PubMed]
2. Baceviciene, M.; Jankauskiene, R.; Emeljanovas, A. Self-perception of physical activity and fitness is related to lower psychosomatic health symptoms in adolescents with unhealthy lifestyles. *BMC Public Health* **2019**, *23*, 980. [CrossRef]
3. Thomas, E.; Bianco, A.; Tabacchi, G.; Marques da Silva, C.; Loureiro, N.; Basile, M.; Giaccone, M.; Sturm, D.J.; Şahin, F.N.; Güler, Ö.; et al. Effects of a Physical Activity Intervention on Physical Fitness of schoolchildren: The Enriched Sport Activity Program. *Int J. Environ. Res. Public Health* **2020**, *17*, 1723. [CrossRef] [PubMed]
4. Mora-Gonzalez, J.; Esteban-Cornejo, I.; Cadenas-Sanchez, C.; Migueles, J.H.; Rodriguez-Ayllon, M.; Molina-García, P.; Hillman, C.H.; Catena, A.; Pontifex, M.B.; Ortega, F.B. Fitness, physical activity, working memory, and neuroelectric activity in children with overweight/obesity. *Scand. J. Med. Sci. Sports* **2019**, *29*, 1352–1363. [CrossRef] [PubMed]
5. Fernández-Bustos, J.G.; Pastor-Vicedo, J.C.; González-Martí, I.; Cuevas-Campos, R. Physical Fitness and Peer Relationships in Spanish Preadolescents. *Int. J. Environ. Res. Public Health* **2020**, *17*, 1890. [CrossRef] [PubMed]
6. Chaddock, L.; Pontifex, M.; Hillman, C.; Kramer, A.F. A Review of the Relation of Aerobic Fitness and Physical Activity to Brain Structure and Function in Children. *J. Int. Neuropsychol. Soc.* **2011**, *17*, 975–985. [CrossRef]
7. Hillman, C.H.; Kamijo, K.; Scudder, M. A review of chronic and acute physical activity participation on neuroelectric measures of brain health and cognition during childhood. *Prev. Med.* **2011**, *52*, S21–S28. [CrossRef] [PubMed]
8. Abdelkarim, O.; Ammar, A.; Chtourou, H.; Wagner, M.; Knisel, E.; Hökelmann, A.; Bös, K. Relationship between motor and cognitive learning abilities among primary school-aged children. *Alex. J. Med.* **2017**, *53*, 325–331. [CrossRef]
9. Chen, W.; Hammond-Bennett, A.; Hypnar, A.; Mason, S. Health-related physical fitness and physical activity in elementary school students. *BMC Public Health* **2018**, *18*, 195. [CrossRef] [PubMed]
10. Esteban-Cornejo, I.; Rodriguez-Ayllon, M.; Román, J.V.; Cadenas-Sanchez, C.; Mora-Gonzalez, J.; Chaddock-Heyman, L.; Raine, L.B.; Stillman, C.M.; Kramer, A.; Erickson, K.I.; et al. Physical Fitness, White Matter Volume and Academic Performance in Children: Findings from the ActiveBrains and FITKids2 Projects. *Front. Psychol.* **2019**, *10*, 208. [CrossRef]
11. Rodriguez-Ayllon, M.; Cadenas-Sanchez, C.; Esteban-Cornejo, I.; Migueles, J.; Mora-Gonzalez, J.; Henriksson, P.; Martín-Matillas, M.; Mena-Molina, A.; Molina-Garcia, P.; Estévez-López, F.; et al. Physical fitness and psychological health in overweight/obese children: A cross-sectional study from the ActiveBrains project. *J. Sci. Med. Sport* **2018**, *21*, 179–184. [CrossRef]
12. Gerber, M.; Endes, K.; Herrmann, C.; Colledge, F.; Brand, S.; Donath, L.; Faude, O.; Pühse, U.; Hanssen, H.; Zahner, L. Fitness, Stress, and Body Composition in Primary Schoolchildren. *Med. Sci. Sports Exerc.* **2017**, *49*, 581–587. [CrossRef]
13. Golle, K.; Muehlbauer, T.; Wick, D.; Granacher, U. Physical Fitness Percentiles of German Children Aged 9–12 Years: Findings from a Longitudinal Study. *PLoS ONE* **2015**, *10*, e0142393.
14. Casonatto, J.; Fernandes, R.A.; Batista, M.B.; Cyrino, E.S.; Coelho-e-Silva, M.J.; de Arruda, M.; Vaz Ronque, E.R. Association between health-related physical fitness and body mass index status in children. *J. Child Health Care* **2016**, *20*, 294–303. [CrossRef] [PubMed]
15. Abdelkarim, O.; Ammar, A.; MA Soliman, A.; Hökelmann, A. Prevalence of overweight and obesity associated with the levels of physical fitness among primary school age children in Assiut city. *Egypt. Pediatr. Assoc. Gaz.* **2017**, *65*, 43–48. [CrossRef]
16. Emeljanovas, A.; Mieziene, B.; Cesnaitiene, V.J.; Fjortoft, I.; Kjønniksen, L. Physical Fitness and Anthropometric Values Among Lithuanian Primary School Children: Population-Based Cross-Sectional Study. *J. Strength Cond. Res.* **2020**, *34*, 414–421. [CrossRef] [PubMed]
17. De Moraes, A.C.F.; Vilanova-Campelo, R.C.; Torres-Leal, F.L.; Carvalho, H.B. Is Self-Reported Physical Fitness Useful for Estimating Fitness Levels in Children and Adolescents? A Reliability and Validity Study. *Medicina* **2019**, *55*, 286. [CrossRef]
18. Eberhardt, T.; Niessner, C.; Oriwol, D.; Buchal, L.; Worth, A.; Bös, K. Secular Trends in Physical Fitness of Children and Adolescents: A Review of Large-Scale Epidemiological Studies Published after 2006. *Int. J. Environ. Res. Public Health* **2020**, *17*, 5671. [CrossRef] [PubMed]
19. Cleven, L.; Krell-Roesch, J.; Nigg, C.R.; Woll, A. The association between physical activity with incident obesity, coronary heart disease, diabetes and hypertension in adults: A systematic review of longitudinal studies published after. *BMC Public Health* **2020**, *20*, 1–15. [CrossRef]
20. Bös, K.; Mechling, H. *International Physical Performance Test Profile for Boys and Girls from 9–17 Years (IPPTP 9–17)*; International Council of Sport Science and Physical Education: Cologne, Germany, 1985.
21. Cratty, B.J. *Motorisches Lernen und Bewegungsverhalten*; Limpert: Bad Homburg, Germany, 1979.
22. Fleishman, E.A. Dimensional analysis of psychomotor abilities. *J. Exp. Psychol.* **1954**, *48*, 437–454. [CrossRef] [PubMed]
23. Guilford, J.P. A System of the Psychomotor Abilities. *Am. J. Psychol.* **1958**, *71*, 164. [CrossRef]
24. Powell, A.; Katzko, M.; Royce, J.R. A Multifactor-Systems Theory of The Structure and Dynamics of Motor Functions. *J. Mot. Behav.* **1978**, *10*, 191–210. [CrossRef] [PubMed]
25. Roth, K. *Strukturanalyse Koordinativer Fähigkeiten*; Limpert: Bad Homburg, Germany, 1982.
26. Fleishman, E.; Quaintance, M.L. *Taxonomies of Human Performance*; Academic Press: New York, NY, USA, 1984.
27. Corbin, C.B. A multidimensional hierarchical model of physical fitness: A basis for integration and collaboration. *Quest* **1991**, *43*, 296–306. [CrossRef]

28. Fetz, F. Motorische Grundeigenschaften. *Leibeserziehung* **1965**, *14*, 200–207.
29. Hollmann, W.; Strüder, H. *Sportmedizin*; Schattauer: Stuttgart, Germany, 2009.
30. Bös, K.; Mechling, H. *Dimensionen Sportmotorischer Leistungen*; Hofmann: Schorndorf, Germany, 1983.
31. Bös, K. *Handbuch Sportmotorischer Tests*; Hogrefe: Göttingen, Germany, 1987.
32. Bös, K.; Worth, A.; Heel, J.; Opper, E.; Romahn, N.; Tittlbach, S.; Wank, V.; Woll, A. *Testmanual des Motorik-Moduls im Rahmen des Kinder und Jugendgesundheitssurveys des Robert Koch-Instituts*; Bundesarbeitsgemeinschaft für Haltungs- und Bewegungsförderung: Wiesbaden, Germany, 2004.
33. Bös, K. *Handbuch Motorischer Tests*; Hogrefe: Göttingen, Germany, 2001.
34. Bös, K. Sport international-the relevance of fitness tests and fitness programs in European countries results from a questionnaire with fitness experts. *Int J. Phys. Educ.* **1992**, *29*, 37–39.
35. Cole, T.J.; Bellizzi, M.C.; Flegal, M.; Dietz, W. Establishing a standard definition for child overweight and obesity worldwide: International survey. *BMJ* **2000**, *320*, 1240. [CrossRef] [PubMed]
36. Bös, K. *German Motor Test 6-18 (DMT 6-18): Manual and Internet-Based Evaluation Software*; Developed by the ad hoc committee [Motor tests for children and young people] of the German Association for Sports Science (dvs); Feldhaus Verlag GmbH+ Co: Hamburg, Germany, 2016.
37. Lämmle, L.; Tittlbach, S.; Oberger, J.; Worth, A.; Bös, K. A two-level model of motor performance ability. *J. Exerc. Sci. Fit.* **2010**, *8*, 41–49. [CrossRef]
38. Abdelkarim, O.; Ammar, A.; Trabelsi, K.; Cthourou, H.; Jekauc, D.; Irandoust, K.; Taheri, M.; Bös, K.; Woll, A.; Bragazzi, N.L.; et al. Prevalence of Underweight and Overweight and Its Association with Physical Fitness in Egyptian Schoolchildren. *Int. J. Environ. Res. Public Health* **2020**, *17*, 75. [CrossRef]
39. Arbuckle, J. *Amos User's Guide: Version 26*; IBM Corp: Armonk, NY, USA, 2019.
40. Jekauc, D.; Völkle, M.; Lämmle, L.; Woll, A. Fehlende Werte in sportwissenschaftlichen Untersuchungen. *Sportwissenschaft* **2012**, *42*, 126–136. [CrossRef]
41. Barrett, P. Structural equation modelling: Adjudging model fit. *Personal. Individ. Dif.* **2007**, *42*, 815–824. [CrossRef]
42. Byrne, B. *Structural Equation Modeling with AMOS: Basic Concepts, Applications, and Programming*; Routledge/Taylor & Francis Group: New York, NY, USA, 2010.
43. Bentler, P.M.; Bonett, D.G. Significance tests and goodness of fit in the analysis of covariance structures. *Psychol. Bull.* **1980**, *88*, 588. [CrossRef]
44. Browne, M.W.; Cudeck, R. Alternative ways of assessing model fit. In *Testing Structural Equation Models*; Bollen, K.A., Long, J.S., Eds.; Sage: Newbury Park, CA, USA, 1993; pp. 136–162.
45. Bös, K.; Schlenker, L.; Büsch, D.; Lämmle, L.; Müller, H.; Oberger, J.; Seidel, I.; Tittlbach, S. *Deutscher Motorik Test 6–18*; Czwalina: Hamburg, Germany, 2009.
46. Fjørtoft, I.; Pedersen, A.V.; Sigmundsson, H.; Vereijken, B. Measuring physical fitness in children who are 5 to 12 years old with a test battery that is functional and easy to administer. *Phys. Ther.* **2011**, *91*, 1087–1095. [CrossRef] [PubMed]
47. Karim, O.A.; Ammar, A.; Chtourou, H.; Wagner, M.; Schlenker, L.; Parish, A.; Gaber, T.; Hökelmann, A.; Bös, K. A Comparative Study of Physical Fitness among Egyptian and German Children Aged Between 6 and 10 Years. *Adv. Phys. Educ.* **2015**, *5*, 7–17. [CrossRef]
48. WHO. *Global Status Report on Noncommunicable Diseases*; WHO/NMH/NVI/15; World Health Organization: Geneva, Switzerland, 2014.
49. Ruiz, J.R.; Castro-Piñero, J.; España-Romero, V.; Artero, E.G.; Ortega, F.B.; Cuenca, M.M.; Jiménez-Pavón, D.; Chillón, P.; Girela-Rejón, M.J.; Mora, J.; et al. Field-based fitness assessment in young people: The ALPHA health-related fitness test battery for children and adolescents. *Br. J. Sports Med.* **2011**, *45*, 518–524. [CrossRef]
50. Federica, F.; Bravo, G.; Parpinel, M.; Messina, G.; Malavolta, R.; Lazzer, S. Relationship between body mass index and physical fitness in Italian prepubertal schoolchildren. *PLoS ONE* **2020**, *15*, e0233362.
51. Lee, P.H.; Macfarlane, D.J.; Lam, T.H.; Stewart, S.M. Validity of the international physical activity questionnaire short form (IPAQ-SF): A systematic review. *Int. J. Behav. Nutr. Phys. Act.* **2011**, *8*, 115. [CrossRef]
52. Armstrong, T.; Fiona, C.B. Development of the world health organization global physical activity questionnaire (GPAQ). *J. Public Health* **2006**, *14*, 66–70. [CrossRef]
53. Guthold, R.; Gretchen, A.S.; Leanne, M.R.; Fiona, C.B. Worldwide trends in insufficient physical activity from 2001 to 2016: A pooled analysis of 358 population-based surveys with 1.9 million participants. *Lancet Glob. Health* **2018**, *6*, e1077–e1086. [CrossRef]
54. WHO. *Guidelines on Physical Activity and Sedentary Behavior*; World Health Organization: Geneva, Switzerland, 2020.

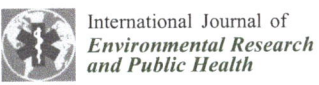

Article

Relative Handgrip Strength as Marker of Cardiometabolic Risk in Women with Systemic Lupus Erythematosus

Sergio Sola-Rodríguez [1,2,*], José Antonio Vargas-Hitos [3], Blanca Gavilán-Carrera [4], Antonio Rosales-Castillo [3], José Mario Sabio [3], Alba Hernández-Martínez [1,2], Elena Martínez-Rosales [1,2], Norberto Ortego-Centeno [5] and Alberto Soriano-Maldonado [1,2]

[1] Department of Education, Faculty of Education Sciences, University of Almería, 04120 Almería, Spain; ahm137@ual.es (A.H.-M.); emr809@ual.es (E.M.-R.); asoriano@ual.es (A.S.-M.)
[2] SPORT Research Group (CTS-1024), CERNEP Research Center, University of Almería, 04120 Almería, Spain
[3] Systemic Autoimmune Diseases Unit, Department of Internal Medicine, Virgen de las Nieves University Hospital, 18014 Granada, Spain; joseantoniovh@hotmail.com (J.A.V.-H.); anrocas90@hotmail.com (A.R.-C.); jomasabio@gmail.com (J.M.S.)
[4] Department of Physical Education and Sport, Faculty of Sport Sciences, University of Granada, 18071 Granada, Spain; bgavilan@ugr.es
[5] Systemic Autoimmune Diseases Unit, Department of Internal Medicine, "San Cecilio" University Hospital, 18016 Granada, Spain; nortego@ugr.es
* Correspondence: sergiosola95@gmail.com; Tel.: +34-675-109-317

Abstract: This study aimed to examine the association of relative handgrip strength (rHGS) with cardiometabolic disease risk factors in women with systemic lupus erythematosus (SLE). Methods: Seventy-seven women with SLE (mean age 43.2, SD 13.8) and clinical stability during the previous six months were included. Handgrip strength was assessed with a digital dynamometer and rHGS was defined as absolute handgrip strength (aHGS) divided by body mass index (BMI). We measured blood pressure, markers of lipid and glucose metabolism, inflammation (high sensitivity C-reactive protein [hs-CRP]), arterial stiffness (pulse wave velocity [PWV]), and renal function. A clustered cardiometabolic risk index (z-score) was computed. Results: Pearson's bivariate correlations revealed that higher rHGS was associated with lower systolic blood pressure (SBP), triglycerides, hs-CRP, PWV, and lower clustered cardiometabolic risk (r_{range} = from -0.43 to -0.23; all $p < 0.05$). Multivariable linear regression analyses adjusted for age, disease activity (SLEDAI), and accrual damage (SDI) confirmed these results (all $p < 0.05$) except for triglycerides. Conclusions: The findings suggest that higher rHGS is significantly associated with lower cardiometabolic risk in women with SLE.

Keywords: autoimmune disease; cardiovascular risk; muscle strength; body mass index; metabolism; cardiovascular disease; lupus; risk factors

1. Introduction

Systemic lupus erythematosus (SLE) is a chronic autoimmune disease marked with a wide variety of organ system dysfunctions, such as damage to joints, lungs, heart, kidneys, brain, blood vessels or skin [1,2]. The SLE prevalence rates are 20 of every 100,000 women [3], and it affects women at a rate of 10:1 more than men [4]. Due to improved diagnostic methods and treatments [5], mortality in SLE patients continues to improve. However, cardiovascular and metabolic diseases are still one of the biggest causes of mortality in SLE [6], and common risk factors cannot fully explain the increased cardiometabolic risk in this population [7].

Traditional cardiometabolic risk factors including hypertension, diabetes, dyslipidemia, and smoking [8,9], and non-traditional cardiometabolic risk factors including abdominal obesity, insulin resistance, lipid profile, arterial stiffness, renal markers, and high-sensitivity C-reactive protein (hs-CRP; as a marker of inflammation [10,11]) levels [8,12,13] are both expensive and difficult to measure outside a clinical environment [14].

Furthermore, patients with SLE are usually treated with corticosteroids, which at high doses interfere with lipid and glycemic metabolism [15].

Muscular strength is reduced in women with SLE [16,17], and low strength levels are associated with higher fatigue, worse quality of life [18], and higher risk of cardiovascular disease and mortality [19,20]. Handgrip strength, a simple and quick method to assess upper body muscular strength, is inversely associated with coronary heart disease [19,21], inflammation (which appears very often in SLE) [22], and mortality risk [23] in the general population. In women with SLE, handgrip strength is negatively related to obesity [13,17,19], and positively associated with quality of life [24].

Relative handgrip strength (rHGS), defined by the summation of both hands' strength divided by body mass index (BMI), is an easy instrument for measuring relative muscular strength in clinical practice and public health [25] and has been recommended in recent research to address the increased strength due to body mass [25–28]. Handgrip strength and BMI have both been linked to cardiometabolic disease risk in the general population [29–32], although the evidence regarding the association of rHGS with cardiometabolic risk in women is scarce [26]. Since rHGS is cost- and time-efficient, it is of clinical interest to understand the extent to which it might be associated with cardiometabolic risk factors in a population at high risk of cardiometabolic diseases, such as women with SLE.

The primary purpose of the current study was to examine the association of rHGS with biomarkers of cardiometabolic disease risk in women with SLE.

2. Materials and Methods

2.1. Design and Participants

In this cross-sectional study, a total of 172 Caucasian patients with SLE were invited to participate. Inclusion criteria were: (i) women aged between 18 and 60 years with (ii) >4 SLE classification criteria provided by the American College of Rheumatology [33]; (iii) a minimum follow-up of one year at our unit; and (iv) clinical stability (i.e., the absence of changes in the systemic lupus erythematosus disease activity index (SLEDAI) and/or treatment) during the previous 6 months. Exclusion criteria were: (i) not being able to read, understand, and/or sign the informed consent; (ii) having cancer; (iii) history of clinical cardiovascular disease and/or lung disease in the last year; and (iv) receiving doses of biological treatment higher than 10 mg/d of prednisone (or equivalent) in the previous 6 months. All participants received detailed information about the study aims and procedures and signed informed consent before being included in the study.

2.2. Measurement of Relative Handgrip Strength

Muscular strength was assessed through the handgrip strength test. The handgrip strength test [34] was assessed using a digital dynamometer (Model T.K.K.540®; Takei Scientific Instruments Co., Ltd., Niigata, Japan) with a precision to the nearest 0.1 kg. Participants performed the trial in a standing position, with the elbow fully extended and the arm relaxed in a neutral position and were encouraged by the evaluators to exert to their maximal effort during a couple of seconds, alternating between the two hands. Participants performed the test twice with a one-minute break between the two attempts of each hand. The aHGS was summed from the best score of each hand. The rHGS was defined as aHGS divided by BMI [25]. Height (cm) was measured using a stadiometer (SECA 222, Hamburg, Germany) and weight (kg) with a bioimpedance device (InBody R20, Biospace, Seoul, Korea). BMI was calculated as weight (kg) divided by height squared (m^2).

2.3. Measurement of Cardiometabolic Risk Factors

Systolic blood pressure (SBP), diastolic blood pressure (DBP), and resting heart rate were measured using the Mobil-O-Graph® 24 h pulse wave analysis monitor (IEM GmbH, Stolberg, Germany) in a sitting position according to the European Society of Hypertension [35], after 5 min of rest.

Arterial stiffness was indirectly assessed through the pulse wave velocity (PWV) [36]. The test was performed in a sitting position after 5 min of rest, using the Mobil-O-Graph® 24 h pulse wave analysis monitor, the operation of which is based on oscillometry recorded by a blood pressure cuff placed on the brachial artery. This instrument is validated for clinical practice [36]. PWV was obtained from a single measurement. The coefficient of variation (CV) of the Mobil-O-Graph for consecutive PWV analyses is 3.4%, and its intraclass correlation coefficient is 0.98 (0.96–0.99) [37].

Venous fasting blood samples were collected in the morning with heparin as the anticoagulant. Blood was centrifuged at 3500 rpm for 15 min to separate the plasma, which was subsequently removed. Plasma triglycerides, high-density lipoprotein cholesterol (HDL-c), low-density lipoprotein cholesterol (LDL-c), total cholesterol, glucose, urea, albumin and creatinine concentrations were analyzed enzymatically with an autoanalyzer (Olympus Diagnostic, Hamburg, Germany). Insulin was measured with an enzyme immunoassay kit, and the homeostasis model assessment of insulin resistance (HOMA-IR) was calculated [(fasting insulin (µIU/mL) × fasting glucose (mg/dL))/405]. Apolipoproteins A and B, hs-CRP, and glycosylated hemoglobin were determined by immunoturbidimetry (HORIBA-ABX Diagnostics, Japan) with an autoanalyzer (PENTRA-400, HORIBA-ABX Diagnostics, Japan). The albumin-creatinine ratio was measured from a first-morning urine sample. Values above or equal to 30 mg/g in women were considered pathological. The estimated glomerular filtration rate was determined by the modification of diet in renal disease (MDRD) equation [38]: (GFe (MDRD)):

$$175 \times SCr - 1.154 \times age - 0.203 \times 0.742$$

SCr: serum creatinine

2.4. Other Measurements

All participants filled out a sociodemographic and clinical data questionnaire to gather information, such as age, disease duration, current medication (including antidiabetics and corticosteroids), and tobacco consumption. The systemic lupus erythematosus disease activity index (SLEDAI) was included to assess disease activity [39], considering the presence or absence of several clinical and analytical manifestations in the preceding 10 days. The final score ranges from 0 to 105, where a higher score indicates a higher degree of disease activity. The degree of tissue damage from the onset of the disease was evaluated by the International Collaborating Clinics/American College of Rheumatology's systemic lupus damage index (SLICC-SDI) [40]. The score ranges from 0 to 40, where a higher score indicates greater damage produced by SLE in the last 6 months.

2.5. Sample Size

The sample size was calculated for a clinical trial evaluating the effects of aerobic exercise on arterial stiffness, inflammation, and fitness, which was published earlier [41]. We recruited 58 participants for that trial, although a larger sample ($n = 77$) was used to perform baseline evaluations for cross-sectional analyses.

2.6. Statistical Analysis

The descriptive characteristics of the study participants are presented as means and standard deviations for continuous variables, and as frequencies and percentages for categorical variables, unless otherwise indicated in Table 1. Due to the presence of outliers, hs-CRP was winsorized. Normality was assessed through histograms, the Kolmogorov–Smirnov Test, and Q–Q plots, with muscular strength and cardiometabolic risk factors showing a normal distribution. Pearson's bivariate correlations were used to explore the raw association between rHGS and cardiometabolic risk factors, and we additionally assessed the crude association of aHGS and BMI with cardiometabolic risk factors. Regression models were built including each cardiometabolic risk factor as dependent variables in separate models. rHGS, age, SLEDAI, and SDI were entered as independent variables in all models (enter method). Age, SLEDAI, and SDI were entered as covariables due to their potential role as confounders [42]. Menopause, statins or corticosteroids were initially included, but they did not alter the coefficients, and thus they were not included in final models to avoid overfitting [43].

Table 1. Descriptive characteristics of the study participants (n = 77).

	Mean	SD
Age (years)	43.2	1.57
Weight (kg)	65.1	1.27
Height (cm)	160.1	0.77
Body Mass Index (kg/m^2)	25.5	0.51
Absolute Handgrip Strength (kg)	47.2	1.24
Relative Handgrip Strength (kg/BMI)	1.89	0.05
SLEDAI	0.6	0.17
Duration of SLE (years)	13.9	1.15
Systolic Blood Pressure (mmHg)	118	1.29
Diastolic Blood Pressure (mmHg)	76.5	1.18
Pulse Wave Velocity (m/s)	6.47	0.17
Fasting Glucose (mg/dL)	76.3	2.17
Glycosylated Hemoglobin (%)	5.31	
High Density Lipoprotein (mg/dL)	57.8	1.57
Low Density Lipoprotein (mg/dL)	100.7	2.88
Total Cholesterol (mg/dL)	177.5	3.56
Triglycerides (mg/dL)	93.6	4.85
Homeostatic Model Assessment	1.45	0.09
hs-CRP (mg/L)	2.73	0.17
Glomerular Filtration (mL/min/1.73 m^2)	92.6	3.33
Microalbuminuria (%)	28	
Cumulative Prednisone dose (mg)	2875	2677
Daily Prednisone dose (mg)	3.99	0.57
Prednisone use (%)	65	
Immunosuppressants (%)	45	
Antimalarials (%)	89	

For absolute and relative handgrip strength the total sample size was n = 75 due to missing data. SLEDAI: systemic lupus erythematosus disease activity index; hs-CRP: high-sensitivity C-reactive protein.

A clustered cardiometabolic risk index (z-score) [12] was created using the mean of the standardized scores [(value-mean)/standard deviation] for SBP, fasting glucose, triglycerides, HOMA-IR, total cholesterol/HDL-c, and hs-CRP. Statistical significance was set at $p < 0.05$.

3. Results

The flowchart of the study participants is presented in Figure 1. From a total of 172 patients initially invited, 81 refused to participate (41 patients reported living very far from the hospital, 36 were not able to find time to perform the evaluations, and 4 were not interested), 12 patients did not present clinical stability during the previous 6 months to the beginning of the study, and 2 patients had cardiovascular disease during the previous year. A total of 77 women with SLE (mean age 43.2, SD 13.8) complied with the inclusion criteria, agreed to participate, and were assessed in two waves (49 women in October 2016 and 28 women in February 2017). Both evaluations were identical. Two women did not perform the handgrip strength test due to a wrist injury.

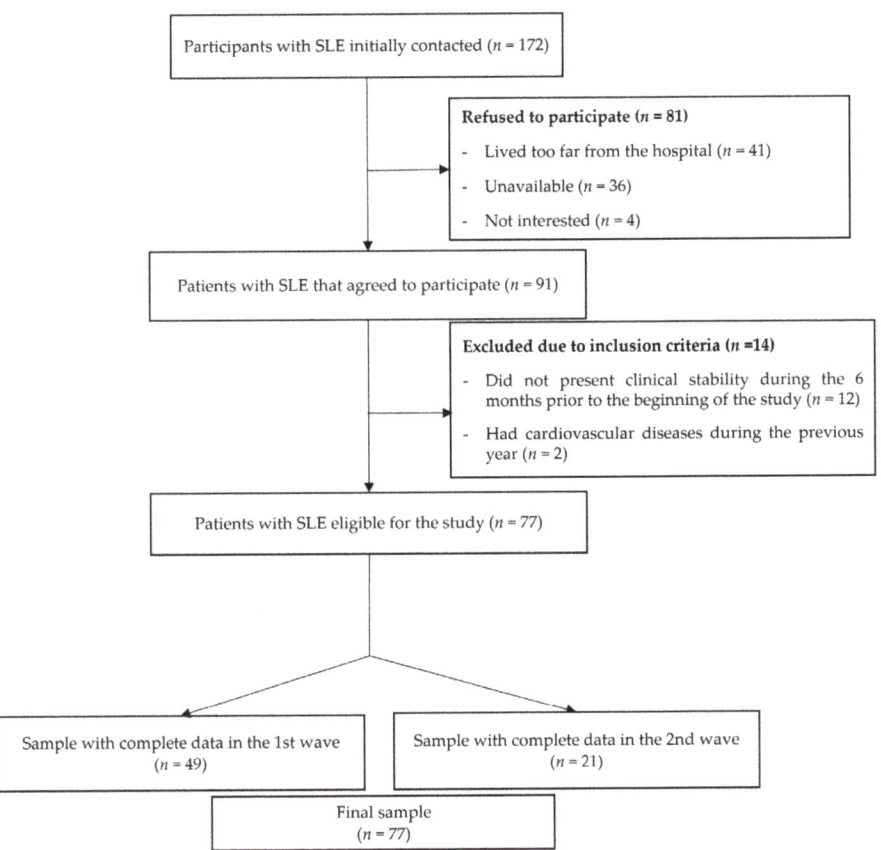

Figure 1. Flow diagram of the inclusion of women with systemic lupus erythematosus (SLE) for the present study.

The descriptive characteristics of the study participants are presented in Table 1. The average BMI was 25.5 (SD 0.51) kg/m^2. The average aHGS was 47.2 (SD 1.24) kg and for rHGS was 1.89 (SD 0.05) units. Regarding cardiometabolic risk variables, the average SBP was 118 (SD 1.29) mmHg, the average DBP was 76.5 (SD 1.18) mmHg, and the average fasting glucose levels were 76.3 (SD 2.17) mg/dL. Average total cholesterol was 177.5 (SD 3.56) mg/dL, the average hs-CRP levels were 2.73 (SD 0.35) mg/L and the average PWV was 6.47 (SD 0.17) m/s.

Table 2 represents the raw association of rHGS, aHGS, and BMI with cardiometabolic risk factors. rHGS was negatively associated with SBP, triglycerides, hs-CRP, PWV, and z-score (r_{range} = from −0.43 to −0.23; all $p < 0.05$). aHGS was negatively associated with triglycerides and PWV (r_{range} = from −0.34 to −0.23; all $p < 0.05$). Finally, BMI was positively associated with SBP, DBP, fasting glucose, HOMA-IR, PWV, and z-score (r_{range} = from 0.23 to 0.44; all $p < 0.05$). A graphic representation of the crude association of rHGS and cardiometabolic risk factors is presented in Figure 2. The linear regression models evaluating the association of rHGS and cardiometabolic risk factors are presented in Table 3. rHGS was inversely associated with SBP (unstandardized coefficient (B) = −6.58; 95% confidence interval (CI) −11.91 to −1.26; $p = 0.016$), hs-CRP (B = −1.67; 95% CI −3.11 to −0.23; $p = 0.023$), PWV (B = −0.34; 95% CI −0.58 to −0.09; $p = 0.007$) and z-score (B = −0.30; 95% CI −0.54 to −0.06; $p = 0.014$). These results were consistent even when statins and corticosteroids were included as covariates.

Table 2. Pearson's bivariate correlations analysis evaluating the raw association between relative handgrip strength, absolute handgrip strength and body mass index with cardiometabolic risk components in women with systemic lupus erythematosus.

	rHGS (n = 75)	aHGS (n = 75)	BMI
SBP	−0.34 **	−0.15	0.40 **
DBP	−0.13	0.01	0.32 **
Fasting Glucose	−0.06	0.08	0.23 *
Glycosylated Hemoglobin	−0.13	−0.07	0.11
HDL	0.04	0.08	0.04
LDL	0.04	0.04	−0.00
Total Cholesterol	0.01	0.03	0.04
Triglycerides	−0.28 *	−0.23 *	0.15
HOMA-IR	−0.15	0.11	0.43 **
hs-CRP	−0.23 *	−0.15	0.17
PWV	−0.43 **	−0.34 **	0.24 *
Glomerular Filtration	0.11	0.08	−0.10
Microalbumin	0.05	−0.04	−0.15
z−score	−0.32 **	−0.09	0.44 **

SBP: systolic blood pressure; DBP: diastolic blood pressure; HDL: high-density lipoprotein; LDL: low-density lipoprotein; HOMA-IR: homeostatic model assessment of insulin resistance; hs-CRP: high-sensitivity C-reactive protein; PWV: pulse wave velocity. Notes: * $p < 0.05$; ** $p < 0.01$.

Table 3. Multivariable linear regression analysis evaluating the association of relative handgrip strength with cardiometabolic risk components in women with systemic lupus erythematosus (n = 75).

	Beta	B	Std Error	95% CI		p	R²
SBP	−0.29	−6.58	2.67	−11.91	−1.26	**0.016**	0.20
DBP	−0.10	−2.02	2.63	−7.27	3.23	0.445	0.03
Fasting Glucose	−0.09	−3.58	5.00	−13.55	6.39	0.476	0.01
Glycosylated Hemoglobin	−0.02	−0.02	0.11	−0.25	0.20	0.846	0.10
HDL	0.10	2.77	3.56	−4.33	9.89	0.438	0.02
LDL	0.16	8.06	6.08	−4.06	20.20	0.189	0.14
Total Cholesterol	0.15	9.03	7.25	−5.44	23.50	0.218	0.18
Triglycerides	−0.23	−19.41	10.50	−40.35	1.52	0.069	0.12
HOMA-IR	−0.19	−0.34	0.22	−0.79	0.10	0.127	0.03
hs-CRP	−0.29	−1.67	0.72	−3.11	−0.23	**0.023**	0.09
PWV	−0.11	−0.34	0.12	−0.58	−0.09	**0.007**	0.91
Glomerular Filtration	−0.14	−7.68	5.75	−19.16	3.80	0.187	0.37
Microalbumin	−0.11	−0.01	0.11	−0.23	0.21	0.925	0.10
z-score	−0.30	−0.30	0.12	−0.54	−0.06	**0.014**	0.15

B: unstandardized coefficient; SBP: systolic blood pressure DBP: diastolic blood pressure; HDL: high-density lipoprotein; LDL: low-density lipoprotein; HOMA-IR: homeostatic model assessment of insulin resistance; hs-CRP: high-sensitivity C-reactive protein; PWV: pulse wave velocity. All regression models were adjusted for age, SLEDAI, and SDI. Regression models were built including each cardiometabolic risk factor as dependent variables in separate models. Relative handgrip strength was entered as the independent variable in all models (enter method) where age, SLEDAI, and SDI were entered as confounders in order to adjust the independent variable. Statistically significant associations ($p < 0.05$) are highlighted in bold.

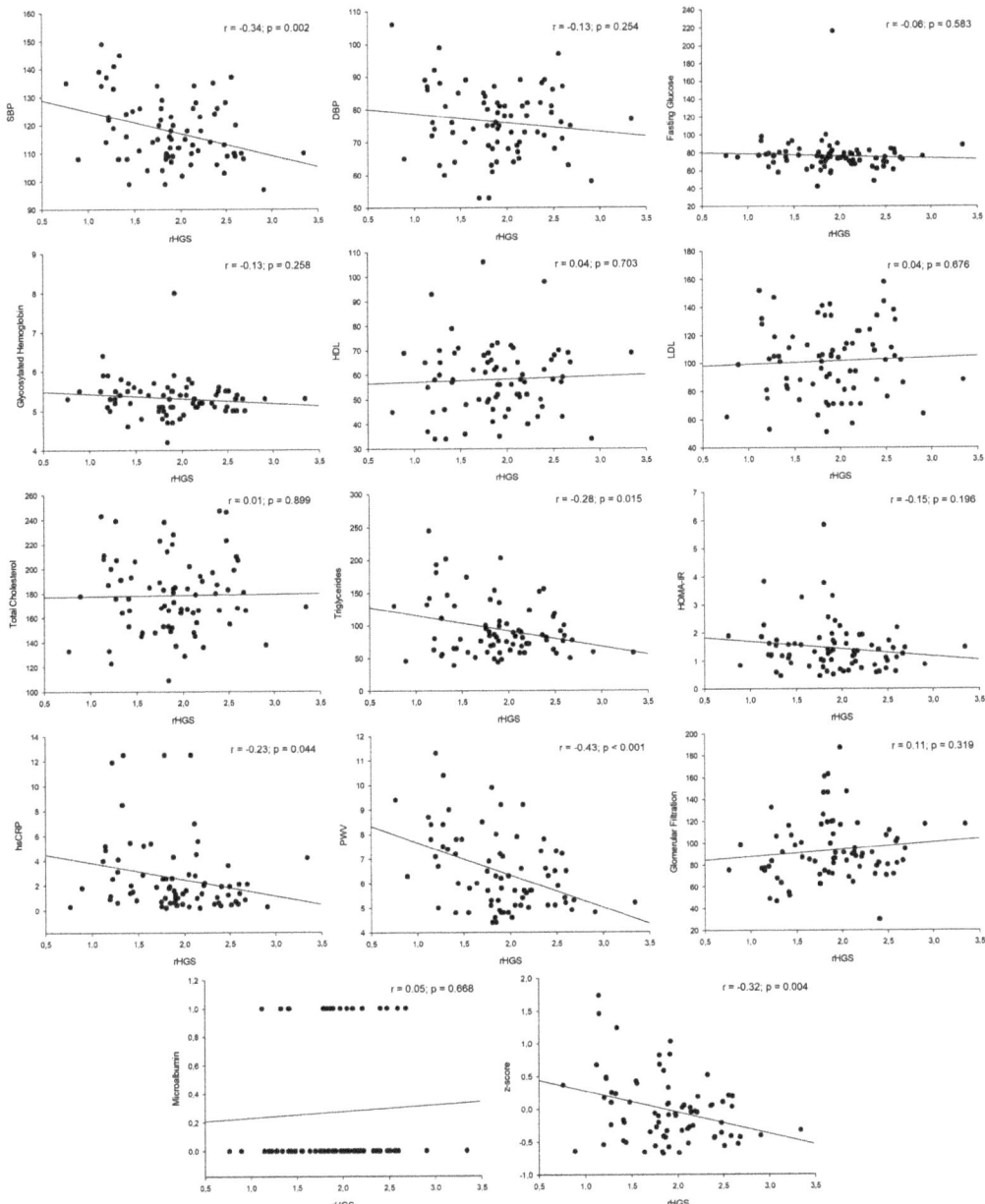

Figure 2. Graphic representation of the crude association of rHGS and cardiometabolic risk factors.

4. Discussion

The main finding of this study is that a higher rHGS was associated with lower SBP, triglycerides, hs-CRP, PWV, and clustered cardiometabolic risk index (z-score) in women with SLE. Furthermore, rHGS could be an alternative to aHGS when evaluating cardiometabolic risk. Our results were consistent despite adjusting for multiple potential confounders such as age, SLEDAI, SDI, statins, menopause, smoking or corticosteroids.

The association of aHGS and cardiometabolic risk has been previously studied in the general population. Lee et al. [27] found that a higher aHGS was associated with lower cardiovascular risk in older Korean adults. Similar findings were described by Leong et al. [21], who found that aHGS was inversely associated with all-cause death in a prospective cohort study with 140,000 men and women. However, Gregorio-Arenas et al. [44] found no association of aHGS with cardiometabolic risk in a sample of 228 perimenopausal women. In line with this, Gubelmann, Vollenweider and Marques-Vidal [45] observed no association between aHGS and cardiovascular risk in healthy adults. Regarding rHGS, previous studies have assessed its association with cardiometabolic risk, although not in rheumatological or autoimmune populations. Choquette et al. found that rHGS could be an indicator of cardiometabolic risk in 1793 community-dwelling men and women [25]. Moreover, Lawman et al. [28] found that higher rHGS was significantly associated with lower SBP, triglycerides, glucose, and higher HDL in both healthy men and women. Finally, Campa et al. [46] demonstrated that resistance training is effective in improving both cardiometabolic risk factors and rHGS in obese women, but improvements regarding rHGS are only achieved if training frequency is high and prolonged over time [47]. Our results are overall in line with these findings derived from other populations and extend current knowledge on potential indicators of cardiometabolic risk in SLE, as well as agreeing with recent literature.

The novel approach of this study is the concurrent analysis of the association of rHGS, aHGS and BMI itself with cardiometabolic risk factors. Although no statistical test can compare the strength of their independent association with the outcomes, these analyses provide the opportunity to determine which of these markers of risk is more worthwhile in clinical practice. Overall, rHGS and BMI were clearly better indicators of cardiometabolic risk than aHGS. However, when comparing BMI with rHGS, the results were less clear. While BMI was associated with markers of insulin resistance and the association with the clustered cardiometabolic risk score was stronger than with rHGS, rHGS was more strongly associated with arterial stiffness and, more importantly, with hs-CRP. As inflammation is a hallmark of autoimmune diseases including SLE, these results should not be taken into consideration when deciding whether to include the assessment of handgrip strength in clinical practice. The relatively low sample size precludes making strong arguments either in favor of or against this, although further research on this topic seems warranted. In practical terms, it is obvious that BMI is the simplest way to obtain a strong marker of cardiometabolic risk. However, it must be considered that adding a handgrip strength assessment takes approximately 2 min (including double assessment of both hands), which, depending on the context, might be feasible or not.

This study has potential limitations. Although other widely used tools to measure CV risk have been proposed, these tools could underestimate CV risk in patients with SLE. Our study provides a greater knowledge of CV risk using individual factors and a cluster score. The cross-sectional design precludes the establishment of causal relationships; therefore, our results must be corroborated in future prospective and experimental research. The sample size was relatively small, and we do not know whether these results apply to men or to women with medium or high disease activity, as only women with mild disease activity were included.

5. Conclusions

The findings suggest that higher rHGS is significantly associated with lower cardiometabolic risk in women with SLE. Although assessing rHGS might add relevant information regarding the potential cardiometabolic risk of SLE patients, BMI alone is a rather good indicator of cardiometabolic risk that might be preferred under time-constrained situations.

Author Contributions: Conceptualization, S.S.-R., J.A.V.-H. and A.S.-M.; data curation, J.A.V.-H. and A.S.-M.; formal analysis, S.S.-R., B.G.-C. and A.S.-M.; funding acquisition, J.A.V.-H. and A.S.-M.; investigation, S.S.-R., J.A.V.-H., B.G.-C., A.R.-C., A.H.-M., E.M.-R., J.M.S. and A.S.-M. methodology, B.G.-C., A.S.-M. and J.A.V.-H.; project administration, J.A.V.-H.; resources, A.R.-C.,

A.H.-M., E.M.-R., N.O.-C., J.M.S. and A.S.-M. supervision J.A.V.-H. and A.S.-M.; visualization, A.R.-C.; writing—original draft, S.S.-R.; writing—review and editing, S.S.-R., J.A.V.-H., B.G.-C., A.R.-C., J.M.S., A.H.-M., E.M.-R., N.O.-C. and A.S.-M. All authors have read and agreed to the published version of the manuscript.

Funding: This work was funded by the Consejería de Salud, Junta de Andalucía (grant numbers: PI-0525-2016 and PIER-0223-2019). B.G.-C. was supported by the Spanish Ministry of Education (FPU15/00002), E.M-R was funded by the Spanish Ministry of Science, Innovation and Universities (FPU18/01107) and A.H.-M. by the Gerty Cory pre-doctoral program for deficit areas at the University of Almería. The funders had no role in study design, data collection and analysis decision to publish, or preparation of the manuscript.

Institutional Review Board Statement: The Research Ethics Committee of Granada reviewed and approved the study protocol on 31 October 2016 (reference number: 09/2016).

Informed Consent Statement: All participants received detailed information about the study aims and procedures and signed informed consent before being included in the study.

Acknowledgments: The authors would like to thank the members of the Autoimmune Diseases Unit at the "Virgen de las Nieves" University Hospital (i.e., Luis Manuel Sáez-Urán, Nuria Navarrete-Navarrete, Mónica Zamora-Pasadas, and Juan Jiménez-Alonso) as well as Cristina Montalbán-Méndez for their support during data collection and study design. The study participants are also gratefully acknowledged for their collaboration.

Conflicts of Interest: The funders had no role in the design of the study; in the collection, analyses, or interpretation of data; in the writing of the manuscript, or in the decision to publish the results.

References

1. Rees, F.; Doherty, M.; Grainge, M.J.; Lanyon, P.; Zhang, W. The worldwide incidence and prevalence of systemic lupus erythematosus: A systematic review of epidemiological studies. *Rheumatology* **2012**, *56*, 1945–1961. [CrossRef]
2. Fatoye, F.; Gebrye, T.; Svenson, L.W. Real-world incidence and prevalence of systemic lupus erythematosus in Alberta, Canada. *Rheumatol. Int.* **2018**, *38*, 1721–1726. [CrossRef]
3. Somers, E.C.; Marder, W.; Cagnoli, P.; Lewis, E.E.; DeGuire, P.; Gordon, C.; Helmick, C.G.; Wang, L.; Wing, J.J.; Dhar, J.P.; et al. Population-based incidence and prevalence of systemic lupus erythematosus: The Michigan Lupus Epidemiology and Surveillance program. *Arthritis Rheum.* **2014**, *66*, 369–378. [CrossRef] [PubMed]
4. Renau, A.I.; Isenberg, D.A. Male versus female lupus: A comparison of ethnicity, clinical features, serology and outcome over a 30 year period. *Lupus* **2012**, *21*, 1041–1048. [CrossRef] [PubMed]
5. Kiriakidou, M.; Ching, C.L. Systemic Lupus Erythematosus. *Ann. Intern. Med.* **2020**, *172*, ITC81–ITC96. [CrossRef] [PubMed]
6. Fors Nieves, C.E.; Izmirly, P.M. Mortality in Sistemic Lupus Erythematosus: An Updated Review. *Curr. Rheumatol. Rep.* **2016**, *18*, 121–128. [CrossRef]
7. Esdaile, J.M.; Abrahamowicz, M.; Grodzicky, T.; Li, Y.; Panaritis, C.; Berger, R.D.; Côté, R.; Grover, S.A.; Fortin, P.R.; Clarke, A.E.; et al. Traditional Framingham risk factors fail to fully account for accelerated atherosclerosis in systemic lupus erythematosus. *Arthritis Rheum.* **2011**, *44*, 2331–2337. [CrossRef]
8. Chatterjee, A.; Harris, S.B.; Leiter, L.A.; Fitchett, D.H.; Teoh, H.; Bhattacharyya, O.K. Cardiometabolic Risk Working Group (Canadian). Managing cardiometabolic risk in primary care: Summary of the 2011 consensus statement. *Can. Fam. Physician* **2012**, *58*, 389–393.
9. Mikolasevic, I.; Milic, S.; Racki, S.; Zaputovic, L.; Stimac, D.; Radic, M.; Markic, D.; Orlic, L. Nonalcoholic Fatty Liver Disease (NAFLD). A New Cardiovascular Risk Factor in Peritoneal Dialysis Patients. *Perit. Dial. Int.* **2016**, *36*, 427–432. [CrossRef]
10. Ridker, P.M.; Koenig, W.; Kastelein, J.J.; Mach, F.; Lüscher, T.F. Has the time finally come to measure hsCRP universally in primary and secondary cardiovascular prevention? *Eur. Heart J.* **2018**, *39*, 4109–4111. [CrossRef]
11. Musunuru, K.; Kral, B.G.; Blumenthal, R.S.; Fuster, V.; Campbell, C.Y.; Gluckman, T.J.; Lange, R.A.; Topol, E.J.; Willerson, J.T.; Desai, M.Y.; et al. The use of high sensitivity C-reactive protein in clinical practice. *Nat. Clin. Pr. Cardiovasc. Med.* **2008**, *5*, 621–635. [CrossRef]
12. Soriano-Maldonado, A.; Aparicio, V.A.; Félix-Redondo, F.J.; Fernández-Bergés, D. Severity of obesity and cardiometabolic risk factors in adults: Sex differences and role of physical activity. The HERMEX study. *Int. J. Cardiol.* **2016**, *223*, 352–359. [CrossRef]
13. Hwang, A.C.; Liu, L.K.; Lee, W.J.; Chen, L.Y.; Peng, L.N.; Lin, M.H.; Chen, L.K. Association of Frailty and Cardiometabolic Risk Among Community-Dwelling Middle-Aged and Older People: Results from the I-Lan Longitudinal Aging Study. *Rejuvenation Res.* **2015**, *18*, 564–572. [CrossRef]
14. Kupusinac, A.; Doroslovački, R.; Malbaški, D.; Srdić, B.; Stokić, E. A primary estimation of the cardiometabolic risk by using artificial neural networks. *Comput. Biol. Med.* **2013**, *43*, 751–757. [CrossRef]

15. Ammirati, E.; Bozzolo, E.P.; Contri, R.; Baragetti, A.; Palini, A.G.; Cianflone, D.; Banfi, M.; Uboldi, P.; Bottoni, G.; Scotti, I.; et al. Cardiometabolic and immune factors associated with increased common carotid artery intima-media thickness and cardiovascular disease in patients with systemic lupus erythematosus. *Nutr. Metab. Cardiovasc. Dis.* **2014**, *24*, 751–759. [CrossRef] [PubMed]
16. Stockton, K.A.; Kandiah, D.A.; Paratz, J.D.; Bennell, K.L. Fatigue, muscle strength and vitamin D status, in women with systemic lupus erythematosus compared with healthy controls. *Lupus* **2012**, *21*, 271–278. [CrossRef]
17. Sola-Rodríguez, S.; Gavilán-Carrera, B.; Vargas-Hitos, J.A.; Sabio, J.M.; Morillas-de-Laguno, P.; Soriano-Maldonado, A. Physical Fitness and Body Composition in Women with Sistemic Lupus Erythematosus. *Medicina* **2019**, *55*, 57. [CrossRef] [PubMed]
18. Balsamo, S.; da Mota, L.M.H.; de Carvalho, J.F.; da Cunha Nascimento, D.; Tibana, R.A.; de Santana, F.S.; Moreno, R.L.; Gualano, B.; dos Santos-Neto, L. Low dynamic muscle strength and its associations with fatigue, functional performance, and quality of life in premenopausal patients with systemic lupus erythematosus and low disease activity: A case-control study. *BMC Musculoskelet. Disord.* **2013**, *14*, 1–7. [CrossRef] [PubMed]
19. Artero, E.G.; Lee, D.C.; Lavie, C.J.; España-Romero, V.; Sui, X.; Church, T.S.; Blair, S.N. Effects of muscular strength on cardiovascular risk factors and prognosis. *J. Cardiopulm. Rehabil. Prev.* **2012**, *32*, 351–358. [CrossRef]
20. Farias, D.L.; Tibana, R.A.; Teixeira, T.G.; Vieira, D.C.L.; Tarja, V.; Nascimento, D.D.C.; Silva, A.D.O.; Funghetto, S.S.; Coura, M.A.D.S.; Valduga, R.; et al. Elderly women with metabolic syndrome present higher cardiovascular risk and lower relative muscle strength. *Einstein* **2013**, *11*, 174–179. [CrossRef]
21. Leong, D.P.; Teo, K.K.; Rangarajan, S.; Lopez-Jaramillo, P.; Avezum Jr, A.; Orlandini, A.; Seron, P.; Ahmed, S.H.; Rosengren, A.; Kelishadi, R.; et al. Prognostic value of grip-strength: Findings from the Prospective Urban Rural Epidemiology (PURE) study. *Lancet* **2015**, *386*, 266–273. [CrossRef]
22. Hsu, F.C.; Kritchevsky, S.B.; Liu, Y.; Kanaya, A.; Newman, A.B.; Perry, S.E.; Visser, M.; Pahor, M.; Harris, T.B.; Nicklas, B.J.; et al. Association between inflammatory components and physical function in the health, aging, and body composition study: A principal component analysis approach. *J. Gerontol. A Biol. Sci. Med. Sci.* **2009**, *64*, 581–589. [CrossRef]
23. Sasaki, H.; Kasagi, F.; Yamada, M.; Fujita, S. Grip strength predicts cause-specific mortality in middle-aged and elderly persons. *Am. J. Med.* **2007**, *120*, 337–342. [CrossRef]
24. Gavilán-Carrera, B.; Garcia da Silva, J.; Vargas-Hitos, J.A.; Sabio, J.M.; Morillas-de-Laguno, P.; Rios-Fernández, R.; Delgado-Fernández, M.; Soriano-Maldonado, A. Association of physical fitness components and health-related quality of life in women with systemic lupus erythematosus with mild disease activity. *PLoS ONE* **2019**, *14*, 1–17. [CrossRef] [PubMed]
25. Choquette, S.; Bouchard, D.R.; Doyon, C.Y.; Sénéchal, M.; Brochu, M.; Dionne, I.J. Relative strength as a determinant of mobility in elders 67-84 years of age. A nuage study: Nutrition as a determinant of successful aging. *J. Nutr. Health Aging* **2010**, *14*, 190–195. [CrossRef] [PubMed]
26. Lee, W.J.; Peng, L.N.; Chiou, S.T.; Chen, L.K. Relative Handgrip Strength Is a Simple Indicator of Cardiometabolic Risk among Middle-Aged and Older People: A Nationwide Population-Based Study in Taiwan. *PLoS ONE* **2016**, *25*, 1–11. [CrossRef]
27. Lee, M.R.; Jung, S.M.; Kim, H.S.; Kim, Y.B. Association of muscle strength with cardiovascular risk in Korean adults: Findings from the Korea National Health and Nutrition Examination Survey (KNHANES) VI to VII (2014–2016). *Medicina* **2018**, *97*, 1–7. [CrossRef]
28. Lawman, H.G.; Troaino, R.P.; Perna, F.M.; Wang, C.Y.; Fryar, C.D.; Ogden, C.L. Associations of Relative Handgrip Strength and Cardiovascular Disease Biomarkers in U.S. Adults, 2011-2012. *Am. J. Prev. Med.* **2016**, *50*, 677–683. [CrossRef] [PubMed]
29. Mearns, B.M. Risk factors: Hand grip strength predicts cardiovascular risk. *Nat. Rev. Cardiol.* **2015**, *12*, 379. [CrossRef]
30. Wu, Y.; Wang, W.; Liu, T.; Zhang, D. Association of Grip Strength with Risk of All-Cause Mortality, Cardiovascular Diseases, and Cancer in Community-Dwelling Populations: A Meta-analysis of Prospective Cohort Studies. *J. Am. Med. Dir. Assoc.* **2017**, *18*, 17–35. [CrossRef] [PubMed]
31. Ying, X.; Song, Z.Y.; Zhao, C.J.; Jiang, Y. Body mass index, waist circumference, and cardiometabolic risk factors in young and middle-aged Chinese women. *J. Zhejiang Univ. Sci.* **2010**, *11*, 639–646. [CrossRef]
32. Labraña, A.M.; Duran, E.; Martínez, M.A.; Leiva, A.M.; Garrido-Méndez, A.; Diaz, X.; Salas, C.; Celis-Morales, C. Effects of lower body weight or waist circumference on cardiovascular risk. *Rev. Med. Chile* **2017**, *145*, 585–594. [CrossRef] [PubMed]
33. Hochberg, M.C. Updating the American College of Rheumatology revised criteria for the classification of systemic lupus erythematosus. *Arthritis Rheum.* **1997**, *40*, 1725. [CrossRef]
34. Ruiz-Ruiz, J.; Mesa, J.L.; Gutiérrez, A.; Castillo, M.J. Hand size influences optimal grip span in women but not men. *J. Hand Surg. Am.* **2002**, *27*, 897–901. [CrossRef] [PubMed]
35. Mancia, G.; De Backer, G.; Dominiczak, A.; Cifkova, R.; Fagard, R.; Germano, G.; Grassi, G.; Heagerty, A.M.; Kjeldsen, S.E.; Laurent, S.; et al. 2007 Guidelines for the Management of Arterial Hypertension: The Task Force for the Management of Arterial Hypertension of the European Society of Hypertension (ESH) and of the European Society of Cardiology (ESC). *J. Hypertens.* **2007**, *25*, 1105–1187. [CrossRef] [PubMed]
36. Wei, W.; Tölle, M.; Zidek, W.; van der Giet, M. Validation of the mobil-O-Graph: 24 h-blood pressure measurement device. *Blood Press. Monit.* **2010**, *15*, 225–228. [CrossRef]
37. Grillo, A.; Parati, G.; Rovina, M.; Moretti, F.; Salvi, L.; Gao, L.; Baldi, C.; Sorropago, G.; Faini, A.; Millasseau, S.C.; et al. Short-Term Repeatability of Noninvasive Aortic Pulse Wave Velocity Assessment: Comparison between Methods and Devices. *Am. J. Hypertens.* **2017**, *31*, 80–88. [CrossRef] [PubMed]

38. Levey, A.S.; Coresh, J.; Greene, T.; Stevens, L.A.; Zhang, Y.; Hendriksen, S.; Kusek, J.W.; Van Lente, F. Using standardized serum creatinine values in the modification of diet in renal disease study equation for estimating glomerular filtration rate. *Ann. Intern. Med.* **2006**, *145*, 247–254. [CrossRef] [PubMed]
39. Griffiths, B.; Mosca, M.; Gordon, C. Assessment of patients with systemic lupus erythematosus and use of lupus disease activity indices. *Best Pract. Res. Clin. Rheumatol.* **2005**, *19*, 685–708. [CrossRef]
40. Gladman, D.; Ginzler, E.; Goldsmith, C.; Fortin, P.; Liang, M.; Sanchez-Guerrero, J.; Urowitz, M.; Bacon, P.; Bombardieri, S.; Hanly, J.; et al. The development and initial validation of the systemic lupus international collaborating clinics/American College of Rheumatology Damage Index for Systemic Lupus Erythematosus. *Arthritis Rheum.* **1996**, *39*, 363–369. [CrossRef]
41. Soriano-Maldonado, A.; Morillas-de-Laguno, P.; Sabio, J.M.; Gavilán-Carrera, B.; Rosales-Castillo, A.; Montalbán-Méndez, C.; Sáez-Urán, L.M.; Callejas-Rubio, J.L.; Vargas-Hitos, J.A. Effects of 12-week Aerobic Exercise on Arterial Stiffness, Inflammation, and Cardiorespiratory Fitness in Women with Systemic LUPUS Erythematosus: Non-Randomized Controlled Trial. *J. Clin. Med.* **2018**, *7*, 477. [CrossRef] [PubMed]
42. Kipen, Y.; Briganti, E.M.; Strauss, B.J.; Littlejohn, G.O.; Morand, E.F. Three year follow-up of body composition changes in pre-menopausal women with systemic lupus erythematosus. *Rheumatology* **1999**, *38*, 59–65. [CrossRef] [PubMed]
43. Austin, P.C.; Steyerberg, E.W. The number of subjects per variable required in linear regression analyses. *J. Clin. Epidemiol.* **2015**, *68*, 627–636. [CrossRef] [PubMed]
44. Gregorio-Arenas, E.; Ruiz-Cabello, P.; Camiletti-Moirón, D.; Moratalla-Cecilia, N.; Aranda, P.; López-Jurado, M.; Llopis, J.; Aparicio, V.A. The associations between physical fitness and cardiometabolic risk and body-size phenotypes in perimenopausal women. *Maturitas* **2016**, *92*, 162–167. [CrossRef] [PubMed]
45. Gubelmann, C.; Vollenweider, P.; Marques-Vidal, P. No association between grip strength and cardiovascular risk: The CoLaus population-based study. *Int. J. Cardiol.* **2017**, *236*, 478–482. [CrossRef] [PubMed]
46. Campa, F.; Maietta Latessa, P.; Greco, G.; Mauro, M.; Mazzuca, P.; Spiga, F.; Toselli, S. Effects of Different Resistance Training Frequencies on Body Composition, Cardiometabolic Risk Factors, and Handgrip Strength in Overweight and Obese Women: A Randomized Controlled Trial. *J. Funct. Morphol. Kinesiol.* **2020**, *17*, 51. [CrossRef]
47. Toselli, S.; Badicu, G.; Bragonzoni, L.; Spiga, F.; Mazzuca, P.; Campa, F. Comparison of the Effect of Different Resistance Training Frequencies on Phase Angle and Handgrip Strength in Obese Women: A Randomized Controlled Trial. *Int. J. Environ. Public Health* **2020**, *17*, 1163. [CrossRef] [PubMed]

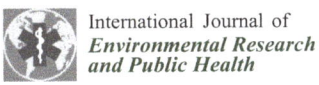

Article

The Combined Effects of Obesity and Cardiorespiratory Fitness Are Associated with Response Inhibition: An ERP Study

Lin Chi [1], Chiao-Ling Hung [2], Chi-Yen Lin [3], Tai-Fen Song [4], Chien-Heng Chu [5,*], Yu-Kai Chang [5,6,*] and Chenglin Zhou [7,*]

[1] School of Physical Education, Minnan Normal University, Zhangzhou 363000, Fujian, China; chilin1215@hotmail.com
[2] Department of Athletics, National Taiwan University, Taipei 106319, Taiwan; musehung@gmail.com
[3] Physical Education Office, National Taiwan Ocean University, Keelung 202301, Taiwan; evalin@ntou.edu.tw
[4] Department of Sport Performance, National Taiwan University of Sport, Taichung 404401, Taiwan; tiffanyfen628@gmail.com
[5] Department of Physical Education, National Taiwan Normal University, Taipei 106209, Taiwan
[6] Institute for Research Excellence in Learning Science, National Taiwan Normal University, Taipei 106209, Taiwan
[7] School of Psychology, Shanghai University of Sport, Shanghai 200438, China
* Correspondence: cchu042@yahoo.com (C.-H.C.); yukaichangnew@gmail.com (Y.-K.C.); Chenglin_600@126.com (C.Z.)

Abstract: Obesity and cardiorespiratory fitness exhibit negative and positive impacts, respectively, on executive function. Nevertheless, the combined effects of these two factors on executive function remain unclear. This study investigated the combined effects of obesity and cardiorespiratory fitness on response inhibition of executive function from both behavioral and neuroelectric perspectives. Ninety-six young adults aged between 18 and 25 years were recruited and assigned into four groups: the high cardiorespiratory fitness with normal weight (NH), high cardiorespiratory fitness with obesity (OH), low cardiorespiratory fitness with normal weight (NL), and low cardiorespiratory fitness with obesity (OL) groups. The stop-signal task and its induced P3 component of event-related potentials was utilized to index response inhibition. The participants with higher cardiorespiratory fitness (i.e., the NH and OH groups) demonstrated better behavioral performance (i.e., shorter response times and higher accuracy levels), as well as shorter stop-signal response times and larger P3 amplitudes than their counterparts with low cardiorespiratory fitness (i.e., the NL and OL groups). The study provides first-hand evidence of the substantial effects of cardiorespiratory fitness on the response inhibition, including evidence that the detrimental effects of obesity might be overcome by high cardiorespiratory fitness.

Keywords: body mass index; fitness; executive control; event-related potential

1. Introduction

The obesity epidemic is increasingly regarded as a global pandemic, as more than 13% of people aged 18 years and over were of excessive weight in 2016 [1]. Obesity is not only linked to a broad range of long-term medical complications, such as cardiovascular disease, type II diabetes, and several types of cancers [2], but is also considered to be a risk factor for healthy lifestyle habits [3] and psychiatric conditions [4], such that it has profound economic consequences.

Obesity also has negative effects on various aspects of executive function (EF) [5], such as inhibition. Inhibition refers to the ability to override a planned, prepotent response or to stop already initiated responses (i.e., response inhibition) [6]. Several studies have utilized a highly theoretically driven cognitive task, the stop-signal task (SST) [7], to assess the efficiency of response inhibition. During the SST, the person being tested is required to response quickly to the go stimuli. Occupationally, the person needs to launch the stop-process induced by the stop stimuli to inhibit the go-process induced by the go stimuli, with that stoppage involving the top-down initiation of the aphasic inhibitory process [7]. Notably, the excessive weight has been attributed to failures to inhibit impulsive or prepotent responses [8]. For instance, individuals with higher BMI scores required longer duration of the reaction time to stop the ongoing response (i.e., stop-signal response time, or SSRT) compared to individuals with normal BMI scores [9]. Similarly, obese young adults have been reported to exhibit greater difficulties in response inhibition, as reflected by having longer SSRTs than normal-weight individuals [10], suggesting a relationship between less efficient response inhibition and obesity in the adult population.

Cardiorespiratory fitness (CRF) may also affect various aspects of EF [11,12]. Cross-sectional research has revealed a positive relationship between CRF and the performance of the tasks involving interference aspect of inhibition in late-middle-aged [13] and older adults [14]. Similarly, studies using laboratory-based and filed-based CRF assessments have indicated positive associations between CRF and task performance involving response inhibition in preadolescent children [15] and young adults [16,17]. Finally, similar positive links between CRF and working memory [11,18] and shifting [18,19] aspects of EF have been reported.

The potential effect of CRF on the association between obesity and EF has been further suggested by the "fat-but-fit" paradigm. Specifically, the fat-but-fit paradigm suggests that higher levels of physical activity or CRF might alleviate some of the adverse effects of obesity (i.e., its effect on all-cause mortality) [20,21]. The fat-but-fit paradigm has been extended to attenuation of the adverse effects of obesity on cognitive function. For instance, Song, et al. [22] compared the performance of interference aspect of inhibition in relation to levels of CRF and BMI, and reported no significant differences in behavioral performance among young adults with high CRF, regardless of their weight status, on the neutral condition of the Stroop task, suggesting that CRF might alleviate the adverse effects of obesity on basic information processing. In another study, Ross, et al. [23] measured CRF, % of body fat, waist-height ratio, and cognitive function in adolescents, and found that the association between obesity and visual working memory was partially mediated by CRF. These studies have explored the interrelationships between CRF, obesity, and various aspects of EF (i.e., the interference aspect of inhibition and working memory), and have provided initial evidence supporting the conclusion that CRF might act to modulate, attenuate, or possibly offset the detrimental effects of obesity in some aspects of EF. Nevertheless, to the best of our knowledge, no research has investigated the interrelationship between CRF and obesity, in terms of their combined effects on response inhibition.

Event-related potential (ERP), a noninvasive measure of brain electrical activity, may provide more insights regarding how response inhibition is associated with CRF and obesity. ERPs represent time-locked neuroelectric activities with sensitive temporal resolution, providing the opportunity for direct and detailed examinations of the neural mechanisms of mental processes [24]. In previous studies, individuals with higher CRF demonstrated larger P3 amplitudes along with shorter response times (RTs) and/or higher response accuracy levels [22,25,26]. Given that the P3 amplitude is regarded as a reflection of the amount of attentional resources allocated [27], such results suggest that higher CRF levels might support the recruitment of attentional resources and contribute to superior behavioral performance. Meanwhile, decreased P3 amplitudes and impaired response inhibition have been reported during the auditory discrimination task paradigm [28] and the Go/NoGo task [29] in obese and/or overweight children.

Taken together, the above findings indicate that obesity and CRF are negatively and positively associated with inhibition, respectively. Nevertheless, the combined effects of CRF and excessive weight on response inhibition remain unknown. The present study was thus conducted to investigate how CRF and excessive weight are simultaneously associated with response inhibition, as assessed by the SST, from both behavioral and neuroelectric perspectives. Given the negative impacts of obesity and the positive effects of CRF reported previously, it was hypothesized that individuals with high CRF and normal weight would exhibit superior response inhibition-related performance and that obese individuals with low CRF would exhibit worse response inhibition-related performance, both in terms of behavioral and neuroelectric measures.

2. Materials and Methods

2.1. Participants

Healthy males aged 18 to 25 years who met the following criteria were recruited: (a) normal or corrected-to-normal vision; (b) no color blindness; (c) no history of neurological disorders, psychiatric disorders, or any brain injury; (d) no current substance abuse; (e) able to complete a CRF assessment based on the Physical Activity Readiness Questionnaire (PAR-Q); (f) body mass index (BMI) within the normal-weight (BMI = 18.5–24 kg/m^2) or within the obese range (BMI > 27 kg/m^2) based on the normative BMI data for Taiwanese adults published by the Ministry of Health and Welfare of Taiwan; (g) CRF level either above the 65th percentile or below the 35th percentile, as reflected by the maximal oxygen uptake (VO_{2max}) index, based on the norms provided by the American College of Sports Medicine [30]; and (h) right-handed. The experimental protocol for the study was approved by the Institutional Review Board of National Taiwan University. Following an initial screening, 92 eligible participants were grouped into four mutually exclusive groups: the high CRF with normal weight (NH, n = 23) group, high CRF with obesity (OH, n = 23) group, low CRF with normal weight (NL, n = 23) group, and low CRF with obesity (OL, n = 23) group. The demographic data and working memory aspect of the intelligence quotient of each participant, as assessed by the Forward and Backward Digit Span Test of the Wechsler Adult Intelligence Scale-Third Edition [31], were collected.

2.2. Submaximal Cardiorespiratory Fitness Assessment

All of the participants completed the YMCA cycling test [32], which is a submaximal CRF test and has been described as effective in predicting VO_{2max} [33]. The test consists of three consecutive 3-min cycling stages. For each participant, the test began with a 3-min warm-up stage involving exercising on a braked cycle ergometer (Ergoselect 100/200 Ergoline GmbH, Germany) at 150 kpm/min (25 W) and pedaling at a constant speed of 50 rpm. The subsequent stages of power output progression were determined by the given participant's steady-state HR recorded during the last 15–30 s of the initial 3-min warm-up stage. An additional 3-min stage was added if the participant's target HR (i.e., 85% of the individual's age-predicted HRmax) was not achieved. The result for the Borg Rating of Perceived Exertion (RPE) scale [34] was recorded at the end of every 3-min stage during the exercise period. Finally, each participant's VO_{2max} was predicted using the extrapolation method.

2.3. Stop-Signal Task (SST)

The SST conducted using the e-prime software was adopted from Johnstone, et al. [35]. The go-trials of the SST consist of leftward- or rightward-pointing black arrows (← or →) with 196 × 42 pixels (hereafter referred to as go stimuli). The probability of a leftward- or rightward-pointing arrow occurring for any trial was 50%. A plus sign was presented as the fixation for 500 ms at the beginning of each trial. Following the plus sign, a blank screen (100 ms) and the go stimuli (500 ms) were presented sequentially. Participants were instructed to press the response button on the response box corresponding to the direction of each presented arrow (that is, they were asked to press the left response button for a leftward-pointing arrow and the right response button for a rightward-pointing arrow) as quickly and accurately as possible.

When presented, the stop stimulus (i.e., a red square superimposed on the go stimulus) was displayed with a certain delay (i.e., the stop-signal delay, SSD) following the go stimulus onset. The given participant was asked to withdraw their response when they detected the presence of the stop-signal stimulus (with each trial involving the stop-signal stimulus hereafter referred to as a stop-trial). The SSD was initially set to 200 ms, and dynamically varied between 50 ms and 450 ms according to each participant's ongoing performance. Specifically, the SSD was increased by 50 ms if the participant could successfully withdraw their response during the previous stop-trial and decreased by 50 ms if the participant failed to withdraw their response during the previous stop-trial. With the dynamic tracking algorithm, success in withholding the response was achieved for approximately 50% of the stop-trials. Presentation of the go- and stop-trials was randomized to prevent subjective expectancy. A low proportion of stop signals (i.e., 25%) was chosen for the trials in order to increase the strength of the conflicting stimuli. Finally, the SSRT of each participant was calculated by subtracting the participant's average SSD from their average response time during the go-trial (i.e., the mean go-trial RT).

2.4. Psychophysiological Recording and Data Analysis

For each participant, the brain electrical activity was recorded continuously from 32 Ag/AgCl scalp electrodes of the international 10-20 system inserted in an elastic cap (Quick-Cap, NeuroScan Inc.) and referenced to the left and right mastoids. The horizontal electrooculogram (HEOG) was recorded from two electrodes attached laterally to each eye to monitor horizontal eye movements. Vertical eye movements and blinks (the VEOG) were recorded from two electrodes attached above and below the left eye. The electrode located on the mid-forehead was used as the ground electrode. The impedance of all the electrodes throughout the recording period was maintained below 10 kΩ. The online EEG signal was digitized at a rate of 500 Hz and amplified by a SynAmps EEG amplifier filtered with a bandpass between 70 Hz and 0.05 Hz and with a 60-Hz notch filter to remove additional electrical noise with the NeuroScan equipment (NeuroScan Inc., El Paso, TX, USA).

The offline EEG data was then analyzed using the Scan software (NeuroScan Inc., El Paso, TX, USA, v4.5). Only the successfully inhibited and corrected response trials were included for further analysis. The offline EEG data was initially processed by correcting the eye movements and blinks using the algorithm proposed by Semlitsch, et al. [36], and an epoch of 1300 ms was segmented starting 100 ms prior to the onset of the go stimulus and lasting until 1200 ms after the go stimulus onset for each trial. The average artifact-free epoch waveforms were computed for both go-trials and stop-trials. The data was then digitized and filtered with a bandpass filter between 0.05 and 30 Hz (12 dB/Oct). The EEG data from poorly recorded channels and trials for which the amplitude exceeded ± 85 μV was excluded from further analysis.

ERP averages were then computed for the successful stop-trials and the correct go-trials for each individual. The initial time windows for the go-P3 (200–700 ms) component during the go-trials were determined based on the grand average waveforms of the four groups. The time windows for the stop-ERP components were determined from the average stop-signal onset time with the consideration of variation in each individual's SSD. That is, the final lower and upper time windows for each participant were equal to the smallest SSD plus the lower limit of the average stop-signal onset time and the largest SSD plus the upper limit of the average stop-signal onset time, respectively. Finally, for each individual P3 time window, the P3 amplitude, defined as the most positive value within the window, was identified by means of an automatic pick-picking program using the Scan software (NeuroScan, v4.5). In a similar manner, the N2 amplitude, which was defined as the most negative value within the final time window, was also identified.

2.5. Experimental Procedure

The participants were required to visit the laboratory located on the National Taiwan Sport University campus individually on two occasions separated by less than seven days from each other. In order to measure the body-weigh accurately, all participants were instructed to avoid having any food for 8 h prior their body-weight measurements. Additionally, they were informed not to consume any food or drink containing caffeine or alcohol and to avoid engaging in any strenuous exercise for 12 h prior to second experimental session in an effort to reduce any effect of stimuli on the cardiovascular system.

During the first visit, the experimental procedure was introduced by the researchers conducting the experiment, and informed written consent was obtained from the given participant. After the informed consent was completed, information regarding the participant's health/physical condition was acquired by filling out the demographic and PAR-Q questionnaires. The participant's BMI was then calculated based on their weight (kg) and height (m), and the participant's score on the Digit Span Test was recorded. Following confirmation that the health condition and BMI status of the participant met the inclusion criteria, the participant was fitted with a Polar heart rate monitor (Sport Tester PE 3000, Polar Electro Oy, Kempele, Finland) and instructed to perform the YMCA cycling test at a room temperature of 20 °C. The resting HR (HR rest) of the participant was measured after the participant sat still for 5 min. The participant's HR during the exercise was recorded every 2 min. Those participants who met the inclusion criteria were invited to return for the second experimental session.

During their second visit, each qualified participant was seated comfortably in a chair in a dimly lit, sound-attenuated, air-conditioned, and electrically shielded room where they then completed the SST. The viewing distance between the participant and the computer screen was set at 70 cm. During the SST, the participant was instructed to focus on a central fixation cross on the screen and to avoid making any body movements during the EEG recording. Prior to being tested with the experimental blocks of the SST, the participant responded to a practice block of 10 trials that allowed the participant to become familiar with the task so that they could keep in mind that they should inhibit their response when the stop signals appeared in the stop-trials. Furthermore, the importance of responding quickly to the go stimuli was emphasized, and the participant was told not to sacrifice response speed by waiting for the occurrence of the stop signals. Time was taken to ensure that each participant clearly understood the test prior to the experimental blocks being presented. After the practice block, two experimental blocks, each containing 200 trials, were presented. A 5-min break was taken halfway through each block, and a 15-min break was taken between the two blocks. EEG recordings were taken throughout the task performance period. The duration of the experiment was about 1.5 h. Each participant received a payment of approximately US $30 for travel expenses incurred.

2.6. Statistical Analysis

The demographic data was analyzed using the one-way analysis of variance (ANOVA) among the four groups (i.e., the NH, OH, NL, and OL groups). For behavioral data, the ANOVA was also conducted for the go RTs, which were defined as the time intervals between the onsets of the go stimuli and the correct responses made by the participants; the accuracy of the go-trials; and the SSRTs. For electrophysiological data, a separate ANOVA was also conducted for the go- and stop-P3 amplitudes at the parietal region (the averaged ERP from the P3, Pz, and P4 electrode locations). Finally, post-hoc Tukey HSD and multiple t-test comparisons with Bonferroni correction were conducted where appropriate. All statistical analyses were carried out using SPSS (version 21.0, IBM, Corp., Armonk, NY, USA). Mean and standard error (SE) values were presented.

3. Results

3.1. Participant Characteristics

The demographic background data of the participants is summarized in Table 1. The ANOVA revealed that there were no significant differences among the four groups in terms of age (years), height (cm), or working memory performance.

Table 1. Demographic and cardiorespiratory fitness for participants (means ± SD).

Variables	NH (n = 23)	OH (n = 23)	NL (n = 23)	OL (n = 23)
Age (years)	20.52 ± 1.65	20.70 ± 2.16	21.47 ± 2.00	21.04 ± 2.16
Height (cm)	173.43 ± 4.86	177.26 ± 7.63	175.91 ± 4.74	174.30 ± 6.27
Weight (kg)	63.91 ± 5.28	91.78 ± 14.54 [b]	66.65 ± 5.36	102.43 ± 19.93 [a]
BMI (kg/m^2)	21.25 ± 1.38	29.08 ± 2.50 [b]	21.53 ± 1.23	33.63 ± 5.93 [a]
Digit span: Forward	14.50 ± 1.30	14.00 ± 1.43	14.68 ± 1.32	14.14 ± 1.08
Digit span: Backward	8.82 ± 3.10	8.23 ± 2.10	9.60 ± 2.67	8.55 ± 2.76
VO$_{2max}$ (mL/kg/min)	55.19 ± 4.73 [a]	53.28 ± 4.29 [a]	41.66 ± 9.60	36.04 ± 3.63

NH = High cardiorespiratory fitness (CRF) with normal weight; OH = high CRF with obesity; NL = low CRF with normal weight; and OL = low CRF with obesity. [a] and [b] = $p < 0.05$.

In terms of weight status (kg), significant differences between the groups were observed ($ps < 0.05$). Follow-up analyses indicated that the OL group was significantly heavier than all three other groups ($ps < 0.05$), while the OH group was significantly heavier than the NH and NL groups ($ps < 0.01$). Meanwhile, no difference in weight status between the NL and NH groups was observed. In terms of BMI scores, significant differences between the groups were observed ($ps < 0.05$). Follow-up analyses indicated that the OL group had significantly higher BMI scores than the other three groups ($ps < 0.01$), while the OH group had higher BMI scores than the NL and NH groups ($ps < 0.01$). No differences were observed, meanwhile, between NL and NH groups.

With regard to the CRF levels, significant differences in VO$_{2max}$ scores were observed among the groups ($ps < 0.05$). Follow-up analysis indicated that both the NH group and the OH group had higher VO$_{2max}$ scores than the NL group, and that the OL group had the smallest VO$_{2max}$ scores.

3.2. Behavioral Data

Response time: One-way ANOVA analysis revealed a main effect of group [$F (3, 88) = 12.78$, $p < 0.01$] (Figure 1a). The follow-up analysis revealed that both the NH group (493.54 ± 26.39 ms) and the OH group (514.27 ± 20.99 ms) had significantly shorter RTs than the NL and OL groups (683.00 ± 27.87 ms and 631.54 ± 26.58 ms, $ps < 0.05$). No significant differences were observed, however, between the NH group and the OH group, or between the NL group and the OL group.

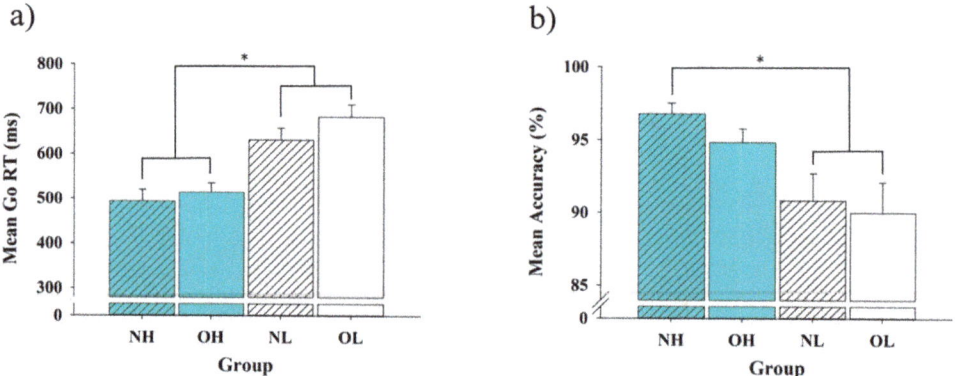

Figure 1. A comparison of the (**a**) response time (RT) and the (**b**) accuracy (means ± SE) on the Stop-Signal task during go-trials for the four groups. NH = High CRF with normal weight; OH = high CRF with obesity; NL = low CRF with normal weight; and OL = low CRF with obesity. * $p < 0.05$.

Accuracy: One-way ANOVA analysis revealed a main effect of group [F (3, 88) = 4.41, $p < 0.01$] (Figure 1b). The follow-up analysis revealed that the NH group (97 ± 0.75 %) had a significantly higher accuracy rate than the NL and OL groups (90 ± 2.1 % and 91 ± 1.9, $ps < 0.05$). No other significant differences among the OH, the NL, and the OL groups were observed ($p > 0.05$).

SSRT: One-way ANOVA analysis revealed a main effect of group [F (3, 88) =14.648, $p < 0.01$] (Figure 2). The post-hoc analysis revealed that both the NH group (223.55 ± 5.31 ms) and the OH group (235.15 ± 5.98 ms) exhibited shorter SSRTs than the NL and OL groups (300.55 ± 13.91 ms and 280.82 ± 10.42 ms, $ps < 0.05$). Furthermore, the mean SSRT of the OH group (235.15 ± 5.98 ms) was also significantly shorter than the mean SSRTs of the OL and NL groups ($p < 0.05$).

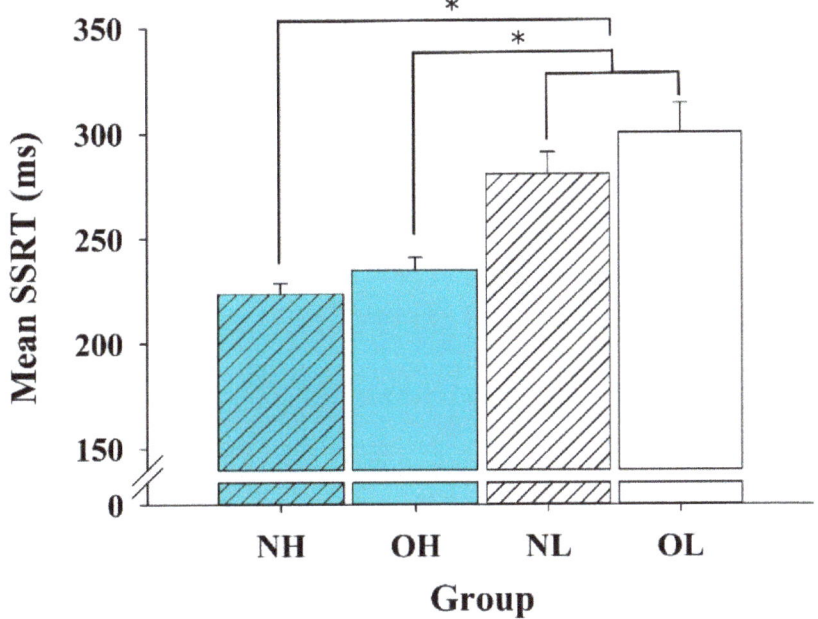

Figure 2. Comparisons of the stop-signal response time (SSRT) across the four groups (means ± SE). NH = High CRF with normal weight; OH = high CRF with obesity; NL = low CRF with normal weight; and OL = low CRF with obesity. * $p < 0.05$.

3.3. ERP Data: P3 Amplitudes

Regarding the go-P3 amplitude, one-way ANOVA analysis revealed a main effect of group [F (3, 88) = 4.02, $p < 0.05$], with the NH group (7.05 ± 0.94 µV) having a significantly larger mean amplitude than the OH (4.34 ± 0.64 µV), NL (4.34 ± 0.64 µV) and OL (3.99 ± 0.56 µV) groups. There was no significant difference among the OH, NL, and OL groups ($p > 0.05$). Regarding the stop-P3 amplitude, a main effect of group was also revealed [F (3, 88) = 5.71, $p < 0.01$], with the NH group (16.68 ± 1.26 µV) having a significantly larger mean amplitude than those observed for the NL (11.18 ± 0.79 µV) and OL (10.13 ± 1.28 µV) groups. No significant difference between the NH group and the OH group (12.55 ± 1.40 µV) group was observed. The topographic distributions of the P3 amplitude of go- and stop-trials across four groups was also presented in Figure 3.

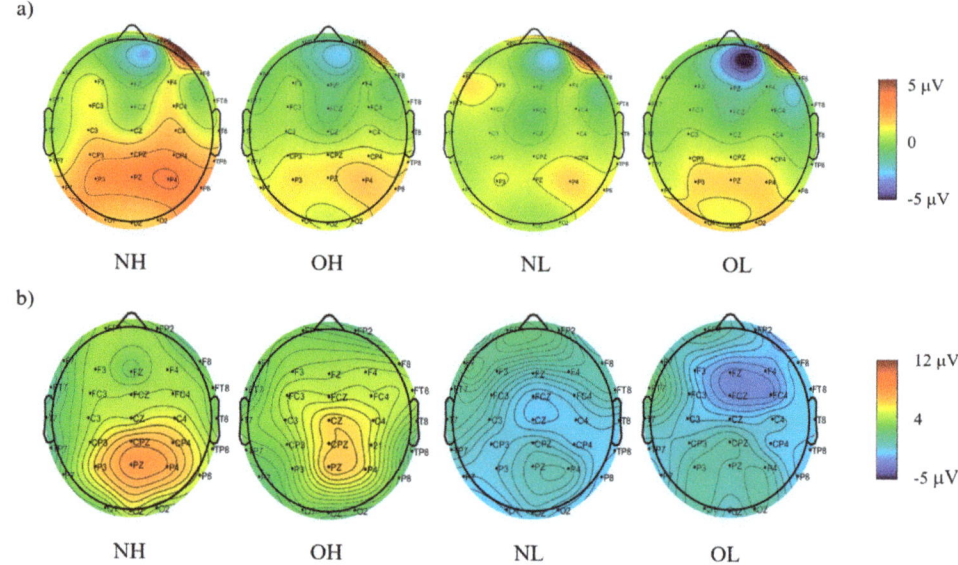

Figure 3. The topographic distributions of the P3 amplitude of (**a**) go- and (**b**) stop-trials across four groups. NH = High CRF with normal weight; OH = high CRF with obesity; NL = low CRF with normal weight; and OL = low CRF with obesity.

4. Discussion

The purpose of the current study was to examine the interrelationship between CRF and excessive weight in terms of their combined effects on response inhibition induced by the SST from both behavioral and ERP perspectives. Our primary behavioral findings revealed that the participants with high CRF levels, regardless of their normal or excessive weight status, had superior response inhibition in comparison to the participants with low CRF levels. Furthermore, the individuals with normal weight and high CRF demonstrated a higher accuracy rate than the other three groups. With regard to ERP indices, the individuals with normal weight and high CRF exhibited significantly larger go- and stop-P3 amplitudes than the obese individuals with low CRF levels, while no significant differences in the P3 amplitudes were observed among the other three groups.

4.1. Behavioral Performance

Superior performance under time pressure reflected by faster response times (in terms of go RTs) was observed among the participants with high CRF (i.e., the NH and OH groups) in comparison to the participants with low CRF (i.e., the NL and OL groups). These findings are consistent with those of prior research reporting that young adults with higher fitness levels had shorter go RTs during the neutral condition of the Stroop task [22], and the congruent condition of the Erickson flanker task [37]. However, similar go RTs for active and non-active young adults have also previously been observed [16,17], which is somewhat inconsistent with our findings in the present study. This inconsistency may be linked to the categories of CRF levels used in the different studies. Specifically, the average CRF levels for the non-active participants in the study by Padilla and colleagues were 44.43 and 48.00 mL/kg/min, respectively, which were higher than those of the low-fitness participants in the current study (35.79 and 36.45 mL/kg/min for the NL and OL groups, respectively). That is, our findings might represent the influence of relatively low CRF levels on the go RT. Given that go RT reflects the time required for the generalized processing needed for stimulus identification, stimulus discrimination, response choice, and response execution [38], CRF may have a positive influence on the general processing speed relative to the weight status during the SST.

Our SSRT results revealed that one difference between the high- and low-fitness participants was in response inhibition ability, with the shorter SSRTs of the participants with high CRF indicating their superior response inhibition compared to their low CRF counterparts. Such superior inhibition on the part of the high CRF participants was in line with previous studies regarding CRF. For example, previous studies have reported that active individuals demonstrated shorter SSRTs in the more executive control-demanding version of the SST compared to their inactive counterparts [16,17]. Other studies using the Erickson flanker task also found that higher CRF is associated with outcomes indicating superior inhibition, such as smaller flanker effects in older adults [39,40], better ability to maintain response accuracy across task conditions [25], and less response variability [41] in children. Consistent with this positive association, prior research has further reported superior performance in the incongruent condition of the Stroop task among older [42] and young adult [22] populations with higher fitness levels.

The covert behavioral response of SST (i.e., success or failure to withhold the on-going go-process) could be interpreted by the "horse-race" model [7], which indicates that the stop performance is determined by the "race" between the go-process and stop-process; that is, a participant will not be able to withhold or terminate their pre-potent response if the "go" process finishes the race before the "stop" process does (i.e., when go RT < (SSRT + SSD)) [7]. Accordingly, successful withholding of the ongoing go-process could be achieved by decreasing the tendency toward executing covert behavioral responses, through either or both of slowing the go RT and shortening the SSRT, for a given SSD [43]. Notably, although faster general cognitive processing speed (i.e., shorter go RTs) observed in individuals with higher CRF (i.e., NH and OH group) might imply a higher tendency toward executing the ongoing go-process, the superior response inhibition (i.e., shorter SSRTs) in the NH and OH groups might suggest greater effects of CRF on the processing of stop-signal detection and the initiating of the response inhibition. Additionally, the higher accuracy rates and shorter go RTs demonstrated by the NH group further indicate that this superior performance was not caused by a speed-accuracy trade-off during the task performance. Taken together, and in addition to the prior findings indicating a positive association between CRF and inhibition, the data collected in the current study thus provide further evidence indicating a beneficial effect of CRF on response inhibition.

Contrary to our predictions, however, our results revealed no differences in response inhibition across weight categories in terms of SSRT performance. While negative associations between the standard SSRT and obesity in adults [10,44] and children [45–47] have previously been reported, non-significant differences in SSRT between normal weight and obese individuals have also been observed [44,48–50]. These inconsistent findings might result from the types of stimuli used [51], as well as the association between obesity and EF being altered by CRF. For instance, Edwards, Dankel, Loenneke and Loprinzi [21] reported that lower executive performance was only related to the present inactivity of older adults, regardless of individuals' past and current weight statuses. Our previous findings also suggested that the inhibition levels assessed by the Stroop task were similar for high-fitness participants with normal weight and high-fitness participants with obesity [22]. As such, the results of the present study extend the current understanding of the interrelationship between CRF and obesity in terms of their combined effects on EF, as well as further supporting the fat-but-fit paradigm in relation to response inhibition.

4.2. ERP

Larger stop-P3 and go-P3 amplitudes were observed in the participants in this study with normal weight and high fitness (i.e., the NH group) than in those with normal weight and low fitness and those with obesity and low fitness (i.e., the NL and OL groups). This observation of a fitness-related difference in P3 amplitudes corroborates the current literature regarding fitness and response inhibition in young adult populations. Specifically, larger P3 amplitudes were previously observed for normal-weight young adults with high CRF levels than for their low-fitness counterparts, along with superior performance across both the neutral and incongruent conditions of the Stroop task [22]. A similar pattern has been reported in preadolescent children, that is, larger P3 amplitudes and superior behavioral performance have been seen in high-fitness as compared to low-fitness healthy preadolescent children [25,26].

Stop-P3 amplitude has previously been reported to be related to the active inhibitory processing of motor responses released by the stop signal [52,53]. Based on the reduced P3 amplitudes in children with attention deficit/hyperactivity disorder during the Erickson flanker task [54] and during the SST [55], it has been suggested that stop-P3 amplitudes involve monitoring of the outcomes of the inhibitory process and its efficiency. In consequence, the larger stop-P3 amplitudes among individuals in the NH group in the current study might reflect a surplus in cognitive control abilities affecting overall performance monitoring. This hypothesis is supported by a previously reported positive association between CRF and the volume of the anterior cingulate cortex (ACC) and reduced ACC activity reflecting better conflict monitoring after aerobic exercise interventions [40,56], as well as studies linking ACC activity with the monitoring of go and stop performance in response inhibition [43]. Therefore, the enhanced modulation of the P3 component observed in the NH group in this study may result from functional and structural changes of the ACC.

P3 amplitude has also been associated with the amount of attentional resources allocated during a cognitive task [27] as well as enhanced go response processing [53]. As a result, the larger stop- and go-P3 amplitudes observed in the NH group might reflect a superior ability to allocate larger amounts of attentional resources, less impulsivity, and faster processing speed for go signals. Given the shorter go RTs and SSRTs, as well as the findings regarding P3 amplitudes, observed for the NH group, it is conceivable that the higher fitness levels of this group cooperated with their normal weight statuses to provide superior abilities in terms of several neuroelectrical processes related to both overall processing speed as well as inhibition.

It is important to note that, while the individuals in the NH group demonstrated the largest P3 amplitudes compared to the participants in the low-fitness groups, the P3 measure itself partly consisted of behavioral performance; that is, despite the OH group demonstrating similar overt stopping performance compared to the NH group, the mean P3 amplitude of the OH group was attenuated and did not differ significantly from those of the NL and OL groups. This finding might indicate that the OH group had, in comparison to the NH group, less attentional resource allocation and/or weaker activation levels that were not observable through their overt behavior alone. Additionally, the finding of no difference in P3 amplitudes for the NL group compared with OH and OL groups was partially consistent with of our prior study [22], in which no difference in behavioral results and P3 amplitudes between NL, OH, and OL groups was reported. However, the findings from both studies might suggest that young adults with normal weight and low CRF levels have lower levels of response inhibition, at least from the neuroelectrical perspective, similar to those of the obese population.

There are several potential mechanisms through which higher CRF might alleviate the adverse effects associated with obesity. Firstly, the reduction of cerebral blood flow associated with obesity [57] might be countered by the improved cerebral blood flow regulation resulting from exercise and/or higher CRF, as both exercise and higher CRF have been associated with better cerebral blood flow regulation in young adults [58] and older adults [59]. Another mechanism might be related to the ameliorating effects of CRF on the chronic systematic inflammation associated with obesity [60]. This systematic inflammation might lead to neuroinflammation in certain brain regions (i.e., the hypothalamus), and inflammatory biomarkers (i.e., interleukin-1 beta) have also been associated with the suppression of brain-derived neurotrophic factor signaling [61], which has vital importance in neuronal repair, neuronal survival, neurogenesis, and neuroplasticity [62]. In contrast,

CRF has been associated with reduced levels of inflammatory biomarkers and enhanced BDNF levels [63]. Therefore, CRF might alleviate the adverse effects of obesity and ultimately enhance cognitive function. Finally, prior research has also provided evidence of an association between higher CRF with larger brain volumes (i.e., prefrontal cortex, basal ganglia, and caudate nucleus volumes) and superior cognitive function [64–66]. This might also contribute to alleviation of the negative impacts of obesity on brain volumes and cognitive function [67–69].

4.3. Limitations and Future Directions

Due to various limitations, the findings of the current study should be interpreted with some caution. Firstly, the study's cross-sectional design prevents any interpretations regarding causality [70]. However, the current study took an initial step in identifying the interrelationships among CRF, obesity, and response inhibition, thereby providing a basis from which to determine the associated cause-effect relationships. Another limitation of this study, meanwhile, is related to its generalizability in terms of population given that only young male adults were recruited. Females have been demonstrated to have superior behavioral inhibitory performance, as well as shorter latencies and larger amplitudes in several ERP components, than males [71], implying that gender differences should also be taken into consideration. Finally, the establishment of obesity status in this study was based only on BMI scores, and although BMI scores have been widely utilized in studies of obesity, BMI is a measure of body fatness rather than exact body fat. As such, measures of body composition or biochemical indices might provide more accurate classifications of obesity and reveal different results [72].

5. Conclusions

The current study provides empirical evidence regarding the interrelationships among CRF, obesity, and response inhibition. Additionally, by employing ERPs, it allowed us to further identify the potential underlying neuronal mechanisms. In brief, young adults with higher levels of CRF, regardless of their weight status, were found to exhibit superior performance in terms of response inhibition. Moreover, the high CRF participants were also observed to have superior attentional resource allocation and inhibitory processing speeds, as well as higher efficiency in terms of the executive control system. Future research employing randomized controlled trials is thus warranted to examine how CRF and weight status changes might be related to the degree of EF benefits achieved.

Author Contributions: Conceptualization, L.C., C.-L.H., C.-Y.L., T.-F.S., C.-H.C., Y.-K.C., and C.Z.; data curation, L.C. and Y.-K.C.; formal analysis, L.C., C.-H.C., and Y.-K.C.; investigation, L.C., C.-H.C., and C.Z.; methodology, L.C.; project administration, T.-F.S., Y.-K.C., and C.Z.; validation, C.-Y.L. and T.-F.S.; writing—original draft, L.C., C.-L.H., C.-H.C., Y.-K.C., and C.Z.; writing—review & editing, L.C., C.-L.H., C.-Y.L., T.-F.S., C.-H.C., Y.-K.C., and C.Z. All authors have read and agreed to the published version of the manuscript.

Funding: This work was supported by part of a grant from Ministry of Science and Technology in Taiwan (MOST 107-2628-H-003-003-MY3) and National Taiwan Normal University from the Higher Education Sprout Project by the Ministry of Education (MOE) in Taiwan to Y.-K.C. This work was also supported by the Major Program of National Fund of Philosophy and Social Science of China (grant number 17ZDA330) to C.Z.

Institutional Review Board Statement: The study was conducted according to the guidelines of the Declaration of Helsinki, and approved by the Ethics Committee of National Taiwan University (NTU-REC No.: 201303HS015 and date of approval on 14 May 2013).

Informed Consent Statement: Informed consent was obtained from all subjects involved in the study.

Data Availability Statement: All datasets generated for this research are included in this published article.

Conflicts of Interest: The authors declare no conflict of interest.

References

1. World Health Organization. Obesity and Overweight. Available online: https://www.who.int/news-room/fact-sheets/detail/obesity-and-overweight (accessed on 21 March 2021).
2. Pantalone, K.M.; Hobbs, T.M.; Chagin, K.M.; Kong, S.X.; Wells, B.J.; Kattan, M.W.; Bouchard, J.; Sakurada, B.; Milinovich, A.; Weng, W.; et al. Prevalence and recognition of obesity and its associated comorbidities: Cross-sectional analysis of electronic health record data from a large US integrated health system. *BMJ Open* **2017**, *7*, e017583. [CrossRef]
3. Moral-García, J.E.; Agraso-López, A.D.; Ramos-Morcillo, A.J.; Jiménez, A.; Jiménez-Eguizábal, A. The influence of physical activity, diet, weight status and substance abuse on students' self-perceived health. *Int. J. Environ. Res. Public Health* **2020**, *17*, 1387. [CrossRef]
4. Pereira-Miranda, E.; Costa, P.R.F.; Queiroz, V.A.O.; Pereira-Santos, M.; Santana, M.L.P. Overweight and obesity associated with higher depression prevalence in adults: A systematic review and meta-analysis. *J. Am. Coll. Nutr.* **2017**, *36*, 223–233. [CrossRef]
5. Favieri, F.; Forte, G.; Casagrande, M. The executive functions in overweight and obesity: A systematic review of neuropsychological cross-sectional and longitudinal studies. *Front. Psychol.* **2019**, *10*, 2126. [CrossRef]
6. Nigg, J.T. Annual research review: On the relations among self-regulation, self-control, executive functioning, effortful control, cognitive control, impulsivity, risk-taking, and inhibition for developmental psychopathology. *J. Child Psychol. Psychiatry* **2017**, *58*, 361–383. [CrossRef] [PubMed]
7. Logan, G.D.; Cowan, W.B.; Davis, K.A. On the ability to inhibit simple and choice reaction time responses: A model and a method. *J. Exp. Psychol. Hum. Percept. Perform.* **1984**, *10*, 276–291. [CrossRef]
8. Yang, Y.; Shields, G.S.; Guo, C.; Liu, Y. Executive function performance in obesity and overweight individuals: A meta-analysis and review. *Neurosci. Biobehav. Rev.* **2018**, *84*, 225–244. [CrossRef]
9. Sellaro, R.; Colzato, L.S. High body mass index is associated with impaired cognitive control. *Appetite* **2017**, *113*, 301–309. [CrossRef]
10. Chamberlain, S.R.; Derbyshire, K.L.; Leppink, E.; Grant, J.E. Obesity and dissociable forms of impulsivity in young adults. *CNS Spectr.* **2015**, *20*, 500–507. [CrossRef]
11. Zhan, Z.; Ai, J.; Ren, F.; Li, L.; Chu, C.H.; Chang, Y.K. Cardiorespiratory fitness, age, and multiple aspects of executive function among preadolescent children. *Front. Psychol.* **2020**, *11*, 1198. [CrossRef]
12. Chen, J.; Li, Y.; Zhang, G.; Jin, X.; Lu, Y.; Zhou, C. Enhanced inhibitory control during re-engagement processing in badminton athletes: An event- related potential study. *J. Sport Health Sci.* **2019**, *8*, 585–594. [CrossRef] [PubMed]
13. Chu, C.H.; Yang, K.T.; Song, T.F.; Liu, J.H.; Hung, T.M.; Chang, Y.K. Cardiorespiratory fitness is associated with executive control in late-middle-aged adults: An event-related (De) sychronization (ERD/ERS) study. *Front. Psychol.* **2016**, *7*, 1135. [CrossRef]
14. Dupuy, O.; Gauthier, C.J.; Fraser, S.A.; Desjardins-Crèpeau, L.; Desjardins, M.; Mekary, S.; Lesage, F.; Hoge, R.D.; Pouliot, P.; Bherer, L. Higher levels of cardiovascular fitness are associated with better executive function and prefrontal oxygenation in younger and older women. *Front. Hum. Neurosci.* **2015**, *9*, 66. [CrossRef] [PubMed]
15. Hogan, M.; O'Hora, D.; Kiefer, M.; Kubesch, S.; Kilmartin, L.; Collins, P.; Dimitrova, J. The effects of cardiorespiratory fitness and acute aerobic exercise on executive functioning and EEG entropy in adolescents. *Front. Hum. Neurosci.* **2015**, *9*, 538. [CrossRef]
16. Padilla, C.; Perez, L.; Andres, P.; Parmentier, F.B.R. Exercise improves cognitive control: Evidence from the stop signal task. *Appl. Cogn. Psychol.* **2013**, *27*, 505–511. [CrossRef]
17. Padilla, C.; Perez, L.; Andres, P. Chronic exercise keeps working memory and inhibitory capacities fit. *Front. Behav. Neurosci.* **2014**, *8*, 49. [CrossRef]
18. Scott, S.P.; De Souza, M.J.; Koehler, K.; Petkus, D.L.; Murray-Kolb, L.E. Cardiorespiratory fitness is associated with better executive function in young women. *Med. Sci. Sports Exerc.* **2016**, *48*, 1994–2002. [CrossRef]
19. Scudder, M.R.; Lambourne, K.; Drollette, E.S.; Herrmann, S.D.; Washburn, R.A.; Donnelly, J.E.; Hillman, C.H. Aerobic capacity and cognitive control in elementary school-age children. *Med. Sci. Sports Exerc.* **2014**, *46*, 1025–1035. [CrossRef]
20. Barry, V.W.; Baruth, M.; Beets, M.W.; Durstine, J.L.; Liu, J.; Blair, S.N. Fitness vs. fatness on all-cause mortality: A meta-analysis. *Prog. Cardiovasc. Dis.* **2014**, *56*, 382–390. [CrossRef] [PubMed]
21. Edwards, M.K.; Dankel, S.J.; Loenneke, J.P.; Loprinzi, P.D. The association between weight status, weight history, physical activity, and cognitive task performance. *Int. J. Behav. Med.* **2016**. [CrossRef]
22. Song, T.F.; Chi, L.; Chu, C.H.; Chen, F.T.; Zhou, C.; Chang, Y.K. Obesity, cardiovascular fitness, and inhibition function: An electrophysiological study. *Front. Psychol.* **2016**, *7*, 1124. [CrossRef] [PubMed]
23. Ross, N.; Yau, P.L.; Convit, A. Obesity, fitness, and brain integrity in adolescence. *Appetite* **2015**, *93*, 44–50. [CrossRef] [PubMed]
24. Pindus, D.M.; Drollette, E.S.; Raine, L.B.; Kao, S.C.; Khan, N.; Westfall, D.R.; Hamill, M.; Shorin, R.; Calobrisi, E.; John, D.; et al. Moving fast, thinking fast: The relations of physical activity levels and bouts to neuroelectric indices of inhibitory control in preadolescents. *J. Sport Health Sci.* **2019**, *8*, 301–314. [CrossRef]
25. Pontifex, M.B.; Raine, L.B.; Johnson, C.R.; Chaddock, L.; Voss, M.W.; Cohen, N.J.; Kramer, A.F.; Hillman, C.H. Cardiorespiratory fitness and the flexible modulation of cognitive control in preadolescent children. *J. Cogn. Neurosci.* **2011**, *23*, 1332–1345. [CrossRef]
26. Hillman, C.H.; Buck, S.M.; Themanson, J.R.; Pontifex, M.B.; Castelli, D.M. Aerobic fitness and cognitive development: Event-related brain potential and task performance indices of executive control in preadolescent children. *Dev. Psychol.* **2009**, *45*, 114–129. [CrossRef]
27. Polich, J. Updating P300: An integrative theory of P3a and P3b. *Clin. Neurophysiol.* **2007**, *118*, 2128–2148. [CrossRef]

28. Tascilar, M.E.; Turkkahraman, D.; Oz, O.; Yucel, M.; Taskesen, M.; Eker, I.; Abaci, A.; Dundaroz, R.; Ulas, U.H. P300 auditory event-related potentials in children with obesity: Is childhood obesity related to impairment in cognitive functions? *Pediatr. Diabetes* **2011**, *12*, 589–595. [CrossRef]
29. Reyes, S.; Peirano, P.; Peigneux, P.; Lozoff, B.; Algarin, C. Inhibitory control in otherwise healthy overweight 10-year-old children. *Int. J. Obes.* **2015**, *39*, 1230–1235. [CrossRef] [PubMed]
30. American College of Sports Medicine. *ACSM's Guidelines for Exercise Testing and Prescription*, 11th ed.; Lippincott Williams and Wilkins: New York, NY, USA, 2021.
31. Wechsler, D. *WAIS-III, Wechsler Adult Iintelligence Scale: Administration and Scoring Manual*; Psychological Corporation: New York, NY, USA, 1997.
32. Golding, L.A.; Myers, C.R.; Sinning, W.E. *The Y's Way to Physical Fitness*; Human Kinetics Publishers: Champaign, IL, USA, 1989.
33. Beekley, M.D.; Brechue, W.F.; Dehoyos, D.V.; Garzarella, L.; Werber-Zion, G.; Pollock, M.L. Cross-validation of the YMCA submaximal cycle ergometer test to predict VO_{2max}. *Res. Q. Exerc. Sport* **2004**, *75*, 337–342. [CrossRef] [PubMed]
34. Borg, G.A. Psychophysical bases of perceived exertion. *Med. Sci. Sports Exerc.* **1982**, *14*, 377–381. [CrossRef]
35. Johnstone, S.J.; Dimoska, A.; Smith, J.L.; Barry, R.J.; Pleffer, C.B.; Chiswick, D.; Clarke, A.R. The development of stop-signal and go/nogo response inhibition in children aged 7–12 years: Performance and event-related potential indices. *Int. J. Psychophysiol.* **2007**, *63*, 25–38. [CrossRef]
36. Semlitsch, H.V.; Anderer, P.; Schuster, P.; Presslich, O. A solution for reliable and valid reduction of ocular artifacts, applied to the P300 ERP. *Psychophysiology* **1986**, *23*, 695–703. [CrossRef] [PubMed]
37. Alderman, B.L.; Olson, R.L. The relation of aerobic fitness to cognitive control and heart rate variability: A neurovisceral integration study. *Biol. Psychol.* **2014**, *99*, 26–33. [CrossRef]
38. Schall, J.D. On building a bridge between brain and behavior. *Annu. Rev. Psychol.* **2004**, *55*, 23–50. [CrossRef]
39. Hillman, C.H.; Motl, R.W.; Pontifex, M.B.; Posthuma, D.; Stubbe, J.H.; Boomsma, D.I.; de Geus, E.J. Physical activity and cognitive function in a cross-section of younger and older community-dwelling individuals. *Health Psychol.* **2006**, *25*, 678–687. [CrossRef] [PubMed]
40. Colcombe, S.J.; Kramer, A.F.; Erickson, K.I.; Scalf, P.; McAuley, E.; Cohen, N.J.; Webb, A.; Jerome, G.J.; Marquez, D.X.; Elavsky, S. Cardiovascular fitness, cortical plasticity, and aging. *Proc. Natl. Acad. Sci. USA* **2004**, *101*, 3316–3321. [CrossRef]
41. Wu, C.T.; Pontifex, M.B.; Raine, L.B.; Chaddock, L.; Voss, M.W.; Kramer, A.F.; Hillman, C.H. Aerobic fitness and response variability in preadolescent children performing a cognitive control task. *Neuropsychology* **2011**, *25*, 333–341. [CrossRef]
42. Smiley-Oyen, A.L.; Lowry, K.A.; Francois, S.J.; Kohut, M.L.; Ekkekakis, P. Exercise, fitness, and neurocognitive function in older adults: The "selective improvement" and "cardiovascular fitness" hypotheses. *Ann. Behav. Med.* **2008**, *36*, 280–291. [CrossRef] [PubMed]
43. Verbruggen, F.; Logan, G.D. Models of response inhibition in the stop-signal and stop-change paradigms. *Neurosci. Biobehav. Rev.* **2009**, *33*, 647–661. [CrossRef]
44. Grant, J.E.; Derbyshire, K.; Leppink, E.; Chamberlain, S.R. Obesity and gambling: Neurocognitive and clinical associations. *Acta Psychiatr. Scand.* **2015**, *131*, 379–386. [CrossRef] [PubMed]
45. Verbeken, S.; Braet, C.; Claus, L.; Nederkoorn, C.; Oosterlaan, J. Childhood obesity and impulsivity: An investigation with performance-based measures. *Behav. Chang.* **2012**, *26*, 153–167. [CrossRef]
46. Nederkoorn, C.; Jansen, E.; Mulkens, S.; Jansen, A. Impulsivity predicts treatment outcome in obese children. *Behav. Res. Ther.* **2007**, *45*, 1071–1075. [CrossRef] [PubMed]
47. Kulendran, M.; Vlaev, I.; Sugden, C.; King, D.; Ashrafian, H.; Gately, P.; Darzi, A. Neuropsychological assessment as a predictor of weight loss in obese adolescents. *Int. J. Obes.* **2014**, *38*, 507–512. [CrossRef]
48. Nederkoorn, C.; Smulders, F.T.Y.; Havermans, R.C.; Roefs, A.; Jansen, A. Impulsivity in obese women. *Appetite* **2006**, *47*, 253–256. [CrossRef] [PubMed]
49. Hendrick, O.M.; Luo, X.; Zhang, S.; Li, C.S. Saliency processing and obesity: A preliminary imaging study of the stop signal task. *Obesity* **2012**, *20*, 1796–1802. [CrossRef] [PubMed]
50. Menzies, L.; Achard, S.; Chamberlain, S.R.; Fineberg, N.; Chen, C.H.; del Campo, N.; Sahakian, B.J.; Robbins, T.W.; Bullmore, E. Neurocognitive endophenotypes of obsessive-compulsive disorder. *Brain* **2007**, *130 Pt 12*, 3223–3236. [CrossRef]
51. Bartholdy, S.; Dalton, B.; O'Daly, O.G.; Campbell, I.C.; Schmidt, U. A systematic review of the relationship between eating, weight and inhibitory control using the stop signal task. *Neurosci. Biobehav. Rev.* **2016**, *64*, 35–62. [CrossRef] [PubMed]
52. Kok, A.; Ramautar, J.R.; De Ruiter, M.B.; Band, G.P.; Ridderinkhof, K.R. ERP components associated with successful and unsuccessful stopping in a stop-signal task. *Psychophysiology* **2004**, *41*, 9–20. [CrossRef] [PubMed]
53. Ramautar, J.R.; Kok, A.; Ridderinkhof, K.R. Effects of stop-signal probability in the stop-signal paradigm: The N2/P3 complex further validated. *Brain Cogn.* **2004**, *56*, 234–252. [CrossRef]
54. Tsai, Y.J.; Hung, C.L.; Tsai, C.L.; Chang, Y.K.; Huang, C.J.; Hung, T.M. The relationship between physical fitness and inhibitory ability in children with attention deficit hyperactivity disorder: An event-related potential study. *Psychol. Sport Exerc.* **2017**, *31*, 149–157. [CrossRef]
55. Liotti, M.; Pliszka, S.R.; Higgins, K.; Perez, R., 3rd; Semrud-Clikeman, M. Evidence for specificity of ERP abnormalities during response inhibition in ADHD children: A comparison with reading disorder children without ADHD. *Brain Cogn.* **2010**, *72*, 228–237. [CrossRef] [PubMed]

56. Hayes, S.M.; Hayes, J.P.; Cadden, M.; Verfaellie, M. A review of cardiorespiratory fitness-related neuroplasticity in the aging brain. *Front. Aging Neurosci.* **2013**, *5*, 31. [CrossRef] [PubMed]
57. Selim, M.; Jones, R.; Novak, P.; Zhao, P.; Novak, V. The effects of body mass index on cerebral blood flow velocity. *Clin. Auton. Res.* **2008**, *18*, 331. [CrossRef]
58. Guiney, H.; Lucas, S.J.; Cotter, J.D.; Machado, L. Evidence cerebral blood-flow regulation mediates exercise–cognition links in healthy young adults. *Neuropsychology* **2015**, *29*, 1. [CrossRef] [PubMed]
59. Brown, A.D.; McMorris, C.A.; Longman, R.S.; Leigh, R.; Hill, M.D.; Friedenreich, C.M.; Poulin, M.J. Effects of cardiorespiratory fitness and cerebral blood flow on cognitive outcomes in older women. *Neurobiol. Aging* **2010**, *13*, 2047–2057. [CrossRef]
60. Hong, S.; Dimitrov, S.; Pruitt, C.; Shaikh, F.; Beg, N. Benefit of physical fitness against inflammation in obesity: Role of beta adrenergic receptors. *Brain Behav. Immun.* **2014**, *39*, 113–120. [CrossRef] [PubMed]
61. Tong, L.; Balazs, R.; Soiampornkul, R.; Thangnipon, W.; Cotman, C.W. Interleukin-1 beta impairs brain derived neurotrophic factor-induced signal transduction. *Neurobiol. Aging* **2008**, *29*, 1380–1393. [CrossRef]
62. Voss, M.W.; Vivar, C.; Kramer, A.F.; van Praag, H. Bridging animal and human models of exercise-induced brain plasticity. *Trends Cogn. Sci.* **2013**, *17*, 525–544. [CrossRef]
63. Hwang, J.; Castelli, D.M.; Gonzalez-Lima, F. The positive cognitive impact of aerobic fitness is associated with peripheral inflammatory and brain-derived neurotrophic biomarkers in young adults. *Physiol. Behav.* **2017**, *179*, 75–89. [CrossRef]
64. Weinstein, A.M.; Voss, M.W.; Prakash, R.S.; Chaddock, L.; Szabo, A.; White, S.M.; Wojcicki, T.R.; Mailey, E.; McAuley, E.; Kramer, A.F. The association between aerobic fitness and executive function is mediated by prefrontal cortex volume. *Brain Behav. Immun.* **2012**, *26*, 811–819. [CrossRef] [PubMed]
65. Chaddock, L.; Erickson, K.I.; Prakash, R.S.; VanPatter, M.; Voss, M.W.; Pontifex, M.B.; Raine, L.B.; Hillman, C.H.; Kramer, A.F. Basal ganglia volume is associated with aerobic fitness in preadolescent children. *Dev. Neurosci.* **2010**, *32*, 249–256. [CrossRef] [PubMed]
66. Verstynen, T.D.; Lynch, B.; Miller, D.L.; Voss, M.W.; Prakash, R.S.; Chaddock, L.; Basak, C.; Szabo, A.; Olson, E.A.; Wojcicki, T.R.; et al. Caudate nucleus volume mediates the link between cardiorespiratory fitness and cognitive flexibility in older adults. *J. Aging Res.* **2012**, *2012*, 939285. [CrossRef] [PubMed]
67. Ward, M.A.; Carlsson, C.M.; Trivedi, M.A.; Sager, M.A.; Johnson, S.C. The effect of body mass index on global brain volume in middle-aged adults: A cross sectional study. *BMC Neurol.* **2005**, *5*, 23. [CrossRef]
68. Raji, C.A.; Ho, A.J.; Parikshak, N.N.; Becker, J.T.; Lopez, O.L.; Kuller, L.H.; Hua, X.; Leow, A.D.; Toga, A.W.; Thompson, P.M. Brain structure and obesity. *Hum. Brain Mapp.* **2010**, *31*, 353–364. [CrossRef]
69. Taki, Y.; Kinomura, S.; Sato, K.; Inoue, K.; Goto, R.; Okada, K.; Uchida, S.; Kawashima, R.; Fukuda, H. Relationship between body mass index and gray matter volume in 1428 healthy individuals. *Obesity* **2008**, *16*, 119–124. [CrossRef] [PubMed]
70. Jepsen, P.; Johnsen, S.P.; Gillman, M.W.; Sørensen, H.T. Interpretation of observational studies. *Heart* **2004**, *90*, 956–960. [CrossRef]
71. Yuan, J.; He, Y.; Qinglin, Z.; Chen, A.; Li, H. Gender differences in behavioral inhibitory control: ERP evidence from a two-choice oddball task. *Psychophysiology* **2008**, *45*, 986–993. [CrossRef]
72. Adab, P.; Pallan, M.; Whincup, P.H. Is BMI the best measure of obesity? *BMJ* **2018**, *360*, k1274. [CrossRef] [PubMed]

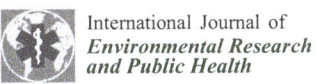

Article

Effects of an African Circle Dance Programme on Internally Displaced Persons with Depressive Symptoms: A Quasi-Experimental Study

Dauda Salihu, Eliza M. L. Wong and Rick Y. C. Kwan *

Centre for Gerontological Nursing, School of Nursing, The Hong Kong Polytechnic University, Kowloon, Hong Kong 999077, China; dauda.salihu@connect.polyu.hk (D.S.); eliza.wong@polyu.edu.hk (E.M.L.W.)
* Correspondence: rick.kwan@polyu.edu.hk; Tel.: +852-2766-6546

Abstract: *Background*: Internally Displaced Persons (IDPs) are people who have been forced to flee their homes due to disasters. Depressive symptoms, at over 31–67%, are prevalent in IDPs in Africa. Despite the evidence for the benefits of the promotion of dance interventions on psychological health, supporting information is needed to outline the benefits of an African Circle Dance (ACD) intervention for IDPs in Africa. *Methods*: A quasi-experimental design (pre-/post-test) was employed. Two IDP camps were randomized into the intervention group (psychoeducation and ACD intervention) and the control group (psychoeducation). Adults aged ≥18 years, living in an IDP camp, able to perform brisk walking, and who scored ≥10 on a depressive symptoms subscale were recruited. The intervention group received an 8-week ACD dance intervention and two 1-h psychoeducation sessions on stress management; the controls only received the psychoeducation sessions. Outcomes were depressive symptoms, stress, and anxiety. Data were collected at baseline (T0), immediately after the intervention at week 8 (T1), and at week 12 (T2) at the post-intervention and follow-up session. A generalized estimating equation was used to test the effects of the ACD intervention, with a 0.05 significance level. *Results*: 198 IDPs completed the study ($n_{control}$ = 98; $n_{intervention}$ = 100). The intervention group reported significantly greater improvements in depressive symptoms (v = 0.33, p < 0.001) and stress (v = 0.15, 0.008) than did the control group. *Conclusions*: ACD could be a valuable complementary intervention in health promotion but more research is needed.

Keywords: internally displaced persons; African circle dance; stress; anxiety; depressive symptoms

Citation: Salihu, D.; Wong, E.M.L.; Kwan, R.Y.C. Effects of an African Circle Dance Programme on Internally Displaced Persons with Depressive Symptoms: A Quasi-Experimental Study. *Int. J. Environ. Res. Public Health* **2021**, *18*, 843. https://doi.org/10.3390/ijerph18020843

Received: 24 November 2020
Accepted: 15 January 2021
Published: 19 January 2021

Publisher's Note: MDPI stays neutral with regard to jurisdictional claims in published maps and institutional affiliations.

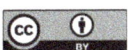

Copyright: © 2021 by the authors. Licensee MDPI, Basel, Switzerland. This article is an open access article distributed under the terms and conditions of the Creative Commons Attribution (CC BY) license (https://creativecommons.org/licenses/by/4.0/).

1. Introduction

Internally Displaced Persons (IDPs) are defined as people who are forced by disasters to flee their places of residence and go elsewhere within the borders of their country [1]. The internal displacement of people through violence is a globally prevalent issue that affects approximately 45.7 million people, equivalent to around 0.6% of the world's population [2]. They are more frequently found in several countries, including Syria, Democratic Republic of Congo, Ethiopia, Burkina Faso, and Afghanistan [2]. A majority of them are African [3]. Displaced people face numerous challenges, including psychological trauma; however, mental health problems (e.g., stress, anxiety, and depressive symptoms) are commonly neglected [4].

Traumatic experiences are inevitable throughout human life [5]. Traumatic experiences in some populations are often the result of disasters such as conflicts, tsunamis, and earthquake [6]. Recently, internal displacement as a result of conflicts is increasingly prevalent [7]. In general, evidence has shown that victims of traumatic experiences were prone to psychoemotional problems such as anxiety and depressive symptoms [8].

Depressive symptoms are the manifestation of sadness, disruptive patterns of sleep, poor appetite, depressed mood, loss of pleasure or interest, and low self-worth or feelings of guilt, resulting in impaired functioning or psychological distress [9]. Stress is strongly associated with the development of depressive symptoms [10]. When left unmanaged, stress could cause anxiety [11]. Depressive symptoms are found in 5–80% of globally dispersed IDPs [12], with 31–67% in Africa, and 80.3% in Asia [3,13]. Such symptoms are associated with functional impairment, low quality of life, short life expectancies, substance abuse, reduced work productivity, and suicidal deaths [14].

To date, conventional treatments for depressive symptoms had depended on pharmacological approaches, despite the known association between the use of drugs and adverse effects, including erectile dysfunction, anxiety, and insomnia [15]. Non-pharmacological approaches are arguably preferable because of their limited adverse effects [16]. Non-pharmacological strategies involving psychological health interventions such as psychotherapy (e.g., cognitive behavioural therapy), physical health interventions (e.g., Tai Chi), physical activity (e.g., moderate-to-vigorous intensity aerobic exercise) and digital health and dietary health interventions have been shown to be effective at reducing depressive symptoms [17–20]. However, many of the interventions require cultural adaptations if they are to be practiced [21]. The implementation of certain non-pharmacological interventions (e.g., psychotherapy) might be compromised because these interventions demand highly trained specialists. Systematic reviews showed that exercise is effective to reduce depressive symptoms in many populations, including older people [22], adolescents [23], people with various chronic illnesses, such as major depressive disorder [24], and neurologic disorder [25]. In particular, aerobic exercises demonstrated a larger effect compared to other forms of exercises (e.g., stretching) [26]. The benefits of physical activity demands intensive physical activities, but adults with depression have barriers against exercises, most commonly exemplified by their lack of motivation, exhaustion, and lack of access to adequate exercising environments [27], plausibly explaining their high attrition rates [28]. However, psychoeducation can help people strengthen their coping strategies which are needed to manage stress and preserve mental health. A systematic review with a meta-analysis indicated that psychoeducation is both effective in reducing stress (d = 0.27) [29], and in helping people to manage stress due to trauma. There is a need to develop a cost-effective and culturally-adapted non-pharmacological intervention for African IDPs. A dance intervention refers to the use of body movements in response to musical sounds [30]. The intervention can be performed individually with a dance partner or in a group. Dance interventions have been proven to strengthen empowerment, acceptance and embodied self-trust [31], and to effectively reduce depressive symptoms [30]. Dance interventions have been found to effectively reduce depressive symptoms in adult populations [31]. A circle is frequently used in the profession of dance/movement therapy, and a circle dance may be using healing elements of dance/movement therapy [32]. An African Circle Dance (ACD) is an African traditional dance that is performed ceremonially as well as on other occasions, where a group of people dance in a circle with the accompaniment of drums [33,34]. ACD may be more readily acceptable to the general African population than other forms of using dance as a therapy [33,34].

Dance interventions have been shown in the literature to have favourable effects on many mental health symptoms (e.g., depressive symptoms) [30,35]. Dance intervention for the disadvantaged adults with depression was found to be acceptable (e.g., with opportunity to connect with others, subjects do not want it to stop) [36]. African dance is a conduit of individual and community healing as Africans conceptualize illness and health as an integration of the social, physical and mental realms: which all of these could be impacted by trauma [37]. Because of its potential healing effect, it is adopted and modified purposefully as a therapeutic modality to treat mental health symptoms in African people facing adversity. ACD is not novel as a ceremonial activity, but its effect on treating mental health symptoms in African IDP is novel. However, its healing effects on mental symptoms have never been examined among IDPs.

Folkman and Lazarus' stress and coping theory is widely used and was chosen to guide this study because it is able to guide the development of many creative arts interventions for the management of stress and related emotional outcomes (e.g., anxiety and depression) [38,39]. Many research indicated that dancing intervention is effective in addressing moderate and mild depression but they are limited to high attrition rate in some studies [40]. IDPs often experience anxiety and stress from having to deal with unfamiliar environments, a loss of family, and previous trauma. Stress is known to be associated with negative affections (e.g., symptoms of anxiety and depression) [41]. Coping is an individual's effort to manage internal/external demands by marshalling available resources [42]. When confronted by this stressor (e.g., displacement), IDPs choose available measures to decrease their stress and enhance their ability to cope. In this study, ACD was chosen as the intervention component because (a) it is widely accepted in IDP people, (b) could be applied to people with a traumatic experience, and (c) is in line with the needs for psychological rehabilitation in trauma-informed care as it evokes abnormal responses [40]. In this study, we employed psychoeducation and an ACD intervention as components to promote the psychological wellbeing of IDPs [43]. Psychoeducation is evidently an effective strategy to enhance psychological wellbeing [44]. For the content, we included the essential knowledge of daily stress management tips and available resources to seek necessary help to enhance the IDPs' coping skills in the camps. Suggestions on positive health behaviour such as physical activities, environmental management, self-care, and other coping techniques were also made to enhance their psychological wellbeing (The contents of the psychoeducation will be further described below).

In the ACD intervention, dancing processes were employed to cope with the stressors. ACD comprises two major therapeutic components, which are body movement and music. They interplay with one another through dancing (e.g., tapping the rhythm of music) to stimulate interoception, which is the process of sensory information inside the body being transmitted and communicated to the brain and other body structures that occurs with or without conscious attention [45]. Interoception acts as distractors to shift a person's attention away from the negative experience and replace it with positive thoughts [46]. This shifting of attention serves as one of the emotion-focused coping strategies allowing the person to cope with stress. As a result, stress and negative emotions could be healed [46]. There is evidence showing that dance interventions, including African dance, reduce physiological stress, perceived stress, and negative affect in various populations (e.g., older people and college students) [47,48].

2. Methods

A quasi-experimental design was adopted. Two IDP camps of similar size and run under the same government were chosen and randomised into an intervention group and a control group. This study was reported using the Transparent Reporting of Evaluations with Non-randomized Designs (TREND) reporting guideline [49] (Supplementary Material). The study was conducted between 7th December 2019 and 15th March 2020.

2.1. Ethical Considerations

Ethical approval was obtained from The Hong Kong Polytechnic University (HSEARS-20190802005), the Borno State Ministry of Health (MOH/GEN/6679/1), and the State Emergency Management Agency (BO/SEMA/56/VOL.II/33). After being given an explanation of the study, eligible clients were invited to participate, giving their signed written consent. The participation of the clients was voluntary, and they were well-informed about the purpose, nature, and procedure of the study. The anonymity of the participants and confidentiality of their data were closely monitored.

2.2. Participants

Subjects were recruited using convenience sampling. All participants were recruited from their respective camp of residence. With the approval of the camp management office, the officers of the psychosocial support units of the IDP camps approached the potential participants and the officers refer them to the research assistants for eligibility screening. The principal researcher placed the information leaflet about the programme in places between the two centres in order to invite people to come for a dance programme screening. Potential participants were told about the ACD programme, potential risks and benefits, as well as their ethic rights (e.g., rights to withdraw) as stipulated on the consent form. The criteria for inclusion in the study were those: (1) aged ≥ 18 years, (2) who lived in one of the two IDP camps, (3) exhibited depressive symptoms, as defined by a Depression Anxiety Stress Scale (DASS-21) score of ≥ 20 [50], and (4) had good mobility, as defined by a score of 7 in the modified Functional Ambulatory Classification (mFAC) [51]. Exclusion criteria were those (1) with a history of disabling diseases such as chronic arthritis, primary pulmonary diseases (requiring long-term oxygen therapy), and cardiac diseases (e.g., end-stage heart failure), which might limit their ability to participate in dancing, and (2) who were unable to communicate in the Nigerian Hausa language.

The displaced individuals involved in this study lived with their family members in the Muna Garage and Teachers Village IDP camps [52,53]. They fled their homes because of an on-going ethno-religious crisis, and a significant proportion of them suffered from mental distress (e.g., depressive symptoms, stress [54]. The two camps each held between 31,019 and 39,560 people [53,55]. Both camps were managed by the State Emergency Management Agency (SEMA) and supported by Non-Governmental Organizations (NGOs).

2.3. Interventions

2.3.1. Development of Psychoeducation Talks

Since psychoeducation has proven to be an effective strategy to help people cope with stress [29], we adopted it as the standard care for stress management. It was provided to both groups to ensure that subjects who were identified as having depressive symptoms would receive an evidence-based intervention to manage their psychological symptoms [56].

Psychoeducation was delivered by adopting the teaching contents of "10 stress Busters" developed by the National Health System because they were developed for laypeople to self-practice [57]. It does not require healthcare professionals, which are in shortage in IDP camps, to deliver. These items were grouped into (a) Positive health behaviour which includes: (1) avoid unhealthy habits, (2) work smarter, not harder, (3) challenge yourself, (4) be active, and (5) take control. (b) To provide support on how to cope and adjust their daily life in IDPs camp using the resources available: (1) connect with people, (2) have some 'me time', (3) help other people, (4) try to be positive, and (5) accept the things you can't change [57]. They were also advised to seek professional help in terms of sickness or counselling using the camp clinic. To adapt these educational contents for people who might struggle with literacy, we incorporated pictures and posters to guide the teaching process. A mental health nurse delivered psychoeducation at the IDP camps to groups of 20–50 participants. We verbally met camp officers and told them our study plans (protocol plan for intervention, schedule of the programme and psychoeducational contents) were presented.

2.3.2. Development of the ACD Dance Protocol

The ACD programme was developed through a two-stage process: (1) a systematic review of randomised controlled trials and (2) a Delphi process. In the systemic review, trials ($n = 25$) examining the effect of a dance intervention on depressive symptoms in various populations (e.g., dementia, breast cancer) were identified. Guided by the template for intervention description and replication (TIDieR) checklist (e.g., materials, dosage), components of the interventions were extracted from the identified articles [58]. Systematic reviews showed that an effective dance intervention is comprised of the following features: (1) administered by a dance therapist or specialist, (2) delivered face-to-face, (3) the dance load of each session ≥ 30 min, (4) 1–4 sessions per week, (5) and with a duration of 6–12 weeks [59,60]. We subsequently consulted a panel of experts and potential participants ($n = 8$), including professors with experience in designing a study with music or educational intervention (*n* = 2), a dance specialist (*n* = 1), a nurse (*n* = 1), a psychologist (*n* = 1), a psychiatrist (*n* = 1), and IDPs (*n* = 2). Finally, we revised the intervention protocol according to the panel's comments and finalized the intervention protocol after achieving a full consensus in the second round of consultations through a Delphi process [61].

2.3.3. Intervention Group

The participants of the intervention group received the same psychoeducation, in addition to a 75-min ACD session weekly for eight weeks. Table 1 showed the details of the ACD session: a 5-min briefing session, subjects were given the opportunity to introduce themsleves briefly, after which the day activity was introduced. At this stage, the physical condition of the subjects was seen, followed by a 10-min warm-up session of stretching exercises. A 50-min ACD session was then led by a dance specialist. During the dancing period, a band of musicians (i.e., two drummers and one flautist) employed Ganga Kura drums and an Algaita (i.e., a traditional African flute) to play the African music. The participants danced alongside the music in a circle made up of a group of participants. The dance type was called Maliki, which is a popular Kanuri (i.e., name of a tribe in North-Eastern Nigeria) traditional dance. The dance movements began at a point of a circle and it ended at the same point of the circle. The participants partnered with another participant of the opposite sex and danced together in the circle. The dancing movements involved multiple body parts (i.e., legs, hands, heads, fingers and torso). The rhythm is key to the dance movements and the participants dance in response to the music that it is like a conversation between the participants and music, and vice-versa. A 10 min cool-down session was followed. In this phase, the musical rhythm and dancing movement faded gradually towards the end. The same set dancing procedures (i.e., dancing pattern and music) repeated every week. A dance specialist is an expert with a definitive knowledge of a particular dance that is required by others, and was able to show essential dance standards by act demonstration [62]. The dance specialist, who is registered at the Borno State Ministry of Art and Culture, Nigeria, delivered the ACD intervention for the intervention group for the whole eight weeks. Eight sub-group sessions with 12–13 participants were conducted according to the protocol.

Table 1. ACD Programme.

Time	Session Name	Contents
Psychoeducation (60-min)		
5 min	Check-in session	Self-introduction, activity introduction
40 min	Education session	Lecture on facts relating to the psychological effect of stress, how to cope in an IDP camp, resources available in the IDP camp, and coping skills depicted on the "10 stress Busters" [57].
5 min	Clarification session	Answer questions raised by the participants
10 min	Oral quiz session	Evaluate the participants' knowledge
Dance intervention (75-min)		
5 min	Check-in session	Self-introduction, activity introduction
10 min	Warm-up session	Preparation for the dance
50 min	ACD session	Dance exercise under the teaching and supervision of a dance specialist
10 min	Cool-down session	Preparation to end the dance

ACD: African Circle Dance.

2.3.4. Control Group

The participants in the control group received psychoeducation only. As shown in Table 1, each session lasted for 60 min, including a 5-min check-in process, a 40-min educational session, a 5-min clarification session, and a 10-min oral quiz session. The psychoeducation delivered by the mental health nurse was conducted on week 1 and week 4

(Table 2). The week 4 materials were the same as those of week 1 and were for the purpose of reinforcement.

Table 2. Trial Process of the ACD programme.

Tasks	Baseline	Treatment Phase								Follow-Up
	Week									
	−2 to 0	1	2	3	4	5	6	7	8	9 to 12
Informed consent	X									
Obtain participant's Assent	X									
Intervention										
ACD Dance		X	X	X	X	X	X	X	X	
Psychoeducation		X			X					
Control										
Psychoeducation		X			X					
Outcomes										
#Depression	X								X	X
#Anxiety	X								X	X
#Stress	X								X	X
Process monitoring										
Compliance		X	X	X	X	X	X	X	X	
Reasons for withdrawal		X	X	X	X	X	X	X	X	
Adverse events/safety		X	X	X	X	X	X	X	X	

ACD: African Circle Dance, #measured by Depression, Anxiety Stress Scale (DASS-21).

2.3.5. Trial Process

The whole ACD programme lasted for a period of 12 weeks, excluding two weeks baseline period. Eight weeks was used as the treatment phase, and four weeks follow-up period (Table 2). At week 1 and 4, psychoeducation was delivered. Outcomes were assessed at baseline, week 8 and 12. During the treatment phase, compliance, withdrawals, and adverse events/safety were assessed.

2.4. Objective

The objective of this study was, therefore, to evaluate the effects of ACD on the depressive symptoms, anxiety, and stress of IDPs who display depressive symptoms. We hypothesised that depressive symptoms, stress and anxiety reduce more in the intervention group than in the control group.

2.5. Outcomes

Demographic data (i.e., age, gender, education, employment, marital status, use of anti-depressive drugs) and clinical data (i.e., depressive symptoms, stress, anxiety, social support, and coping) were collected at T0. The primary outcome of this study was depressive symptoms, and the secondary outcomes were anxiety and stress. Trained research assistants collected data at baseline (T0), in the week immediately after the completion of the 8-week intervention (T1), and four weeks after the completion of the intervention (T2).

A Hausa-language version of the Depression Anxiety Stress Scale—short form (DASS-21) was employed to measure the three outcome variables because it comprises of three constructs (i.e., depression, anxiety, and stress) and 21 items [63]. Each construct is measured by seven items and each item assessing an emotional state is quantified using a 4-point scale (i.e., 0 = never, and 3 = almost always). Each subscale score of DASS-21 ranged from 0 to 21. To obtain a score similar to the DASS—full form which is comprised of 42 items, each DASS-21 subscale score was doubled so that each subscale score ranged from 0 to 42 [64]. The depression subscale score was interpreted as normal (0–9), mild (10–13), moderate (14–20), severe (21–27), and extremely severe (28+); the anxiety subscale score was interpreted as normal (0–7), mild (8–9), moderate (10–14), severe (15–19), and extremely severe (20+); the stress subscale score was interpreted as normal (0–14), mild (15–18), moderate (19-25), severe (26–33), and extremely severe (34+) [65]. DASS-21 was found to have good internal consistency (α = 0.82–0.93) and inter-rater reliability (ICC = 0.82–0.86) [66]. With regards to convergent and discriminant validity, the DASS-21 has a positive correlation with Beck's Anxiety Inventory (BAI) and Beck's Depression Inventory (BDI) (r = 0.5–0.8) [67]. It is negatively associated with positive affectivity and positively correlated with negative affectivity scales [68]. The DASS-21 scale has an inverse correlation with quality of life measures [69]. The concurrent validity of the DASS-21 is good as it shows adequate discrimination of both clinical and non-clinical samples and other specific groups [70]. This tool was translated into the Hausa African language, culturally adapted, and psychometrically tested. It was found to have an overall internal consistency of 0.8, and 0.7 for stress, depression, and anxiety, respectively [63].

2.6. Sample Size

The sample size was estimated using GLIMMPSE, based on an a priori power analysis employing a general linear mixed model [71]. We estimated the effect size from a similar study that evaluated the effect of a dance intervention on depression in the intervention group at T0 (mean = 16.00, SD = 12.35) and T1 (mean = 8.76, SD = 9.64); and in the control group at T0 (mean = 18.62, SD = 11.98) and T1 (mean = 16.92, SD = 9.74) [72]. Given that the attrition rate of a similar study was about 10% at 3 months [72], the minimum total sample size needed was 182 at a 0.05 level of significance and 0.8 power.

2.7. Assignment Methods

This study was conducted in two IDP camps: Muna Garage and Teacher's Village, North-Eastern Nigeria. One camp was assigned to one single group to prevent effect contamination within the same venue. The group assignment was determined by simple randomisation using the coin flipping method [73]. Muna Garage camp was assigned as the intervention group and Teacher's Village camp as the control group.

2.8. Blinding

The outcome assessors were only blinded to the group label of the study because it was not possible to blind the interventionist and participants. Due to the nature of the intervention, it was difficult to blind the participants and the interventionists.

2.9. Unit of Analysis

Groups of individuals were assigned to study conditions. (i.e., intervention and control groups). The analyses were performed at the group level, where mixed effects models (via generalised estimating equations) were employed to account for random subject effects within each group.

2.10. Statistical Methods

We used IBM SPSS statistical software version 20 (IBM Corp, Armonk, NY, USA) to analyse the data. The demographic and clinical profiles of the participants at baseline were described using mean with standard deviation and frequency with percentage according to their level of measurement. The balance of the baseline characteristics was compared through either a Chi-square or independent t-test according to their level of measurement. Outcomes at different time points were described by groups using mean and standard error.

To evaluate the effects of the ACD programme, generalized estimating equations (GEE) were employed. The dependent variables were depressive symptoms, stress, and anxiety. The independent variables were groups (i.e., intervention vs control), time (i.e., baseline, week 8, and week 12), and group x time. All equations were adjusted for potential confounding factors, which were determined by two principles:

(1) Demographic variables that are known to be associated with dependent variables in the literature (i.e., age, gender, education, marital status, and employment) [74], and
(2) Outcome variables (i.e., depression, anxiety, and stress) that were not balanced between groups at baseline because they are known to be associated [75].

The results of both adjusted values were reported. Due to unbalanced characteristics between groups, we adjusted the equations because this was not a randomised controlled trial in which potential confounding factors could alter the effects of the intervention on the outcomes. We set the level of significance at 0.05. The effect size was reported using the Cramer's V [76]. The score was interpreted as very weak (0–0.04), weak (0.05–0.09), moderate (0.10–0.14), strong (0.15–0.25), and very strong (>0.25) [77]. Missing data were handled using an inverse-probability weight GEE if the assumption of missing-at-random was fulfilled [78].

3. Results

3.1. Participant Flow

As can be seen in Figure 1, 280 subjects were approached for screening. Fifteen of them were not eligible, and 67 declined to participate. In the end, 198 participants were recruited and allocated to either the experimental ($n = 100$) or the control ($n = 98$) group. The recruitment rate was 70.7% (i.e., 198/280). All of the subjects received the interventions and data collection was completed at T1. The attrition rate was 17% ($n = 17$) for the intervention group and 10.2% ($n = 10$) for the control group at T2. All the eight dance subgroups have completed their sessions 100%. However, subjects did not attend to all the sessions. Therefore, the average dance attendance per subject in the intervention group was 79.5%; and the overall attendance rate for the intervention group is 74.9%. For the control group with only psychoeducational intervention, all subjects attended the two sessions at week 1 and 4 (i.e., 100%). We only have missing data at T2 in twenty-seven subjects on the outcome variables. The reasons for the loss of follow-up were "change of camp" ($n = 25$) and "being arrested" ($n = 2$). The analysis included all subjects as assigned to the intervention and control groups, respectively.

3.2. Recruitment

The recruitment period was during 21st November 2019 to 5th December 2019 and the follow-up period was during 9th to 15th March 2020.

3.3. Baseline Data

Demographic and Clinical Profiles at Baseline

As shown Table 3, the majority of participants were 18–29 years of age ($n = 102$, 51.5%), female ($n = 127$, 64.1%), unemployed ($n = 184$, 92.9%), uneducated ($n = 147$, 74.2%), and married ($n = 114$, 57.6%). Less than 10% of the subjects were taking an anti-depressant ($n = 19$, 9.6%).

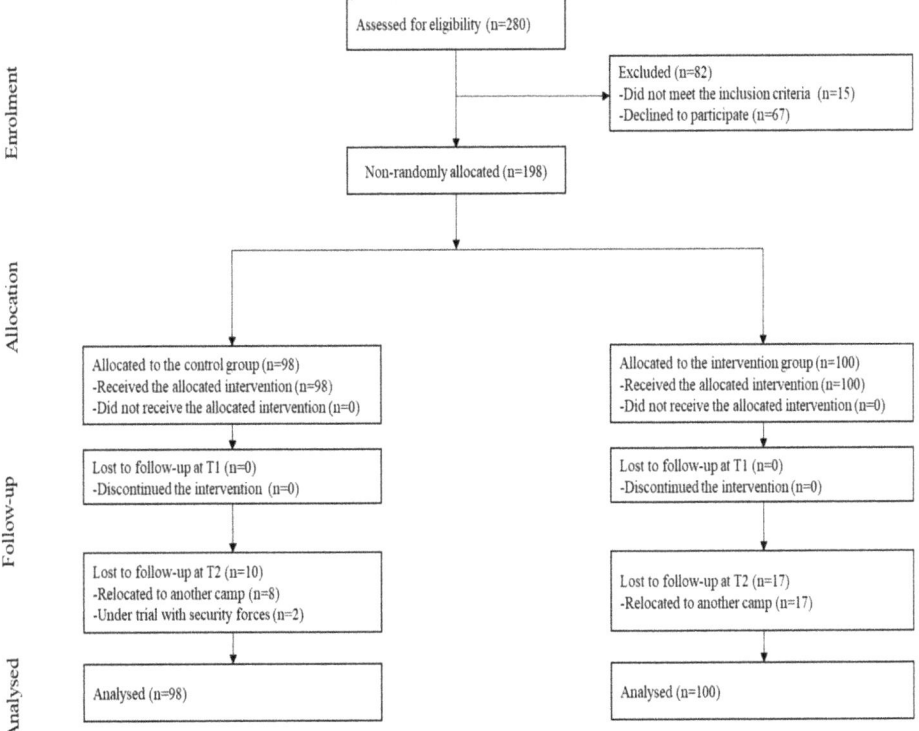

Figure 1. Flowchart.

Table 3. Demographic and clinical characteristics.

Participants' Characteristics	All (*n* = 198)	Control (*n* = 98)	Intervention (*n* = 100)	*p*-Value
Age, n (%)				0.195
18–29 years	102 (51.5)	60 (61.2)	42 (42.0)	
30–49 years	80 (40.4)	32 (32.7)	48 (48.0)	
50 years above	16 (8.1)	6 (6.1)	10 (10.0)	
Gender, n (%)				0.582
Male	71 (35.9)	37 (37.8)	34 (34.0)	
Female	127 (64.1)	61 (62.2)	66 (66.0)	
Education, n (%)				0.038 *
No formal education	147 (74.2)	65 (66.3)	82 (82.0)	
Primary education	19.0 (9.6)	13 (13.3)	6 (6.0)	
High school or above	32.0 (16.2)	20 (20.4)	12 (12.0)	
Marital status, n (%)				<0.001 **
Married	114 (57.6)	49 (50.0)	65 (65.0)	
Widowed	25 (12.6)	9 (9.2)	16 (16.0)	
Divorced	22 (11.1)	10 (10.2)	12 (12)	
Never married	37 (18.7)	30 (30.6)	7 (7.0)	
Employment, n (%)				0.174
Employed	8 (4.0)	5 (5.1)	3 (3.0)	
Unemployed	184 (93.0)	88 (89.8)	96 (96.0)	
Retired	6 (3.0)	5 (5.1)	1 (1.0)	

Table 3. *Cont.*

Participants' Characteristics	All (n = 198)	Control (n = 98)	Intervention (n = 100)	p-Value
Anti-depressant, n (%)				0.774
Yes	19 (9.6)	10 (10.2)	9 (9.0)	
No	179 (90.4)	88 (89.8)	91 (91.0)	
Retired	6 (3.0)	5 (5.1)	1 (1.0)	
DASS-21, mean (SD)				
Depression	26.5 (4.1)	25.2 (3.6)	27.7 (4.2)	<0.001 **
Anxiety	23.4 (6.9)	23.2 (8.1)	23.6 (5.6)	0.645
Stress	21.5 (6.5)	21.8 (6.8)	21.2 (6.1)	0.532

* $p < 0.05$, ** $p < 0.001$; DASS-21 scale: Depression Anxiety Stress Scale-21 SD: Standard Deviation.

3.4. Baseline Equivalence

The baseline group differences were assessed using the Chi-square test and independent t-test for categorical and continuous variables. The groups were not balanced in terms of education ($p = 0.038$), marital status ($p < 0.001$), and depression ($p < 0.001$). However, there was no group differences for gender ($p = 0.582$), age ($p = 0.195$), employment status ($p = 0.174$), and use of anti-depressant ($p = 0.774$) (Table 3).

3.5. Numbers Analysed

The analysis of ACD effects included all subjects that completed the interventions at T1. Although we lost 27 subjects at follow-up, they were all included in the analysis (i.e., 100 for the intervention group and 98 for control).

3.6. Outcomes and Estimation

Effects of the ACD Intervention

As shown in Table 4, in the adjusted model, the depressive symptoms reduced after the completion of the intervention at both T1 and T2 significantly in both groups. The reduction of depression in the intervention was larger than that of the control group with a very strong group*time interaction effect ($v = 0.33$, $p < 0.001$). The reduction was greater in the intervention group than in the control group at both T1 ($\beta = -6.6$, 95% CI = -8.73, -4.41) and T2 ($\beta = -3.4$, 95% CI = -5.46, -1.39). The interpretation of results did not differ between the adjusted and unadjusted models.

Table 4. Effects of the ACD intervention on depression, anxiety, and stress.

Variables	Time	Control (n = 98) Mean (SE)	Intervention (n = 100) Mean (SE)	GxT Interaction Effects β (95% CI)	p-Value
Depressive symptoms—Unadjusted					
	T0	25.2 (0.4)	27.7 (0.4)		
	T1	13.8 (0.7) *	9.7 (0.7) *	−6.6 (−8.73, −4.41)	<0.001
	T2	12.7 (0.8) *	11.6 (0.4) *	−3.5 (−5.51, −1.47)	0.001
Depressive symptoms—Adjusted					
	T0	24.8 (2.7)	26.1 (2.6)		
	T1	13.4 (2.7) *	8.1 (2.7) *	−6.6 (−8.73, −4.41)	<0.001
	T2	12.3 (2.7) *	10.2 (2.8) *	−3.4 (−5.46, −1.39)	0.001
Anxiety—Unadjusted					
	T0	23.2 (0.8)	23.6 (0.6)		
	T1	13.9 (0.8) *	15.8 (0.7) *	1.4 (−1.53, 4.26)	0.355
	T2	12.4 (0.8) *	14.9 (0.6) *	2.0 (−0.74, 4.71)	0.153
Anxiety—Adjusted					
	T0	21.3 (4.4)	21.5 (4.3)		
	T1	12.1 (4.5) *	13.6 (4.3) *	1.4 (−1.53, 4.26)	0.355
	T2	10.5 (4.5) *	12.7 (4.4) *	2.0 (−0.69, 4.75)	0.143
Stress—Unadjusted					
	T0	21.8 (0.7)	21.2 (0.6)		
	T1	5.5 (0.3) *	3.0 (0.3) *	−1.9 (−3.94, 0.11)	0.064
	T2	9.6 (0.5) *	5.7 (0.4) *	−3.3 (−5.46, −1.15)	0.003
Stress—Adjusted					
	T0	21.4 (3.6)	20.5 (3.7)		
	T1	5.2 (3.6) *	2.6 (3.5) *	−1.9 (−3.94, 0.11)	0.064
	T2	9.3 (3.6) *	5.3 (3.6) *	−3.3 (−5.45, −1.14)	0.003

* Significant; M: Mean; SE: Standard Error; β (Beta coeficient); GxT: Group*Time; CI: Confidence Interval.

As shown in Table 4, in the adjusted model, the anxiety reduced after the completion of the intervention at both T1 and T2 significantly in both groups. However, the reduction of anxiety in the intervention was not significantly different from that of the control group with a very weak group*time interaction effect ($v = 0.08$, $p = 0.315$). The interpretation of the results did not differ between the adjusted and unadjusted models.

As show in Table 4, in the adjusted model, the stress reduced after the completion of the intervention at both T1 and T2 significantly in both groups. The reduction of stress in the intervention was larger than that of the control group with a strong group*time interaction effect ($v = 0.15$, $p = 0.008$). The reduction was greater in the intervention group than in the control group at T2 ($β = −3.3$, 95% CI = −5.45, −1.14), but not at T1. The interpretation of results did not differ between the adjusted and unadjusted models.

3.7. Adverse Events

No adverse effects (e.g., injuries and falls) were reported.

4. Discussion

4.1. Interpretation

To the best of our knowledge, this is the first study to investigate on the effects of an ACD programme (i.e., ACD in addition to psychoeducation) on mental health outcomes (i.e., depressive symptoms, stress, and anxiety) among African IDPs. It is also the first study to enquire whether ACD would enhance the effects of psychoeducation. This study showed that the intervention could reduce depressive symptoms from severe to mild level, reduce anxiety from extremely severe to moderate level, and reduce stress from moderate level to normal. The effects in the intervention group were very strong in depressive symptoms, and strong in stress than those in the control group. However, the effect in anxiety was very weak.

ACD is a form of dance intervention. The literature suggests that dancing, including African dance, is effective in reducing stress, as measured by perceived stress and salivary cortisol [79]. Previous studies revealed that a reduction in stress is strongly associated with a reduction in depressive symptoms [75]. The findings of this study provide preliminary support for the view that ACD possibly reduces stress and depressive symptoms through a mechanism different from that employed in psychoeducation, since this study showed that ACD yields effects beyond psychoeducation. In addition, the music component has the ability to adjust emotional states and promote mind–body interactions and is widely accepted for promoting relaxation in healthcare. As an exercise with moderate intensity, dance movements may release endorphins that help people feel relaxed after exercise [80]. The mechanism for stress and emotional adjustment could be that the dance and music elements might regulate states of emotions through mind-body interactions which occur due to the effects of the released neurotransmitters making participants feel entertained and happy [81–83]. Interoception is another critical maturational element of dance whose effects might play a role in mood regulation and the promotion of the emotional state [46]. ACDs' elements of music and body movement stimulate interoception and act as distractors to shift a person's attention away from negative experiences and replace them with positive thoughts [40,41,84]. The group element of the dance on its own also has a positive curative effect on the participants while moving in a circle; the therapeutic factors of the group might advance exchange, universality, instillation of hope on an individual, activates collective unconsciousness, corrective recapitulation and mirror reaction [32]. The group effect was found to have a short-term effect on the global values which fosters social integration [32,85]. Another possible explanation for stress reduction in the current study is that the ACD intervention was undertaken in the social environment [85]. Further studies should purposefully examine the mediation effect of stress between dancing and depressive symptoms. Clinically, an ACD programme (i.e., ACD plus psychoeducation) holds promise to contribute in the management of stress, and depressive symptoms in IDPs.

This study demonstrated that psychoeducation is effective in reducing anxiety, and that dance does not exert any additional effects. Unlike anxiety disorder, post-traumatic stress is associated with a different circuitry in the brain with diminished responsivity in the anterior cingulate cortex [86]. People who have undergone a traumatic experience might not benefit in terms of anxiety from the therapeutic mechanism employed by a dance intervention. Further studies should clarify the effects of dance interventions on anxiety in people with traumatic experiences.

The ACD was highly feasible with high recruitment and low drop-out rates. The acceptability of the ACD in terms of attendance rate was also high. However, the level of satisfaction and barriers of the ACD were not measured in this study. Possible barriers may include space and security. In our study, the camp sites were highly spacious and there were limited number of terrorist attacks during the intervention period. However, some other camp sites may not provide adequate space for group dancing. Terrorist attacks could be more often that the continuity of the programme might be hindered. Further studies should explore the level of satisfaction and barriers of ACD to be implemented in the IDPs.

4.2. Generalizability

There are several limitations to this study. First, it was not a truly randomised controlled trial because of the non-random subject allocation. It is a quasi-experimental design, not a true randomised controlled trial due to the consideration of subjects' contamination in the IDP camps. Due to the non-random subjects' allocation to the groups, it was challenging to know how well the IDPs population were represented, limiting generalisability of this study to other populations with traumatic experiences outside Nigeria [87]. Second, the lack of balance in the baseline characteristics of the subjects could indicate that unobserved confounders might have affected the level of confidence in the effect of the dance intervention, although the models were adjusted for known unbalanced covariates observed at baseline. The baseline scores showed higher depressive symptoms in the intervention group compared to the control group. Sub-analysis proved that there was a regression to the mean, in particular with those in the intervention group who showed a greater reduction because they were higher at baseline. There is a risk that the treatment effect is overestimated by solely looking at changes in scores [88]. Third, the use of a specialist, not a dance/movement therapist was adopted due to resource constraint in Africa. We, therefore recommended the employment of a registered specialist with experience in leading African dance for future studies. The effect could possibly be due to the amount of attention between groups because there was no interaction in the control group after psychoeducation. Without a control group of usual care, the anxiety-reducing effects observed in the psychoeducation group might possibly be caused by other confounding factors. The intervention of this study was not delivered by dance therapists. Nonetheless, this protocol delivered by the dance specialist also demonstrated promising therapeutic effects. We adopted the "10 Stress-buster" as the psychoeducation contents. Although the contents were developed by National Health System, its effects have not been empirically evaluated. This study, therefore, could not confidently conclude that ACD is more superior to psychoeducation. Therefore, in future studies, we recommend that a cluster randomised controlled trial should be employed to ensure for the comparability between groups; one more passive control group should be added to provide better understanding of the effects between ACD and psychoeducation, as well as that efficiency and cost effectiveness of the ACD delivered by dance specialists and dance therapists should be compared.

4.3. Overall Evidence

Compared to psychoeducation, ACD has additional effects on depressive symptoms and stress but not on anxiety in African IDPs with traumatic experience. ACD might be a valuable complementary intervention in health promotion because it may be more readily acceptable to general African population. An ACD programme (i.e., ACD in addition to psychoeducation) holds promise to contribute to the management of stress for people living in IDPs with traumatic experiencess. Further studies should clarify how this ACD programme could be generalised to other IDP camps or other healthy people in Africa.

Supplementary Materials: The following are available online at https://www.mdpi.com/1660-4601/18/2/843/s1, TREND Statement Checklist.

Author Contributions: Conceptualization: D.S., E.M.L.W., and R.Y.C.K.; Design: D.S., E.M.L.W., and R.Y.C.K.; Data collection D.S.; data management and analysis: D.S., E.M.L.W., and R.Y.C.K.; manuscript first draft preparation, D.S.; manuscript Revision: D.S., E.M.L.W. and R.Y.C.K. All authors read and agreed with the published version of the manuscript.

Funding: The School of Nursing of the Hong Kong Polytechnic University funded this research study, under a studentship for Dauda SALIHU, as part of his PhD project.

Institutional Review Board Statement: The study was conducted according to the guidelines of the Declaration of Helsinki, and approved by the Ethics Committee of Hong Kong Polytechnic University (HSEARS20190802005, 11-Oct-2019).

Informed Consent Statement: Informed consent was obtained from all subjects involved in the study.

Data Availability Statement: The data presented in this study are available on request from the corresponding author. The data are not publicly available due to ethical restrictions.

Acknowledgments: Authors wish to acknowledge the staffs of the Borno State Council of Arts and Culture, State Emergency Management Agency (SEMA) in both Muna Garage and Teachers' Village camps, and other staffs of the Non-Governmental Organisations working in the mental health and psychosocial safe space unit of both camps and those who participated in the study. We equally wish to acknowledge Lydia Suen and Mankei Tse for providing technical support to the editing of the manuscript.

Conflicts of Interest: The authors declare that they have no conflicts of interest in connection with this study.

References

1. Mooney, E. The concept of internal displacement and the case for internally displaced persons as a category of concern. *Refug. Surv. Q.* **2005**, *24*, 9–26. [CrossRef]
2. Internal Displacement Monitoring Centre Webpage. Global Report on Internal Displacement. Available online: https://www.internal-displacement.org/global-report/grid2020/ (accessed on 25 November 2020).
3. Owoaje, E.; Uchendu, O.; Ajayi, T.; Cadmus, E. A review of the health problems of the internally displaced persons in Africa. *Niger. Postgrad. Med J.* **2016**, *23*, 161–171. [CrossRef] [PubMed]
4. Hamid, A.A.; Musa, S.A. Mental health problems among internally displaced persons in Darfur. *Int. J. Psychol.* **2010**, *45*, 278–285. [CrossRef] [PubMed]
5. Martinec, R. Dance movement therapy in the wider concept of trauma rehabilitation. *J. Trauma Rehabil.* **2018**, *1*, 2.
6. Makwana, N. Disaster and its impact on mental health: A narrative review. *J. Fam. Med. Prim. Care* **2019**, *8*, 3090–3095. [CrossRef]
7. Bohnet, H.; Cottier, F.; Hug, S. Conflict-induced IDPs and the Spread of Conflict. *J. Confl. Resolut* **2018**, *62*, 691–716. [CrossRef]
8. Kamara, J.K.; Cyril, S.; Renzaho, A.M.N. The social and political dimensions of internal displacement in Uganda: Challenges and opportunities-a systematic review. *Afr. Stud.* **2017**, *76*, 444–473. [CrossRef]
9. Manea, L.M.S.; Gilbody, S.P.D.; McMillan, D.P.D. A diagnostic meta-analysis of the Patient Health Questionnaire-9 (PHQ-9) algorithm scoring method as a screen for depression. *Gen. Hosp. Psychiat.* **2015**, *37*, 67–75. [CrossRef]
10. Tafet, G.E.; Nemeroff, C.B. The Links Between Stress and Depression: Psychoneuroendocrinological, Genetic, and Environmental Interactions. *J. Neuropsychiatry Clin. N.* **2016**, *28*, 77–88. [CrossRef]
11. Khan, S.; Khan, R.A. Chronic stress leads to anxiety and depression. *Ann. Psychiatry Ment. Health* **2017**, *5*, 1091.
12. Morina, N.; Akhtar, A.; Barth, J.; Schnyder, U. Psychiatric disorders in refugees and internally displaced persons after forced displacement: A systematic review. *Front. Psychiatry* **2018**, *9*, 433. [CrossRef] [PubMed]
13. Thapa, S.B.; Hauff, E. Psychological distress among displaced persons during an armed conflict in Nepal. *Soc. Psychiatry Epidemiol.* **2005**, *40*, 672–679. [CrossRef] [PubMed]
14. Henderson, J.; Henderson, G.; Lavikainen, J.; McDaid, D. *Actions against Depression: Improving Mental Health and Well Being by Combating the Adverse Health, Social and Economic Consequences of Depression*; Commission of the European Communities, Health and Consumer Protection Directorate: Luxembourgh, 2004; Available online: http://eprints.lse.ac.uk/id/eprint/13833 (accessed on 15 December 2020).
15. Elias, A.K.; Georgia, L.; Malone, D.A., Jr. Side effects of antidepressants: An overview. *Clevel Clin. J. Med.* **2006**, *73*, 351–361. [CrossRef]
16. Haviland, M.G.; MacMurray, J.P.; Cummings, M.A. The relationship between alexithymia and depressive symptoms in a sample of newly abstinent alcoholic inpatients. *Psychother. Psychosom.* **1988**, *49*, 37–40. [CrossRef] [PubMed]
17. Kandola, A.; Ashdown-Franks, G.; Hendrikse, J.; Sabiston, C.M.; Stubbs, B. Physical activity and depression: Towards understanding the antidepressant mechanisms of physical activity. *Neurosci. Biobehav. Rev.* **2019**, *107*, 525–539. [CrossRef] [PubMed]
18. Rebar, A.L.; Stanton, R.; Geard, D.; Short, C.; Duncan, M.J.; Vandelanotte, C. A meta-meta-analysis of the effect of physical activity on depression and anxiety in non-clinical adult populations. *Health Psychol. Rev.* **2015**, *9*, 366–378. [CrossRef] [PubMed]
19. Bolton, P.; Bass, J.; Betancourt, T.; Speelman, L.; Onyango, G.; Clougherty, K.F.; Neugebauer, R.; Murray, L.; Verdeli, H. Interventions for Depression Symptoms Among Adolescent Survivors of War and Displacement in Northern Uganda: A Randomized Controlled Trial. *JAMA-J. Am. Med. Assoc.* **2007**, *298*, 519–527. [CrossRef]
20. Sonderegger, R.; Rombouts, S.; Ocen, B.; McKeever, R.S. Trauma rehabilitation for war-affected persons in northern Uganda: A pilot evaluation of the EMPOWER programme. *Br. J. Clin. Psychol.* **2011**, *50*, 234–249. [CrossRef]
21. Sit, H.F.; Ling, R.; Lam, A.I.F.; Chen, W.; Latkin, C.A.; Hall, B.J. The Cultural Adaptation of Step-by-Step: An intervention to address depression among Chinese young adults. *Front. Psychiatry* **2020**, *11*, 650. [CrossRef]
22. Catalan-Matamoros, D.; Gomez-Conesa, A.; Stubbs, B.; Vancampfort, D. Exercise improves depressive symptoms in older adults: An umbrella review of systematic reviews and meta-analyses. *Psychiatry Res.* **2016**, *244*, 202–209. [CrossRef]
23. Carter, T.; Morres, I.D.; Meade, O.; Callaghan, P. The effect of exercise on depressive symptoms in adolescents: A systematic review and meta-analysis. *J. Am. Acad. Child. Adolesc. Psychiatry* **2016**, *55*, 580–590. [CrossRef] [PubMed]

24. Krogh, J.; Hjorthøj, C.; Speyer, H.; Gluud, C.; Nordentoft, M. Exercise for patients with major depression: A systematic review with meta-analysis and trial sequential analysis. *BMJ Open* **2017**, *7*, e014820. [CrossRef]
25. Adamson, B.C.M.S.; Ensari, I.E.; Motl, R.W.P. Effect of Exercise on Depressive Symptoms in Adults With Neurologic Disorders: A Systematic Review and Meta-Analysis. *Arch. Phys. Med. Rehab.* **2015**, *96*, 1329–1338. [CrossRef] [PubMed]
26. Morres, I.D.; Hatzigeorgiadis, A.; Stathi, A.; Comoutos, N.; Arpin-Cribbie, C.; Krommidas, C.; Theodorakis, Y. Aerobic exercise for adult patients with major depressive disorder in mental health services: A systematic review and meta-analysis. *Depress. Anxiety* **2019**, *36*, 39–53. [CrossRef] [PubMed]
27. Glowacki, K.; Duncan, M.J.; Gainforth, H.; Faulkner, G. Barriers and facilitators to physical activity and exercise among adults with depression: A scoping review. *Ment. Health Phys. Act.* **2017**, *13*, 108–119. [CrossRef]
28. Jancey, J.; Lee, A.; Howat, P.; Clarke, A.; Wang, K.; Shilton, T. Reducing Attrition in Physical Activity Programs for Older Adults. *J. Aging Phys. Act.* **2007**, *15*, 152–165. [CrossRef]
29. Van Daele, T.; Hermans, D.; Van Audenhove, C.; Van den Bergh, O. Stress reduction through psychoeducation: A meta-analytic review. *Health Educ. Behav.* **2012**, *39*, 474–485. [CrossRef]
30. Meekums, B.; Karkou, V.; Nelson, E.A. Dance movement therapy for depression. *Cochrane Database Syst. Rev.* **2015**. [CrossRef]
31. Duberg, A.; Möller, M.; Sunvisson, H. "I feel free": Experiences of a dance intervention for adolescent girls with internalizing problems. *Int. J. Qual. Stud. Heal.* **2016**, *11*, 31946. [CrossRef]
32. Karampoula, E.; Panhofer, H. The circle in dance movement therapy: A literature review. *Arts Psychother.* **2018**, *58*, 27–32. [CrossRef]
33. Phibion, O.S.; Aedige, T.N. The Basarwa melon throwing circle dance (Siqciru/Sigcuru): The case of Kaudwane village in Kweneng West District of Botswana. *J. Music Danc.* **2019**, *9*, 1–5.
34. Abiola, O. A Historical, Theoretical, and Cultural Analysis of Africana Dance and Theatre. *Evoke* **2019**, *1*, 1.
35. Schwender, T.M.; Spengler, S.; Oedl, C.; Mess, F. Effects of dance interventions on aspects of the participants' self: A systematic review. *Front. Psychol.* **2018**, *9*, 1130. [CrossRef] [PubMed]
36. Murrock, C.J.; Graor, C.H. Depression, Social Isolation, and the Lived Experience of Dancing in Disadvantaged Adults. *Arch. Psychiatr. Nurs.* **2016**, *30*, 27–34. [CrossRef] [PubMed]
37. Monteiro, N.M.; Wall, D.J. African Dance as Healing Modality Throughout the Diaspora: The Use of Ritual and Movement to Work Through Trauma. *J. Pan Afr. Stud.* **2011**, *4*, 234–252.
38. Folkman, S.; Lazarus, R.S. *Stress, Appraisal, and Coping*; Springer Publishing Company: New York, NY, USA, 1984.
39. Martin, L.; Oepen, R.; Bauer, K.; Nottensteiner, A.; Mergheim, K.; Gruber, H.; Koch, S.C. Creative arts interventions for stress management and prevention-a systematic review. *Behav. Sci.* **2018**, *8*, 28. [CrossRef]
40. Bendel-Rozow, T. Recovery-Oriented Dance Movement Therapy: A Controlled Trial in Mental Health Rehabilitation. Ph.D. Thesis, Lesley University, Cambridge, MA, USA, 2020.
41. Daviu, N.; Bruchas, M.R.; Moghaddam, B.; Sandi, C.; Beyeler, A. Neurobiological links between stress and anxiety. *Neurobiol. Stress.* **2019**, *11*, 100191. [CrossRef]
42. Hatfield, A.B.; Lefley, H.P. *Families of the Mentally Ill: Coping and Adaptation*; Guilford Press: New York, NY, USA, 1987.
43. Goodman, R. Contemporary Trauma Theory and Trauma-Informed Care in Substance Use Disorders: A Conceptual Model for Integrating Coping and Resilience. *Adv. Soc. Work.* **2017**, *18*, 186–201. [CrossRef]
44. Al-Sulaiman, R.J.; Bener, A.; Doodson, L.; Al Bader, S.B.; Ghuloum, S.; Lemaux, A.; Bugrein, H.; Alassam, R.; Karim, A. Exploring the effectiveness of crisis counseling and psychoeducation in relation to improving mental well-being, quality of life and treatment compliance of breast cancer patients in Qatar. *Int. J. Womens Health* **2018**, *10*, 285–298. [CrossRef]
45. Hindi, F.S. How attention to interoception can inform dance/movement therapy. *Am. J. Dance Ther.* **2012**, *34*, 129–140. [CrossRef]
46. Dieterich-Hartwell, R. Dance/movement therapy in the treatment of post traumatic stress: A reference model. *Arts Psychother.* **2017**, *54*, 38–46. [CrossRef]
47. Vrinceanu, T.; Esmail, A.; Berryman, N.; Predovan, D.; Vu, T.T.M.; Villalpando, J.M.; Pruessner, J.C.; Bherer, L.J.S. Dance your stress away: Comparing the effect of dance/movement training to aerobic exercise training on the cortisol awakening response in healthy older adults. *Stress* **2019**, *22*, 687–695. [CrossRef] [PubMed]
48. Duberg, A.; Jutengren, G.; Hagberg, L.; Möller, M. The effects of a dance intervention on somatic symptoms and emotional distress in adolescent girls: A randomized controlled trial. *J. Int. Med. Res.* **2020**, *48*, 300060520902610. [CrossRef] [PubMed]
49. Fuller, T.; Pearson, M.; Peters, J.L.; Anderson, R. Evaluating the impact and use of Transparent Reporting of Evaluations with Non-randomised Designs (TREND) reporting guidelines. *BMJ Open* **2012**, *2*, e002073. [CrossRef]
50. Parkitny, L.; McAuley, J. The Depression Anxiety Stress Scale (DASS). *J. Physiother.* **2010**, *56*, 204. [CrossRef]
51. Rosanna Chau, M.W.; Chan, S.P.; Wong, Y.W.; Lau, M.Y.P. Reliability and validity of the Modified Functional Ambulation Classification in patients with hip fracture. *Hong Kong Physiother. J.* **2013**, *31*, 41–44. [CrossRef]
52. Turner, S. What Is a Refugee Camp? Explorations of the Limits and Effects of the Camp. *J. Refug. Stud.* **2016**, *29*, 139–148. [CrossRef]
53. Displacement Tracking Matrix, International Organization for Migration Webpage. Nigeria—Teachers' Village and Stadium Camp Biometric Registration Update. Available online: https://dtm.iom.int/reports/nigeria-%E2%80%94-teachers-village-and-stadium-camp-biometric-registration-update-april-2019 (accessed on 20 November 2019).
54. Aluh, D.O.; Okoro, R.N.; Zimboh, A. The prevalence of depression and post-traumatic stress disorder among internally displaced persons in Maiduguri, Nigeria. *JPMH* **2019**, *19*, 19–168. [CrossRef]

55. United Nations Office for the Coordination of Humanitarian Affairs Webpage. North-East Nigeria: Flash Update Fire at Muna Garageel-Badawe IDP Camp, Jere LGA, Borno State. Available online: https://reliefweb.int/sites/reliefweb.int/files/resources/OCHA_NGA_FlashUpdate_MunaGarageFireOutbreak_26052020.pdf (accessed on 15 November 2020).
56. Donker, T.; Griffiths, K.M.; Cuijpers, P.; Christensen, H. Psychoeducation for depression, anxiety and psychological distress: A meta-analysis. *BMC Med.* **2009**, *7*, 1–9. [CrossRef]
57. National Health System Webpage. 10 Stress Busters. Available online: https://www.nhs.uk/conditions/stress-anxiety-depression/reduce-stress/ (accessed on 15 October 2019).
58. Hoffmann, T.C.; Glasziou, P.P.; Boutron, I.; Milne, R.; Perera, R.; Moher, D.; Altman, D.G.; Barbour, V.; Macdonald, H.; Johnston, M. Better reporting of interventions: Template for intervention description and replication (TIDieR) checklist and guide. *BMJ* **2014**, *348*, 1–12. [CrossRef]
59. Strassel, J.K.; Cherkin, D.C.; Steuten, L.; Sherman, K.J.; Vrijhoef, H.J. A systematic review of the evidence for the effectiveness of dance therapy. *Altern. Health Med.* **2011**, *17*, 50–59.
60. Dauda, S.K.; Cho, R.Y.; Wong, E. The Effect of Dance Intervention on Stress in Adults Living with Depression: A Systematic Review. In Proceedings of the 23rd East. Asian Forum of Nursing Scholars: Advancing Nursing Scholars in the Era of Global Transformation and Disruptive Innovation, Chiang Mai, Thailand, 10–11 January 2020.
61. Hsu, C.-C.; Sandford, B.A. The Delphi technique: Making sense of consensus. *Pr. Assess. Res. Eval.* **2007**, *12*, 10.
62. Academic Invest Webpage. What is a dance specialist? Available online: https://www.academicinvest.com/arts-careers/dance-careers/what-is-a-dance-specialist (accessed on 20 November 2020).
63. Salihu, D.; Wong, E.M.L.; Leung, D.Y.P. Depression Anxiety Stress Scale Hausa version (DASS-21 H). In *Psychology Foundation of Australia*; University of New South Wales: New South Wales, Australia; Available online: http://www2.psy.unsw.edu.au/Groups/Dass/Hausa/Hausa.htm (accessed on 17 October 2020).
64. Beaufort, I.N.; De Weert-Van Oene, G.H.; Buwalda, V.A.; de Leeuw, J.R.J.; Goudriaan, A.E. The depression, anxiety and stress scale (DASS-21) as a screener for depression in substance use disorder inpatients: A pilot study. *Eur. Addict. Res.* **2017**, *23*, 260–268. [CrossRef] [PubMed]
65. Gomez, F.J.C. A guide to the depression, anxiety and stress scale (DASS 21). *Cesphn* **2016**.
66. Da Silva, H.A.; dos Passos, M.H.P.; de Oliveira, V.M.A.; Palmeira, A.C.; Pitangui, A.C.R.; Araújo, R.C. Short version of the Depression Anxiety Stress Scale-21: Is it valid for Brazilian adolescents? *Einstein (São Paulo)* **2016**, *14*, 486–493. [CrossRef]
67. Lovibond, P.F.; Lovibond, S.H. The structure of negative emotional states: Comparison of the Depression Anxiety Stress Scales (DASS) with the Beck Depression and Anxiety Inventories. *Behav. Res.* **1995**, *33*, 335–343. [CrossRef]
68. Norton, P.J. Depression Anxiety and Stress Scales (DASS-21): Psychometric analysis across four racial groups. *Anxiety Stress Coping* **2007**, *20*, 253–265. [CrossRef]
69. Gloster, A.T.; Rhoades, H.M.; Novy, D.; Klotsche, J.; Senior, A.; Kunik, M.; Wilson, N.; Stanley, M.A. Psychometric properties of the Depression Anxiety and Stress Scale-21 in older primary care patients. *J. Affect. Disord.* **2008**, *110*, 248–259. [CrossRef]
70. Antony, M.M.; Bieling, P.J.; Cox, B.J.; Enns, M.W.; Swinson, R.P. Psychometric properties of the 42-item and 21-item versions of the Depression Anxiety Stress Scales in clinical groups and a community sample. *Psychol. Assess* **1998**, *10*, 176. [CrossRef]
71. Kreidler, S.M.; Muller, K.E.; Grunwald, G.K.; Ringham, B.M.; Coker-Dukowitz, Z.T.; Sakhadeo, U.R.; Barón, A.E.; Glueck, D.H. Glimmpse: Online power computation for linear models with and without a baseline covariate. *J. Stat. Softw.* **2013**, *54*, 1–6. [CrossRef]
72. Pinniger, R.; Brown, R.F.; Thorsteinsson, E.B.; McKinley, P. Argentine tango dance compared to mindfulness meditation and a waiting-list control: A randomised trial for treating depression. *Complement. Med.* **2012**, *20*, 377–384. [CrossRef] [PubMed]
73. Suresh, K. An overview of randomization techniques: An unbiased assessment of outcome in clinical research. *J. Hum. Reprod. Sci.* **2011**, *4*, 8. [CrossRef] [PubMed]
74. Akhtar-Danesh, N.; Landeen, J. Relation between depression and sociodemographic factors. *Int. J. Ment. Health Syst.* **2007**, *1*, 4. [CrossRef] [PubMed]
75. Hammen, C. Stress and depression. *Annu. Rev. Clin.* **2005**, *1*, 293–319. [CrossRef]
76. Ialongo, C. Understanding the effect size and its measures. *Biochem. Med.* **2016**, *26*, 150–163. [CrossRef]
77. Akoglu, H. User's guide to correlation coefficients. *Turk. J. Emerg. Med.* **2018**, *18*, 91–93. [CrossRef]
78. Wang, C.; Paik, M.C. A weighting approach for GEE analysis with missing data. *Commun. Stat. Theory Methods* **2011**, *40*, 2397–2411. [CrossRef]
79. West, J.; Otte, C.; Geher, K.; Johnson, J.; Mohr, D.C. Effects of hatha yoga and african dance on perceived stress, affect, and salivary cortisol. *Ann. Behav. Med.* **2004**, *28*, 114–118. [CrossRef]
80. Everly, G.S.; Lating, J.M. *The Anatomy and Physiology of the Human Stress Response*; Springer: New York, NY, USA, 2019; pp. 19–56.
81. Koch, S.C. Arts and health: Active factors and a theory framework of embodied aesthetics. *ArtS Psychother.* **2017**, *54*, 85–91. [CrossRef]
82. Kattenstroth, J.-C.; Kolankowska, I.; Kalisch, T.; Dinse, H.R. Superior sensory, motor, and cognitive performance in elderly individuals with multi-year dancing activities. *Front. Aging Neurosci.* **2010**, *2*. [CrossRef]
83. Wiedenhofer, S.; Hofinger, S.; Wagner, K.; Koch, S.C. Active Factors in Dance/Movement Therapy: Health Effects of Non-Goal-Orientation in Movement. *Am. J. Danc. Ther.* **2017**, *39*, 113–125. [CrossRef]
84. Schmalzl, L.; Crane-Godreau, M.A.; Payne, P. Movement-based embodied contemplative practices: Definitions and paradigms. *Front. Hum. Neurosci.* **2014**, *8*, 205. [CrossRef] [PubMed]

85. Sphere, P. *Humanitarian Charter and Minimum Standards in Humanitarian Response*, 3rd ed.; Sphere Project: Geneva, Switzerland, 2011.
86. Shin, L.M.; Liberzon, I. The Neurocircuitry of Fear, Stress, and Anxiety Disorders. *Neuropsychopharmacology* **2010**, *35*, 169–191. [CrossRef] [PubMed]
87. Vehovar, V.; Toepoel, V.; Steinmetz, S. Non-probability sampling. In *The Sage Handbook Survey Methods*; SAGE: New York, NY, USA, 2016; pp. 329–345.
88. Vickers, A.J.; Altman, D.G. Analysing controlled trials with baseline and follow up measurements. *BMJ* **2001**, *323*, 1123. [CrossRef] [PubMed]

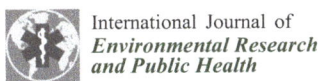 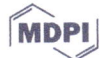

Article

Heart Rate Variability in Women with Systemic Lupus Erythematosus: Association with Health-Related Parameters and Effects of Aerobic Exercise

Elena Martínez-Rosales [1,2,*], Sergio Sola-Rodríguez [1,2], José Antonio Vargas-Hitos [3], Blanca Gavilán-Carrera [4], Antonio Rosales-Castillo [3], Alba Hernández-Martínez [1,2], Enrique G. Artero [1,2], José Mario Sabio [3] and Alberto Soriano-Maldonado [1,2]

[1] Department of Education, Faculty of Education Sciences, University of Almería, 04120 Almería, Spain; sergiosola95@gmail.com (S.S.-R.); albaherzm@ual.es (A.H.-M.); artero@ual.es (E.G.A.); asoriano@ual.es (A.S.-M.)
[2] SPORT Research Group (CTS-1024), CERNEP Research Center, University of Almería, 04120 Almería, Spain
[3] Systemic Autoimmune Diseases Unit, Department of Internal Medicine, Virgen de las Nieves University Hospital, 18014 Granada, Spain; joseantoniovh@hotmail.com (J.A.V.-H.); anrocas90@hotmail.com (A.R.-C.); jomasabio@gmail.com (J.M.S.)
[4] Physical Activity for Health Promotion Research Group (PAHELP), Sport and Health University Research Institute (iMUDS), Department of Physical Education and Sports Faculty of Sport Sciences, University of Granada, 18071 Granada, Spain; bgavilan@ugr.es
* Correspondence: emr809@ual.es

Received: 16 November 2020; Accepted: 12 December 2020; Published: 18 December 2020

Abstract: Abnormal heart rate variability (HRV) has been observed in patients with systemic lupus erythematosus (SLE). In a combined cross-sectional and interventional study approach, we investigated the association of HRV with inflammation and oxidative stress markers, patient-reported outcomes, and the effect of 12 weeks of aerobic exercise in HRV. Fifty-five women with SLE (mean age 43.5 ± 14.0 years) were assigned to either aerobic exercise ($n = 26$) or usual care ($n = 29$) in a non-randomized trial. HRV was assessed using a heart rate monitor during 10 min, inflammatory and oxidative stress markers were obtained, psychological stress (Perceived Stress Scale), sleep quality (Pittsburg Sleep Quality Index), fatigue (Multidimensional Fatigue Inventory), depressive symptoms (Beck Depression Inventory), and quality of life (36-item Short-Form Health Survey) were also assessed. Low frequency to high frequency power (LFHF) ratio was associated with physical fatigue ($p = 0.019$). Sample entropy was inversely associated with high-sensitivity C-reactive protein ($p = 0.014$) and myeloperoxidase ($p = 0.007$). There were no significant between-group differences in the changes in HRV derived parameters after the exercise intervention. High-sensitivity C-reactive protein and myeloperoxidase were negatively related to sample entropy and physical fatigue was positively related to LFHF ratio. However, an exercise intervention of 12 weeks of aerobic training did not produce any changes in HRV derived parameters in women with SLE in comparison to a control group.

Keywords: autonomic nervous system; exercise; inflammation; fatigue; rheumatic disease

1. Introduction

Systemic lupus erythematosus (SLE) is a systemic autoimmune disease with multifactorial etiology that predominantly affects women [1]. In recent years, the diagnosis and treatment of SLE has significantly improved [2], and deaths due to lupus manifestation have decreased [3]. However, cardiovascular disease (CVD) mortality remains one of the leading causes of death in SLE patients [4,5].

The importance of the autonomic nervous system (ANS) on cardiovascular health and prognosis has already been reported [6,7]. In fact, the ANS plays a key role in regulating immune responses to inflammatory stimuli [8]. Heart rate variability (HRV) is a noninvasive and sensitive measure of ANS function [9] and is defined as the physiological variation in the duration of intervals between sinus beats [10]. Autonomic dysfunction is common in autoimmune rheumatic diseases [11], and specifically, increased sympathetic and decreased parasympathetic activity as reported by several studies in patients with SLE [12–14]. In this sense, patients with SLE have shown abnormal HRV, a surrogate marker of cardiac ANS dysfunction [15], which may predispose to the onset of fatal arrhythmias in these patients [16]. Considering that HRV is inversely associated with inflammatory markers in healthy individuals and in patients with CVD [17], it is of clinical interest to: (i) understand the extent to which HRV might be associated to inflammatory markers and patient-reported outcomes (PROs) and (ii) whether HRV can be enhanced through interventions in women with SLE.

Exercise is a potential intervention that significantly increases cardiorespiratory fitness [18,19], improves cardiovascular function and PROs (i.e., fatigue, depression, etc.) [20] in patients with SLE. Although exercise has shown to decrease cardiovascular morbidity and mortality in the general population [21,22], its benefits in SLE population are understudied to the extent that exercise hardly appear in the EULAR guidelines for the management of this chronic disease [23]. Benatti and Pedersen [24] suggested that one of the mechanisms by which exercise might benefit the cardiovascular system in patients with rheumatic diseases is through direct or indirect anti-inflammatory effects. Based on the effects of exercise in the general population [25] and other chronic conditions [26,27], it might be hypothesized that exercise (and particularly aerobic exercise) could also increase HRV and thus regulate the ANS in women with SLE. Although there have been some studies evaluating HRV after an exercise stress test in this population [28,29], to the best of our knowledge, no prior research has evaluated the effects of an aerobic exercise program on HRV in women with SLE.

Therefore, the aims of this study are (1) to cross-sectionally explore the associations of HRV with inflammatory markers and PROs; and (2) to analyze the effect of a 12-week aerobic program in women with SLE on HRV derived parameters.

2. Materials and Methods

2.1. Study Design and Participants

This study included data of 58 women with SLE from a non-randomized controlled trial investigating the effects of a 12-week aerobic exercise program on arterial stiffness, inflammation, and cardiorespiratory fitness [19]. Participants were recruited from the Systemic Autoimmune Diseases Unit of the "Virgen de las Nieves" and "San Cecilio" University Hospitals (Granada, Spain). A comprehensive description of the inclusion and exclusion criteria can be found elsewhere [19]. The study was approved by the Research Ethics Committee of Granada (ref. No.: 10/2016) and registered at clinicaltrials.gov [NCT03107442] with HRV among the pre-established secondary outcomes. All participants signed written informed consent. The baseline data were used for the cross-sectional analyses of the present study.

2.2. Intervention

2.2.1. Exercise Group

The exercise program has been comprehensively described elsewhere [19] following the Consensus on Exercise Reporting Template (CERT) [30]. Participants assigned to the exercise group performed two 75-min sessions per week of moderate to vigorous intensity aerobic exercise on a treadmill (BH, Serie i.RC12 Dual, Vitoria-Gasteiz, Spain) for 12 weeks. All sessions began with a warm-up on the treadmill at about 35–40% of the heart rate reserve (HRR) plus 3–4 min of active stretching, while ending with a cool down of static stretching and relaxation. Exercise was prescribed with training intensity progressively increasing in a range from 40% to 75% of each individual's HRR. In all sessions, heart rate was monitored with a Polar V800 (Polar Inc., Kempele, Finland).

Only continuous exercise was performed during the first half of the program. Continuous sessions comprised several bouts of exertion at constant intensity, followed by a couple of minutes of recovery. At 8 weeks, continuous and interval sessions were alternated, and at 12 weeks, the patients performed only interval training sessions, with periods of lower and higher intensity efforts followed by some minutes of rest for hydration. The progression in volume and/or intensity was undertaken by increasing the treadmill speed or inclination according to the perceived exertion of each patient. Lastly, the exercise intensity progressions had to be slightly modified since several patients perceived a 5% HRR intensity increase as very heavy and difficult-to-follow. Therefore, exercise intensity increased by 2.5% instead of 5% in some weeks.

2.2.2. Control Group

SLE patients assigned to the control (usual care) group received information about a healthy lifestyle, including physical activity guidelines and basic nutritional information.

2.3. Heart Rate Variability

Participants were requested not to drink caffeinated or alcoholic drinks, to fast for at least 3 h, and not to participate in physical activity 24 h before the assessment. R-R intervals were recorded with a Polar V800 (Polar Inc., Kempele, Finland), a validated instrument [31], placed at the sternum level. Participants were place in supine position in a quiet room (temperature 22–24 °C) between 4 p.m. and 7 p.m., and were instructed to breath normally, stay relaxed and not to speak or fidget during the assessment. HRV was recorded for 10 min, after a period of 5 min, at a sampling frequency of 1000 Hz. HRV raw data was analyzed with Kubios (HRV analysis, Finland). After visual inspection for any premature contractions or ectopic beats in the recording, a 5-min period was manually selected by the evaluator. Kubios filters were applied accordingly based on inter-individual variability and if the sample presented more than 5% of interpolated R-R intervals it was discarded as per manufacturer's recommendation [32].

The following HRV derived parameters were analyzed: the standard deviation of the average normal-to-normal (NN) interval (SDNN), the square root of the mean squared differences of successive NN intervals (RMSSD), and percentage of consecutive R-R intervals that differ by more than 50 ms (pNN50), low frequency power (LF: 0.04–0.15 Hz), high frequency power (HF: 0.15–0.4 Hz) and LF to HF power ratio (LFHF) indices (which were computed using the fast Fourier transform), Poincaré Plot were standard deviation 1 (SD1), represents short-term variability, and standard deviation 2 (SD2), the long-term variability (compared with SD1); and sample entropy (SampEn).

2.4. Patient-Reported Outcomes

Health-related quality of life was assessed using the short version of the Spanish version of the 36-item Short-Form Health Survey (SF-36) [33]. Depression was assessed through the Beck Depression Inventory-second edition (BDI-II) [34]. Psychological stress was measured with the Perceived Stress Scale (PSS) [35], and fatigue with the Multidimensional Fatigue Inventory (MFI) [36].

2.5. Inflammatory and Oxidative Stress Markers

Fasting blood samples for biochemical and immunological tests were collected and processed. High-sensitivity CRP (hsCRP), interleukin 6 (IL-6), and tumor necrosis factor α (TNF-α) were measured as markers of inflammation, whereas myeloperoxidase (MPO) was determined as a marker of oxidative stress.

2.6. Other Measurements

Height was measured using a height gauge, weight with a bioimpedance device (InBody R20, Korea), and body mass index (BMI) was calculated (kg/m^2). Blood pressure was measured with Mobil-O-Graph® (IEM GmbH, Stolberg, Germany) [37]. Disease activity was assessed through the Systemic Lupus Erythematosus Disease Activity Index (SELENA-SLEDAI) [38]. Physical activity was self-reported with the International Physical Activity Questionnaire [39]. All participants filled out a socio-demographic and clinical data questionnaire.

2.7. Classification of Responders, Non-Responders, and Adverse Responders

The inter-individual variability of the patients in the response to the intervention was analyzed by categorizing participants from each group as responders, non-responders or adverse responders using the typical error measurement (TE). The TE was calculated using the equation TE = SDdiff/$\sqrt{2}$, where SDdiff is the standard deviation of the difference scores observed between the 2 repeats of each measurement [40]. A responder was defined as an individual who demonstrated an increase (in favor of beneficial changes), an adverse responder was defined as an individual who demonstrated a decrease, and a non-responder was defined as an individual who failed to demonstrate an increase or decrease that was >2 times the TE away from 0. A change more than 2 times the TE means that this response is a true physiological adaptation beyond what might be expected to result from technical and/or biological variability [41].

2.8. Treatment Allocation and Blinding

Randomization was not possible as many participants lived far and were not able to attend the exercise sessions in case of being randomized to exercise. Therefore, participants from the city of Granada were included in the exercise group and participants living outside Granada were included in the control group. To minimize potential selection bias, we aimed to match the groups by age (±2 years), BMI (±1 kg/m^2), and SLEDAI (±1 unit). The data analyzer was blinded to the patient allocation.

2.9. Statistical Analysis

Normality was tested using visual inspection of histograms and Q-Q plots. As HRV-derived parameters were non-normally distributed, their descriptive analysis was presented using median and interquartile range, while non-parametric test was used for the main analysis. Between-group baseline characteristics were compared with the Student t-test (when normally distributed), Kruskal–Wallis test (when non-normally distributed) for continuous variables and the Chi-square test for categorical variables. To explore the associations of HRV with inflammatory and oxidative stress markers (hsCRP, IL-6, TNF-α and MPO) and PROs (aim 1), scatter plots and Spearman's bivariate correlations were used as preliminary analyses to understand raw associations. Subsequently, quantile regression models were built, including each of the above HRV parameters as dependent variables and each inflammatory marker as independent variables in regression models along with age, heart rate, and disease duration as relevant factors that might confound the association of interest. This same procedure was followed with PROs. Other variables included in the regression model were SLEDAI, systemic damage index (SDI), and smoking. However, neither of these variables affected the regression coefficients; therefore, they were not included. Inflammatory markers (hsCRP, IL-6 and TNF–α) and MPO were winsorized to the highest value due to the presence of outliers.

To assess the effects of the exercise intervention (aim 2), the between group differences in the change from baseline in HRV-derived parameters were assessed through quantile regression with baseline values, heart rate, and age as covariables. As we aimed at assessing efficacy, the primary analyses were defined as per-protocol, where patients from the exercise group were included if attendance to the exercise sessions was ≥75%. We additionally performed sensitivity analyses including (i) participants with attendance

≥90%; and (ii) baseline observation carried forward (BOCF). All the analyses were conducted with SPSS v.26 (IBM SPSS Statistics, Chicago, IL, USA). Statistical significance was set at $p < 0.05$.

3. Results

The flowchart of the study participants throughout the trial is presented in Figure 1. A total of 58 patients completed the baseline assessment and were included in aim 1 analysis ($n = 55$).

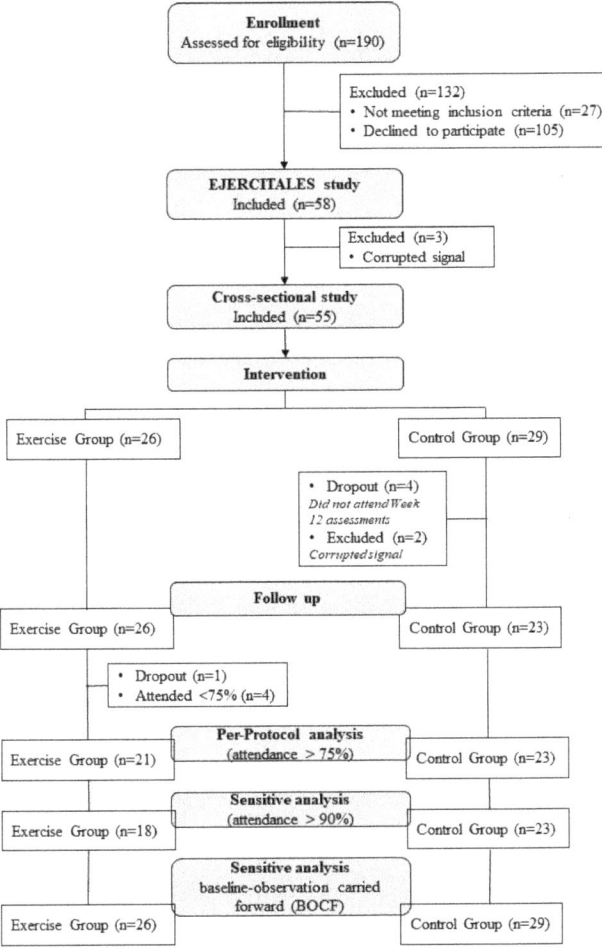

Figure 1. Flowchart of the study participants throughout the study.

For aim 2, participants were assigned to either the exercise group ($n = 26$) or the control group ($n = 32$). At baseline (Tables 1 and 2), the control group showed a higher IL-6 levels (median difference 3.10 pg/mL; $p = 0.018$), lower score in the physical component summary of the SF-36 (mean difference −4.9 units; $p = 0.034$), and higher punctuation in depressive symptoms (mean difference 9.0 units; $p = 0.011$) than the exercise group.

Table 1. Baseline characteristics of the study participants.

	All (n = 55)	Exercise (n = 26)	Control (n = 29)	p
	Mean (SD)	Mean (SD)	Mean (SD)	
Age, years	43.5 (14.0)	42.9 (15.1)	43.9 (13.3)	0.808
BMI, kg/m²	25.4 (4.8)	25.9 (3.4)	25.0 (5.8)	0.491
SBP, mm/Hg	117.5 (10.3)	116.8 (9.9)	118.1 (10.6)	0.653
DBP, mm/Hg	75.3 (9.4)	75.5 (8.7)	75.1 (10.01)	0.843
MBP, mm/Hg	94.6 (8.7)	94.5 (8.3)	94.7 (9.2)	0.937
Mean HR, bpm	76.70 (10.71)	79.11 (9.76)	74.54 (11.23)	0.112
hsCRP, mg/L (median, IQR)	1.6 (2.6–6.5)	2.2 (1.9–7.6)	1.2 (1.5–7.1)	0.218
IL-6, pg/mL (median, IQR)	10.5 (9.4–12.3)	8.2 (7.1–11.7)	11.3 (10.3–14.0)	0.018
TNF-α, pg/mL (median, IQR)	15.6 (15.7–19.8)	16.5 (15.4–21.1)	14.8 (14.3–20.4)	0.385
MPO, ng/mL (median, IQR)	69.6 (79.1–119.6)	60.1 (62.4–126.9)	75.7 (76.3–130.9)	0.385
Smoke (%)	23.6	15.4	31.0	0.237
Menopause (%)	38.2	38.5	37.9	0.968
Dyslipidemia (%)	16.4	19.2	13.8	0.586
Statins (%)	16.4	23.1	10.3	0.203
Immunosuppressants (%)	45.5	46.1	44.8	0.921
Current corticosteroid intake (mg/day)	3.86 (5.1)	4.08 (6.1)	3.70 (4.2)	0.789
Disease duration, years	15.1 (10.1)	14.54 (10.4)	15.6 (9.9)	0.704
Total PA, min/week	94.8 (92.6)	97.5 (95.9)	92.4 (91.1)	0.660
SLEDAI	0.16 (0.764)	0.04 (0.196)	0.28 (1.0)	0.254
SDI	0.42 (1.1)	0.19 (0.63)	0.62 (1.3)	0.145
Psychological Stress (PSS; 0–56; median, IQR)	31.0 (28.9–32.1)	30.0 (27.7–31.6)	31.0 (28.7–33.9)	0.303
Depressive symptoms (BDI-II; 0–63)	12.8 (9.2)	8.0 (6.4–12.7)	17.0 (12.2–19.3)	0.011
Fatigue (MFI-S; 0–20)				
General Fatigue (median, IQR)	15.0 (12.9–15.1)	14.5 (12.1–15.3)	16.0 (12.5–15.9)	0.498
Physical fatigue	12.8 (4.7)	12.4 (4.8)	13.1 (4.7)	0.577
Reduced Activity (median, IQR)	10.0 (8.7–11.5)	8.0 (7.8–11.5)	11.0 (8.4–12.6)	0.741
Reduced Motivation	9.4 (3.7)	8.5 (3.4)	10.1 (3.9)	0.112
Mental Fatigue	12.2 (2.8)	12.04 (3.0)	12.3 (2.6)	0.720
Health-related quality of life (SF-36; 0–00) *				
Physical Component Summary	43.0 (8.2)	45.5 (8.5)	40.6 (7.8)	0.034
Mental Component Summary	44.9 (11.0)	47.5 (11.7)	40.4 (11.0)	0.106

* For SF-36 domains total sample size was n = 45 due to missing data. Values are the mean (standard deviation; SD), unless otherwise indicated. BMI, body mass index; DBP, diastolic blood pressure; HR, heart rate; hsCRP, high sensitivity C-reactive protein; IL-6, interleukin-6; mg, milligrams; MBP, mean blood pressure; MPO, myeloperoxidase; PA, physical activity; SBP, systolic blood pressure; SDI, systemic damage index; SLEDAI, systemic lupus erythematosus disease activity index; TNF-α, tumor necrosis factor alpha.

Table 2. Baseline heart rate variability (HRV) derived parameters of the study participants.

	All (n = 55)	Exercise (n = 26)	Control (n = 29)	p
	Median (IQR)	Median (IQR)	Median (IQR)	
SDNN, ms	19.59 (13.30–25.80)	15.87 (11.34–25.24)	21.42 (14.55–26.36)	0.376
RMSSD, ms	16.20 (11.55–25.07)	14.82 (8.86–24.86)	17.33 (13.61–26.75)	0.292
pNN50 (%)	0.57 (0.21–3.17)	0.42 (0.22–2.78)	0.70 (0.22–3.48)	0.715
LF, ms^2	164.12 (76.51–340.51)	157.23 (76.51–345.26)	198.18 (76.51–345.26)	0.607
HF, ms^2	97.20 (39.31–299.42)	93.65 (29.92–334.81)	100.37 (59.40–216.69)	0.607
LFHF	1.57 (0.93–2.81)	1.31 (0.83–3.29)	1.82 (1.08–2.55)	0.980
SD1, ms	11.48 (8.18–17.75)	10.49 (6.27–17.60)	12.27 (9.64–17.60)	0.292
SD2, ms	25.30 (15.54–30.46)	20.86 (18.28–30.42)	25.80 (18.29–30.42)	0.423
SampEn, au	1.70 (1.55–1.83)	1.70 (1.60–1.82)	1.70 (1.51–1.83)	0.692

Values are the median (IQR, interquartile range). HF, high frequency power in absolute value; LF, low frequency power in absolute value; pNN50, percentage of successive normal sinus RR intervals more than 50 ms; RMSSD, root mean square successive difference; SampEn, sample entropy; ms. milliseconds: SD1, standard deviation—poincaré plot crosswise; SD2, standard deviation—poincaré plot lengthwise; SDNN, standard deviation of NN intervals.

3.1. Associations of HRV with Inflammatory, Oxidative Stress Markers, and PROs (Aim 1)

The raw association of the HRV parameters with inflammatory markers and PROs is presented in abbreviated form in Table 3 (see Table S1 and Figure S1 for more details). SampEn was inversely correlated with hsCRP and MPO ($r = -0.35$, $p < 0.01$ and $r = -0.32$, $p < 0.05$, respectively). LFHF ratio was positively correlated with IL-6 ($r = 0.32$, $p < 0.05$). There was no association of any time-domain derived parameter with inflammatory markers. Regarding PROs, LFHF ratio was positively correlated with the Physical Fatigue dimension of the MFI ($r = 0.30$, $p < 0.05$). There were no other significant correlations.

Table 3. Spearman's correlations between HRV derived parameters, inflammatory markers, and PROs (n = 55).

	hsCRP	IL-6	TNF-α	MPO	SLEDAI	SDI	PSS	BDI	MFI-General Fatigue	MFI-Physical Fatigue	MFI-Reduce Activity	MFI-Reduce Motivation	MFI-Mental Fatigue	SF-36 Physical Component	SF-36 Mental Component
SDNN	−0.05	−0.11	−0.21	0.04	−0.21	−0.14	0.16	−0.11	0.05	−0.14	−0.10	−0.08	−0.06	−0.03	−0.01
RMSSD	−0.09	−0.14	−0.17	−0.01	−0.19	−0.03	0.04	−0.04	0.06	−0.09	0.03	0.03	0.04	0.05	−0.05
pNN50	−0.06	−0.14	−0.14	0.05	−0.09	−0.06	0.16	−0.06	0.10	−0.09	0.05	−0.02	0.04	0.07	−0.04
LF	−0.03	−0.08	−0.23	−0.08	−0.16	−0.17	0.17	−0.13	0.10	−0.08	−0.10	−0.13	−0.05	−0.03	0.01
HF	−0.07	−0.20	−0.23	−0.08	−0.25	−0.15	0.05	−0.14	−0.05	−0.25	−0.13	−0.03	−0.03	0.03	−0.07
LFHF	0.05	0.32 *	0.17	0.20	0.17	0.03	0.08	0.12	0.14	0.30 *	−0.13	−0.05	−0.05	−0.11	0.17
SD1	−0.09	−0.14	−0.17	−0.01	−0.19	−0.03	0.04	−0.04	0.06	−0.09	−0.03	0.04	0.04	0.05	−0.05
SD2	−0.03	−0.09	−0.21	0.09	−0.20	−0.17	0.18	−0.14	0.06	−0.14	0.03	−0.09	−0.09	−0.05	0.00
SampEn	−0.35 **	−0.16	−0.16	−0.32 *	−0.03	−0.05	−0.19	0.15	0.05	0.04	−0.12	0.23	0.23	0.14	0.14

Notes: * p < 0.05; ** p < 0.01. BDI, Beck depression inventory; HF, high frequency power; hsCRP, high sensitivity C-reactive protein; IL-6, interleukin-6; LF, low frequency power; MFI, multidimension fatigue inventory; MPO, myeloperoxidase; pNN50, percentage of successive normal sinus RR intervals more than 50 ms; PSS, perceived stress scale; RMSSD, root mean square successive difference; SampEn, sample entropy; ms. milliseconds; SD1, standard deviation—poincaré plot crosswise; SD2, standard deviation—poincaré plot lengthwise; SDI, systemic damage index; SDNN, standard deviation of NN intervals; SF-36, short form health survey; SLEDAI, systemic lupus erythematosus disease activity index; TNF-α, tumor necrosis factor alpha.

The quantile regression models evaluating the association between HRV parameters, inflammatory markers, and PROs are presented in Table 4 adjusted by age, heart rate and disease duration. Only significant correlations were explored. LFHF ratio was associated with the physical fatigue dimension of the MFI (unstandardized coefficient (B) = 0.89; 95% confidence interval (CI) 0.15 to 1.62; $p = 0.019$) but there was no association with IL-6 (B = 0.48; 95% CI −0.31 to 1.27; $p > 0.05$). SampEn was inversely associated with hsCRP (B = −4.82; 95% CI −8.62 to −1.03; $p = 0.014$) and MPO (B = −106.51; 95% CI −182.54 to −30.50; $p = 0.007$). We did not find associations of HRV derived parameters with SLEDAI or SDI.

Table 4. Quantile regression analysis evaluating the association between different components of heart rate variability, inflammatory markers, and PROs in women with systemic lupus erythematosus ($n = 55$).

	B	SE	CI 95%		p
LFHF					
IL-6	0.48	0.39	−0.31	1.27	0.231
MFI-Physical Fatigue	0.89	0.37	0.15	1.62	0.019
SampEn					
hsCRP	−4.82	1.89	−8.62	−1.03	0.014
MPO	−106.51	37.85	−182.54	−30.50	0.007

hsCRP, high sensitivity C-reactive protein; IL-6, interleukin-6, LFHF, low frequency to high frequency ratio; MFI, multidimensional fatigue inventory; MPO, myeloperoxidase; SampEn, sample entropy; adjusted by age, heart rate and disease duration.

3.2. Effects of the Exercise Intervention on HRV-Derived Parameters (Aim 2)

The HRV signals from 5 participants from the control group were excluded due to excessive interpolated beats (>5%). Full HRV data at baseline and week 12 was obtained from 44 participants (21 exercise and 23 control). The primary analyses revealed no significant between-group differences between changes in HRV derived parameters (Table 5) in all domains, and these results were consistent in sensitivity analyses in which participants from the exercise group were included only when attendance of the exercise sessions was ≥90% (Table S2) and in BOCF analyses (Table S3).

Table 5. Per-protocol (primary) analyses assessing the effects of 12-week progressive aerobic exercise on HRV derived parameters in women with systemic lupus erythematosus (participants in the exercise group were included if attendance was ≥75%).

Change from Baseline at Week 12	Exercise ($n = 21$) Median (SE)	Control ($n = 23$) Median (SE)	Median Difference (95% CI)	p
SDNN	2.70 (2.36)	4.18 (2.91)	−1.48 (−12.00 to 6.37)	0.539
RMSSD	2.03 (3.52)	2.75 (4.33)	−0.72 (−12.05 to 9.74)	0.831
pNN50	0.21 (1.93)	0.28 (2.96)	−0.07 (−5.87 to 6.16)	0.960
LF (ms)	2.50 (81.86)	−22.31 (57.00)	24.81 (−142.07 to 169.88)	0.858
HF (ms)	4.76 (98.31)	6.91 (73.40)	−2.15 (−140.79 to 129.24)	0.932
LFHF	−0.12 (1.30)	0.05 (1.01)	−0.17 (−01.45 to 2.30)	0.652
SD1	1.44 (2.49)	1.95 (3.07)	−0.51 (−8.53 to 6.90)	0.831
SD2	3.10 (2.51)	5.22 (3.04)	−2.45 (−11.91 to 6.33)	0.539
SampEn	0.02 (0.07)	0.01 (0.08)	0.01 (−0.31 to 0.23)	0.741

The analyses were adjusted for baseline values, mean heart rate, and age. Values are the median (standard error). HF, high frequency power in absolute value; LF, low frequency power in absolute value; pNN50, percentage of successive normal sinus RR intervals more than 50 ms; RMSSD, root mean square successive difference; SampEn, sample entropy; ms. milliseconds; SD1, standard deviation—poincaré plot crosswise; SD2, standard deviation—poincaré plot lengthwise; SDNN, standard deviation of NN intervals.

Regarding responders, non-responders, and adverse responders, in the control group we observed significant differences in RMSSD between responders against non-responders and adverse responders ($p = 0.37$ and $p = 0.002$, respectively) and between non-responder and adverse responder ($p = 0.37$). In the exercise group, there was a significant difference in RMSSD between responders and non-responders ($p = 0.001$) Figure 2.

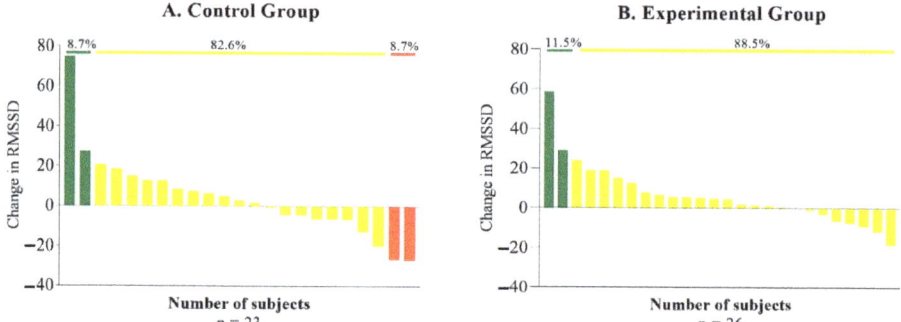

Figure 2. Responders (green line), non-responders (yellow line), and adverse responders (red line) on RMSSD endpoints. RMSSD; root mean square successive difference.

4. Discussion

Our cross-sectional analyses revealed that, among the studied HRV-related variables, sample entropy was inversely associated with hsCRP and MPO and that low frequency and high frequency ratio was directly associated with physical fatigue in women with SLE. The secondary analyses of our clinical trial revealed that 12 weeks of progressive aerobic training did not change HRV-derived parameters in comparison to a control group of SLE patients who received recommendations for a healthy lifestyle.

Imbalance in the sympathetic and parasympathetic divisions of the ANS are associated with increased risk of inflammation [8] which could lead to higher cardiovascular risk [41]. In our study, we observed that higher values of hsCRP and MPO were associated with decreased regularity (SampleEn) but not with any other HRV parameter. Elevated hsCRP and MPO levels have been shown to be increased in this population and associated with inflammation [42]. In addition, MPO and hsCRP accurately predicted cardiovascular mortality risk and risk assessment in coronary angiography patients [43]. Several inflammatory pathways seem to be involved in the relationship with HRV. One of the possible explanations could be changes in the activity of the vagal system that modulates the inflammatory response significantly, which can be blocked or enhanced by transmitter substances (i.e., noradrenaline) or by pro-inflammatory cytokines [44]. A decrease in regularity (SampleEn) could be related to the idea proposed by Goldberger et al. [45], in which nonlinear complexity breaks down with aging and disease reducing the individual's adaptive capabilities. We also found a positive correlation between HRV and IL-6 but not with TNF-α. After adjusting the quantile regression model by age, heart rate, and disease duration we did not find an association between HRV and IL-6. However, it should be noted that both inflammatory markers and ANS have a circadian variation and that the explanatory power of correlating HRV activity and inflammation may be limited by the time frame of the analysis [46]. Given that our HRV data were collected in the afternoon and once at baseline and after the intervention, this could affect our conclusions about these associations.

Regarding PROs, we did not find in our sample associations between HRV and depression, stress or health-related quality of life as previously reported [47]. However, we observed an association between HRV and physical fatigue, as previous findings in other illnesses such as breast cancer [48]. According to Pagani et al. [49], slow autonomic responses to environmental demands or an imbalance between sympathetic and parasympathetic branches may contribute to reduced physical activity, and increased fatigue. It is important to note that fatigue improvements have been described in SLE independently of changes in fitness levels and that fatigue is a multifaceted phenomenon that might be affected by different peripheral and central mechanisms [50]. However, we have observed reductions in general fatigue after our exercise intervention with cardiorespiratory fitness as a mediator [20], which could be related to a better conditioning in these patients.

To the best of our knowledge, no prior research has evaluated the effects of aerobic exercise on HRV in women with SLE. Yorgun et al. [28] studied HRV during 24 h in SLE patients and controls after an exercise stress test finding a higher QT dispersion, along the lines of previous work by Rivera-López et al. [51], and impairments in the autonomic cardiac function in SLE patients compared to controls. A similar study was performed by Bienias et al. [29] controlling the effect of beta-blockers in one of the groups, concluding that impaired heart rate recovery was associated with disease duration and beta-blocker treatment. Our results showed no differences in HRV between groups after an aerobic exercise program. However, as shown in Figure 2, there are some participants that improved their RMSDD after the intervention and, compared to the control group, all participants slightly improved as well even if these differences were not significant. It is important to note that our sample size is small, and we had dropout patients in both groups, although our results were consistent across different sensitivity analyses (Tables S2 and S3). This show that, although our intervention improved CRF in these patients [19], it was not as effective in other secondary parameters such as HRV. Therefore, a more effective or intense intervention program could have had improvements in HRV and other physiological parameters. In fact, HRV as a tool to guide daily training has shown to be superior (at increasing fitness and exercise performance) to other training conventional methods [52].

This study has limitations. First, since our sample size was relatively small, and this study is exploratory and hypotheses-generating in nature, we did not perform corrections for multiple comparisons, which would likely eliminate all the observed associations. Future studies with larger samples should confirm or contrast these findings. Second, only women with mild/inactive disease were included. Therefore, the results are not generalizable to men or even women with medium–high disease. Third, this study comes from the secondary analysis of a non-randomized design, and, despite statistical adjustment, residual confounding cannot be discarded. Four, we did not have a group of healthy subjects performing the exercise program, which would have enabled us to compare the results. However, the study also has some strengths that must be highlighted. First, to our knowledge this is the most comprehensive study done about HRV in women with SLE. Second, we have shown how everyone responded individually to the exercise program based on their HRV.

5. Conclusions

Our study suggests that increases in hsCRP and MPO are related to decreased regularity, and that physical fatigue seems to be related to HRV in women with SLE. Additionally, 12 weeks of progressive aerobic training (75 min twice a week) did not produce any changes in HRV derived parameters compared to a usual care control group in women with mild/inactive disease. Future clinical trials with larger sample sizes and a different training program or with higher intensity are needed to enhance our understanding on how HRV could help monitor inflammation in this population; and how they respond to an exercise intervention using HRV as a guideline to prescribe training on a day-to-day basis.

Supplementary Materials: The following are available online at http://www.mdpi.com/1660-4601/17/24/9501/s1, Figure S1: Correlations between HRV derived parameters and inflammatory markers ($n = 55$), Table S1: Spearman's correlations between HRV derived parameters, inflammatory markers, and PROs ($n = 55$), Table S2: Sensitivity analyses assessing the effects of 12-week progressive aerobic exercise on HRV derived parameters in women with systemic lupus erythematosus (participants in the exercise group were included if attendance ≥90%), Table S3: Sensitivity analyses using baseline-observation carried forward imputation assessing the effects of 12-week progressive aerobic exercise on HRV derived parameters in women with systemic lupus erythematosus.

Author Contributions: Conceptualization, E.M.-R. and A.S.-M.; methodology, S.S.-R. and A.H.-M.; formal analysis, E.M.-R.; resources, S.S.-R., A.H.-M., A.R.-C., and B.G.-C.; data curation, B.G.-C.; writing—original draft preparation, E.M.-R.; writing—review and editing, E.M.-R., S.S.-R., A.H.-M., A.R.-C., B.G.-C., E.G.A., J.A.V.-H., and A.S.-M.; visualization, E.G.A.; supervision, J.A.V.-H.; project administration, J.M.S.; funding acquisition, J.A.V.-H and A.S.-M. All authors have read and agreed to the published version of the manuscript.

Funding: This work was supported by Fundación para la Investigación Biosanitaria de Andalucía Oriental (grant number: PI-0525-2016 and PIER-0223-2019). E.M.-R. was supported by the Spanish Ministry of Universities (FPU18/01107) and A.H.-M. by the Gerty Cory pre-doctoral program for deficit areas at the University of Almería.

Acknowledgments: The authors would like to thank the study participants for their collaboration. We also gratefully acknowledge the members of the Internal Medicine Department for their support during data collection, and the people involved in the supervision of the exercise intervention and suggestions during the design of it.

Conflicts of Interest: The authors declare no conflict of interest. The funders had no role in the design of the study; in the collection, analyses, or interpretation of data; in the writing of the manuscript, or in the decision to publish the results.

References

1. Margery-Muir, A.A.; Bundell, C.; Nelson, D.; Groth, D.M.; Wetherall, J.D. Gender balance in patients with systemic lupus erythematosus. *Autoimmun. Rev.* **2017**, *16*, 258–268. [CrossRef] [PubMed]
2. Lisnevskaia, L.; Murphy, G.; Isenberg, D. Systemic lupus erythematosus. *Lancet* **2014**, *384*, 1878–1888. [CrossRef]
3. Stojan, G.; Petri, M. Epidemiology of systemic lupus erythematosus: An update. *Curr. Opin. Rheumatol.* **2018**, *30*, 144–150. [CrossRef]
4. Ocampo-Piraquive, V.; Nieto-Aristizábal, I.; Cañas, C.A.; Tobón, G.J. Mortality in systemic lupus erythematosus: Causes, predictors and interventions. *Expert Rev. Clin. Immunol.* **2018**, *14*, 1043–1053. [CrossRef]
5. Liu, Y.; Kaplan, M.J. Cardiovascular disease in systemic lupus erythematosus: An update. *Curr. Opin. Rheumatol.* **2018**, *30*, 441–448. [CrossRef]
6. Freeman, J.V.; Dewey, F.E.; Hadley, D.M.; Myers, J.; Froelicher, V.F. Autonomic Nervous System Interaction With the Cardiovascular System During Exercise. *Prog. Cardiovasc. Dis.* **2006**, *48*, 342–362. [CrossRef]
7. Lahiri, M.K.; Kannankeril, P.J.; Goldberger, J.J. Assessment of Autonomic Function in Cardiovascular Disease. Physiological Basis and Prognostic Implications. *J. Am. Coll. Cardiol.* **2008**, *51*, 1725–1733. [CrossRef]
8. Marsland, A.L.; Gianaros, P.J.; Prather, A.A.; Jennings, J.R.; Neumann, S.A.; Manuck, S.B. Stimulated production of proinflammatory cytokines covaries inversely with heart rate variability. *Psychosom. Med.* **2007**, *69*, 709–716. [CrossRef]
9. Task Force Heart rate variability. Standards of measurement, physiological interpretation, and clinical use. Task Force of the European Society of Cardiology and the North American Society of Pacing and Electrophysiology. *Eur. Heart J.* **1996**, *17*, 354–381. Available online: https://www.escardio.org/static-file/Escardio/Guidelines/Scientific-Statements/guidelines-Heart-Rate-Variability-FT-1996.pdf (accessed on 14 December 2020). [CrossRef]
10. Singh, N.; Moneghetti, K.J.; Christle, J.W.; Hadley, D.; Plews, D.; Froelicher, V.; Plews, D. Heart Rate Variability: An Old Metric with New Meaning in the Era of using mHealth Technologies for Health and Exercise Training Guidance. Part One: Physiology and Methods. *Arrhythmia Electrophysiol. Rev.* **2018**, *7*, 193–198. [CrossRef]
11. Stojanovich, L. Autonomic dysfunction in autoimmune rheumatic disease. *Autoimmun. Rev.* **2009**, *8*, 569–572. [CrossRef] [PubMed]
12. Laversuch, C.J.; Seo, H.; Modarres, H.; Collins, D.A.; McKenna, W.; Bourke, B.E. Reduction in heart rate variability in patients with systemic lupus erythematosus. *J. Rheumatol.* **1997**, *24*, 1540–1544. [PubMed]
13. Aydemir, M.; Yazisiz, V.; Basarici, I.; Avci, A.; Erbasan, F.; Belgi, A.; Terzioglu, E. Cardiac autonomic profile in rheumatoid arthritis and systemic lupus erythematosus. *Lupus* **2010**, *19*, 255–261. [CrossRef] [PubMed]
14. Thanou, A.; Stavrakis, S.; Dyer, J.W.; Munroe, M.E.; James, J.A.; Merrill, J.T. Impact of heart rate variability, a marker for cardiac health, on lupus disease activity. *Arthritis Res. Ther.* **2016**, *18*, 197. [CrossRef] [PubMed]
15. Matusik, P.S.; Matusik, P.T.; Stein, P.K. Heart rate variability in patients with systemic lupus erythematosus: A systematic review and methodological considerations. *Lupus* **2018**, *27*, 1225–1239. [CrossRef]
16. Tselios, K.; Gladman, D.D.; Harvey, P.; Su, J.; Urowitz, M.B. Severe brady-arrhythmias in systemic lupus erythematosus: Prevalence, etiology and associated factors. *Lupus* **2018**, *27*, 1415–1423. [CrossRef]
17. Whelton, S.P.; Narla, V.; Blaha, M.J.; Nasir, K.; Blumenthal, R.S.; Jenny, N.S.; Al-Mallah, M.H.; Michos, E.D. Association between resting heart rate and inflammatory biomarkers (high-sensitivity C-reactive protein, interleukin-6, and fibrinogen) (from the Multi-Ethnic Study of Atherosclerosis). *Am. J. Cardiol.* **2014**, *113*, 644–649. [CrossRef]

18. O'Dwyer, T.; Durcan, L.; Wilson, F. Exercise and physical activity in systemic lupus erythematosus: A systematic review with meta-analyses. *Semin. Arthritis Rheum.* **2017**, *47*, 204–215. [CrossRef]
19. Soriano-Maldonado, A.; Morillas-de-Laguno, P.; Sabio, J.M.; Gavilán-Carrera, B.; Rosales-Castillo, A.; Montalbán-Méndez, C.; Sáez-Urán, L.M.; Callejas-Rubio, J.L.; Vargas-Hitos, J.A. Effects of 12-week Aerobic Exercise on Arterial Stiffness, Inflammation, and Cardiorespiratory Fitness in Women with Systemic LUPUS Erythematosus: Non-Randomized Controlled Trial. *J. Clin. Med.* **2018**, *7*, 477. [CrossRef]
20. Gavilán-Carrera, B.; Vargas-Hitos, J.A.; Morillas-de-laguno, P.; Rosales-Castillo, A.; Sola-Rodríguez, S.; Callejas-Rubio, L.; Sabio, M.; Soriano-Maldonado, A. Effects of 12-week aerobic exercise on patient-reported outcomes in women with systemic lupus erythematosus. *Disabil. Rehabil.* **2020**, 1–9. [CrossRef]
21. Sloan, R.A.; Sawada, S.S.; Martin, C.K.; Church, T.; Blair, S.N. Associations between cardiorespiratory fitness and health-related quality of life. *Health Qual. Life Outcomes* **2009**, *7*, 47. [CrossRef] [PubMed]
22. Myers, J.; McAuley, P.; Lavie, C.J.; Despres, J.-P.; Arena, R.; Kokkinos, P. Physical Activity and Cardiorespiratory Fitness as Major Markers of Cardiovascular Risk: Their Independent and Interwoven Importance to Health Status. *Prog. Cardiovasc. Dis.* **2015**, *57*, 306–314. [CrossRef] [PubMed]
23. Fanouriakis, A.; Kostopoulou, M.; Alunno, A.; Aringer, M.; Bajema, I.; Boletis, J.N.; Cervera, R.; Doria, A.; Gordon, C.; Govoni, M.; et al. 2019 Update of the EULAR recommendations for the management of systemic lupus erythematosus. *Ann. Rheum. Dis.* **2019**, *78*, 736–745. [CrossRef] [PubMed]
24. Benatti, F.B.; Pedersen, B.K. Exercise as an anti-inflammatory therapy for rheumatic diseases-myokine regulation. *Nat. Rev. Rheumatol.* **2015**, *11*, 86–97. [CrossRef]
25. Lavie, C.J.; Ozemek, C.; Carbone, S.; Katzmarzyk, P.T.; Blair, S.N. Sedentary Behavior, Exercise, and Cardiovascular Health. *Circ. Res.* **2019**, *124*, 799–815. [CrossRef]
26. Anderson, L.; Thompson, D.R.; Oldridge, N.; Zwisler, A.-D.; Rees, K.; Martin, N.; Taylor, R.S. Exercise-based cardiac rehabilitation for coronary heart disease. *Cochrane Database Syst. Rev.* **2016**, *67*, 1–12.
27. Speck, R.M.; Courneya, K.S.; Mâsse, L.C.; Duval, S.; Schmitz, K.H. An update of controlled physical activity trials in cancer survivors: A systematic review and meta-analysis. *J. Cancer Surviv.* **2010**, *4*, 87–100. [CrossRef]
28. Yorgun, H.; Canpolat, U.; Aytemir, K.; Ateş, A.; Kaya, E.; Akdoğan, A.; Sunman, H.; Canpolat, A.G.; Çalgüneri, M.; Kabakçı, G.; et al. Evaluation of cardiac autonomic functions in patients with systemic lupus erythematosus. *Lupus* **2012**, *21*, 373–379. [CrossRef]
29. Bienias, P.; Ciurzyński, M.; Chrzanowska, A.; Dudzik-Niewiadomska, I.; Irzyk, K.; Oleszek, K.; Kalińska-Bienias, A.; Kisiel, B.; Tłustochowicz, W.; Pruszczyk, P. Attenuated post-exercise heart rate recovery in patients with systemic lupus erythematosus: The role of disease severity and beta-blocker treatment. *Lupus* **2018**, *27*, 217–224. [CrossRef]
30. Slade, S.C.; Dionne, C.E.; Underwood, M.; Buchbinder, R.; Beck, B.; Bennell, K.; Brosseau, L.; Costa, L.; Cramp, F.; Cup, E.; et al. Consensus on Exercise Reporting Template (CERT): Modified Delphi Study. *Phys. Ther.* **2016**, *96*, 1514–1524. [CrossRef]
31. Giles, D.; Draper, N.; Neil, W. Validity of the Polar V800 heart rate monitor to measure RR intervals at rest. *Eur. J. Appl. Physiol.* **2016**, *116*, 563–571. [CrossRef] [PubMed]
32. Tarvainen, M.P.; Lipponen, J.; Niskanen, J.-P.; Ranta-aho, P.O. User's Guide HRV. 2017. Available online: https://www.kubios.com/downloads/Kubios_HRV_Users_Guide.pdf (accessed on 14 December 2020).
33. Alonso, J.; Prieto, L.; Anto, J.M. The Spanish version of the SF-36 Health Survey (the SF-36 health questionnaire): An instrument for measuring clinical results. *Med. Clin.* **1995**, *104*, 771–776.
34. Beck, A.T.; Steer, R.A.; Brown, G. *Manual for the Beck Depression Inventory-II*; Psychological Corporation: San Antonio, TX, USA, 1996.
35. Cohen, S.; Kamarck, T.; Mermelstein, R. A Global Measure of Perceived Stress. *J. Health Soc. Behav.* **1983**, *24*, 385–396. [CrossRef] [PubMed]
36. Smets, E.M.A.; Garssen, B.; Bonke, B.; De Haes, J.C.J.M. The multidimensional Fatigue Inventory (MFI) psychometric qualities of an instrument to assess fatigue. *J. Psychosom. Res.* **1995**, *39*, 315–325. [CrossRef]
37. Weiss, W.; Gohlisch, C.; Harsch-Gladisch, C.; Tölle, M.; Zidek, W.; van der Giet, M. Oscillometric estimation of central blood pressure: Validation of the Mobil-O-Graph in comparison with the SphygmoCor device. *Blood Press. Monit.* **2012**, *17*, 128–131. [CrossRef]
38. Petri, M. Disease activity assessment in SLE: Do we have the right instruments? *Ann. Rheum. Dis.* **2007**, *66*, 61–64. [CrossRef]

39. Craig, C.L.; Marshall, A.L.; Sjöström, M.; Bauman, A.E.; Booth, M.L.; Ainsworth, B.E.; Pratt, M.; Ekelund, U.; Yngve, A.; Sallis, J.F.; et al. International physical activity questionnaire: 12-country reliability and validity. *Med. Sci. Sports Exerc.* **2003**, *35*, 1381–1395. [CrossRef]
40. Hopkins, W.G. Measures of Reliability in Sports Medicine and Science. *Curr. Opin. Sport. Med.* **2000**, *30*, 1–15.
41. Riemann, B.L.; Lininger, M.R. Statistical Primer for Athletic Trainers: The Essentials of Understanding Measures of Reliability and Minimal Important Change. *J. Athl. Train.* **2018**, *53*, 98. [CrossRef]
42. Ndrepepa, G. Myeloperoxidase—A bridge linking inflammation and oxidative stress with cardiovascular disease. *Clin. Chim. Acta* **2019**, *493*, 36–51. [CrossRef]
43. Heslop, C.L.; Frohlich, J.J.; Hill, J.S. Myeloperoxidase and C-Reactive Protein Have Combined Utility for Long-Term Prediction of Cardiovascular Mortality After Coronary Angiography. *J. Am. Coll. Cardiol.* **2010**, *55*, 1102–1109. [CrossRef] [PubMed]
44. Aeschbacher, S.; Schoen, T.; Dörig, L.; Kreuzmann, R.; Neuhauser, C.; Schmidt-Trucksäss, A.; Probst-Hensch, N.M.; Risch, M.; Risch, L.; Conen, D. Heart rate, heart rate variability and inflammatory biomarkers among young and healthy adults. *Ann. Med.* **2017**, *49*, 32–41. [CrossRef] [PubMed]
45. Goldberger, A.L.; Peng, C.K.; Lipsitz, L.A. What is physiologic complexity and how does it change with aging and disease? *Neurobiol. Aging* **2002**, *23*, 23–26. [CrossRef]
46. Haensel, A.; Mills, P.J.; Nelesen, R.A.; Ziegler, M.G.; Dimsdale, J.E. The relationship between heart rate variability and inflammatory markers in cardiovascular diseases. *Psychoneuroendocrinology* **2012**, *76*, 211–220. [CrossRef] [PubMed]
47. Schiweck, C.; Piette, D.; Berckmans, D.; Claes, S.; Vrieze, E. Heart rate and high frequency heart rate variability during stress as biomarker for clinical depression. A systematic review. *Psychol. Med.* **2019**, *49*, 200–211. [CrossRef]
48. Crosswell, A.D.; Lockwood, K.G.; Ganz, P.A.; Bower, J.E. Low heart rate variability and cancer-related fatigue in breast cancer survivors. *Psychoneuroendocrinology* **2014**, *45*, 58. [CrossRef]
49. Pagani, M.; Lucini, D. Chronic fatigue syndrome: A hypothesis focusing on the autonomic nervous system. *Clin. Sci.* **1999**, *96*, 117–125. [CrossRef]
50. Balsamo, S.; Santos-Neto, L. dos Fatigue in systemic lupus erythematosus: An association with reduced physical fitness. *Autoimmun. Rev.* **2011**, *10*, 514–518. [CrossRef]
51. Rivera-López, R.; Jiménez-Jáimez, J.; Sabio, J.M.; Zamora-Pasadas, M.; Vargas-Hitos, J.A.; Martínez-Bordonado, J.; Navarrete-Navarrete, N.; Fernández, R.R.; Sanchez-Cantalejo, E.; Jiménez-Alonso, J. Relationship between QT Interval Length and Arterial Stiffness in Systemic Lupus Erythematosus (SLE): A Cross-Sectional Case-Control Study. *PLoS ONE* **2016**, *11*, e0152291. [CrossRef]
52. Vesterinen, V.; Nummela, A.; Heikura, I.; Laine, T.; Hynynen, E.; Botella, J.; Häkkinen, K. Individual Endurance Training Prescription with Heart Rate Variability. *Med. Sci. Sports Exerc.* **2016**, *48*, 1347–1354. [CrossRef]

Publisher's Note: MDPI stays neutral with regard to jurisdictional claims in published maps and institutional affiliations.

© 2020 by the authors. Licensee MDPI, Basel, Switzerland. This article is an open access article distributed under the terms and conditions of the Creative Commons Attribution (CC BY) license (http://creativecommons.org/licenses/by/4.0/).

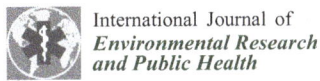
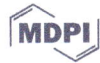

Article

Associations between Health-Related Physical Fitness and Cardiovascular Disease Risk Factors in Overweight and Obese University Staff

Jiangang Chen [1], Yuan Zhou [1], Xinliang Pan [2], Xiaolong Li [1], Jiamin Long [1], Hui Zhang [1] and Jing Zhang [1,*]

[1] Department of Exercise Science, School of Physical Education, Shaanxi Normal University, Xi'an 710119, China; chenjiangang@snnu.edu.cn (J.C.); yuanzhou@snnu.edu.cn (Y.Z.); lixiaolong@snnu.edu.cn (X.L.); longjiamin@snnu.edu.cn (J.L.); 41710161@snnu.edu.cn (H.Z.)
[2] School of Kinesiology, Beijing Sport University, Beijing 100084, China; panxl@snnu.edu.cn
* Correspondence: zhangjiing0578@snnu.edu.cn; Tel.: +86-139-911-920-58

Received: 28 October 2020; Accepted: 1 December 2020; Published: 3 December 2020

Abstract: Purpose: This cross-sectional study examined the associations between health-related physical fitness (HPF) and cardiovascular disease (CVD) risk factors in overweight and obese university staff. Methods: A total of 340 university staff (109 women, mean age 43.1 ± 9.7 years) with overweight ($n = 284$) and obesity ($n = 56$) were included. The HPF indicators included skeletal muscle mass index (SMI), body fat percentage (BFP), grip strength (GS), sit-and-reach test (SRT), and vital capacity index (VCI). CVD risk factors were measured, including uric acid (UA), triglycerides (TG), high-density lipoprotein cholesterol (HDL-C), low-density lipoprotein cholesterol (LDL-C), and glucose (GLU). Results: BFP, SMI, and GS were positively associated with UA level ($\beta = 0.239$, $\beta = 0.159$, $\beta = 0.139$, $p < 0.05$). BFP was positively associated with TG and TG/HDL-C levels ($\beta = 0.421$, $\beta = 0.259$, $p < 0.05$). GS was positively associated with HDL-C level ($\beta = 0.244$, $p < 0.05$). SRT was negatively associated with GLU level ($\beta = -0.130$, $p < 0.05$). Conclusions: In overweight and obese university staff, body composition, muscle strength, and flexibility were associated with CVD risk factors. An HPF test may be a practical nonmedical method to assess CVD risk.

Keywords: university staff; health-related physical fitness; cardiovascular disease; overweight; obesity

1. Introduction

Cardiovascular disease (CVD) is a significant public health issue, as it is the leading cause of adult mortality, accounting for more than 40% of deaths in China [1]. Over the past 30 years, the number of CVD deaths in China has increased from 2.51 million to 3.97 million annually [2]. Although the age-standardized mortality rate remained stable overall from 2002 to 2016, it increased among the young population [3]. Therefore, the early prevention of CVD is essential [4].

The risk factors of CVD include dyslipidemia, diabetes, and obesity [5]. In recent years, hyperuricemia has also been recognized as a potential risk factor for CVD, following the discovery of a causal relationship between uric acid and the adverse outcomes of CVD [6,7]. Among the many risk factors, obesity affects cardiovascular disease in several ways; for instance, obesity affects the morbidity of CVD, and early obesity may increase the risk of future CVD events [8]. Obesity also affects the prognosis of CVD. A meta-analysis showed that overweight and obese individuals had 25% and 42% increased risks of CVD mortality, respectively, compared to those of normal-weight individuals [9]. Furthermore, the duration of obesity may also affect CVD. Abdullah et al. [10] found that every two years of obese living significantly increased the risk of CVD mortality by 7%. This may be because obesity worsens other CVD risk factors such as blood lipid and blood glucose levels [11]. It is necessary, therefore, to assess the risk factors of CVD in overweight and obese individuals.

Common measures of obesity include body mass index (BMI) and body composition. Body composition is one of the components of health-related physical fitness (HPF). In addition to body composition, other HPF components include cardiorespiratory fitness, muscular fitness, and flexibility. HPF reflects not only the ability of the body to participate in exercise, but also the body's ability to reduce the risk of disease. HPF assessment, therefore, may have important implications in the prevention of chronic diseases. Previous studies have shown that HPF can predict multiple risk factors for CVD [12–14]. Body composition is better at distinguishing between fat mass and fat-free mass than BMI. Studies have shown that individuals with the same BMI may differ in body composition, which affects their risks of CVD [15]. Cardiorespiratory fitness (CRF) is one of the most important HPF factors, and it is a strong predictor of CVD [16,17]. The respiratory function, however, also plays an important role in cardiovascular health [18], and it is not clear whether indicators of respiratory function can be used to assess the risk of CVD. In recent years, the relationship between muscular fitness and CVD has gradually attracted attention. Grip strength has a negative correlation with triglyceride and glucose levels [19], and decreased respiratory muscle strength is an independent risk factor for CVD [20]. The relationship between muscle strength and uric acid level may vary between populations. One study reported a negative correlation between grip strength and uric acid in young people but a positive correlation in older people [21]. Flexibility may also be an indicator of CVD risk. Chang et al. found that flexibility was positively correlated with high-density lipoprotein levels among 628 community residents but did not control other variables such as sex and age [22]. Thus, the relationship between flexibility and CVD requires further exploration.

To the best of our knowledge, numerous studies have been conducted on the relationship between HPF and CVD in normal-weight individuals [13,22]. No study, however, has focused on overweight and obese university staff. A cross-sectional study found that 94 percent of university staff were exposed to one or more CVD risk factors [23]. This may indicate that university staff have a higher risk of cardiovascular disease. Furthermore, university staff have a higher prevalence of overweight and obesity than the general population does because of longer working hours and psychosocial factors [24]. Cardiovascular disease risk factors, such as blood lipids, glucose, and uric acid levels, may further worsen among university staff in overweight and obese states. The purpose of this study, therefore, was to explore the associations between HPF and CVD risk factors in overweight and obese university staff and to provide a basis for HPF testing in evaluating the risk of CVD and the development of future exercise intervention strategies.

2. Materials and Methods

2.1. Participants and Study Design

From October 2019 to January 2020, a total of 2800 university staff underwent annual health screenings at the Community Hospital Health Management Center. This cross-sectional study recruited university staff every morning in the breakfast serving area of the Health Management Center. A sample size of 319 was required to achieve 90% statistical power based on the calculation of PASS.11.0, and 412 university staff were actually recruited. Among the 412 participants, 38 participants did not complete HPF tests, and 34 participants were over 60 years. A total of 340 overweight and obese university staff aged between 25 and 60, with a BMI greater than 24.0, were eventually included in the study. The classification criteria for overweight and obesity were from the China Obesity Working Group [25].

Participants first underwent a blood collection procedure, and then height, weight, and body composition were measured. Other HPF tests were performed after participants ate breakfast and took a 15 min break to regain their strength. The participants were informed of the test procedures, requirements, and possible risks before the test, and they signed the informed consent forms. The protocols were approved by the Ethics Committee of Shaanxi Normal University, and the ethical approval code is 202016003.

2.2. Study Variables

2.2.1. Health-Related Physical Fitness Measurement

Health-related physical fitness indicators were measured by trained research assistants according to the National Physical Fitness Standards Manual.

Body height and weight were measured using an all-in-one machine (GK 720, Shandong, China), which combined an ultrasonic stadiometer with an electronic weight scale. The machine was calibrated before each use to ensure accuracy. Participants stood barefoot in a designated position and looked straight ahead. The test results were automatically recorded and reported.

Body composition was assessed with a bioelectrical impedance machine (InBody 230, Seoul, South Korea). Participants stood barefoot on the electrodes of the machine and held the handles with both hands. Participants remained in a natural standing position throughout the test and always kept their hands and feet in contact with the electrodes. The test program took 1 to 2 min, and skeletal muscle mass (SMM) and total body fat mass (BFM) were automatically recorded by the InBody 230. Skeletal muscle mass index (SMI) was determined using SMM divided by height squared. Body fat percentage (BFP) was determined using BFM divided by body weight.

Grip strength was measured using a portable electronic grip strength dynamometer (Hengkangjiaye, Guangzhou, China). Participants stood naturally with their arms slanting down and their palms inward. Participants were not allowed to swing their arms or hold the dynamometer close to their bodies during the test. Each hand was tested twice, and the highest measurements were recorded.

Flexibility was assessed with the sit-and-reach test (SRT). An electronic fleximeter (HKD-1442, Beijing, China) was used to achieve better accuracy. Participants sat barefoot in the required position with their legs straight and their feet together. During each measurement, participants pushed their feet against the front baffle and stretched their arms as far forward as possible. Measurements were recorded to evaluate flexibility as participants tried to push the cursor on the farthest scale with the fingertips of their hands. Participants tried three times, and the largest measurements were recorded.

Vital capacity (VC) was measured using an electronic pneumometer (WCS-1000, Beijing, China). Participants inhaled deeply and then exhaled all the air to assess vital capacity. Participants tried this three times, and the maximum exhalation was recorded. Participants were asked to rest 30–60 s between the three measurements in order to avoid hypoxia. Vital capacity Index (VCI) was determined using VC divided by body weight.

2.2.2. Cardiovascular Disease Factors Measurement

After a night of fasting, blood samples were collected from 8 a.m. to 10 a.m. in the Community Hospital Health Management Center. On the same day, blood specimens were processed and analyzed in the laboratory of the Community Hospital. The automatic analyzer AU480 (Beckman Coulter, California, USA) was used to analyze blood biochemistry. Serum uric acid (UA), triglycerides (TG), total cholesterol (TC), high-density lipoprotein cholesterol (HDL-C), and low-density lipoprotein cholesterol (LDL-C) were measured with enzymatic methods. Blood glucose (GLU) was measured using a hexokinase enzymatic method. TG/HDL-C was, thereafter, used to estimate insulin resistance [26].

2.3. Statistical Analysis

All variables were checked for normality using the Kolmogorov–Smirnov test. Continuous variables with normal distribution were presented by mean ± standard deviation (SD), continuous variables with non-normal distribution were presented by median (interquartile range (IQR)), and categorical variables were presented by number (percentage). Multiple linear regression was used to analyze the associations between HPF and CVD risk factors. Each variable was z-standardized before the regression analysis to compare these values on the same scale. A two-sided p-value < 0.05 was considered statistically significant. SPSS 23.0 software (Chicago, IL, USA) was used for statistical analyses.

3. Results

Table 1 illustrates the baseline characteristics of participants. A total of 340 university staff (109 women, 231 men) were included in this study. Participants' mean age was 43.1 ± 9.7 years, and 9.1% of participants were 25–30 years, 35.6% were 31–40 years, 26.8% were 41–50 years, and 28.5% were 51–60 years old. Participants' mean BMI was 26.2 ± 1.9 kg/m^2, 83.5% of participants were overweight, and 16.5% were obese.

Table 1. Baseline characteristics of the participants.

	Men	Women	All
Sample size (n, %)	231 (67.9%)	109 (32.1%)	340 (100%)
Age (n, %)			
≤30 years	20 (8.7%)	11 (10.1%)	31 (9.1%)
31–40 years	80 (34.6%)	41 (37.6%)	121 (35.6%)
41–50 years	60 (26.0%)	31 (28.4%)	91 (26.8%)
51–60 years	71 (30.7%)	26 (23.9%)	97 (28.5%)
BMI (n, %)			
24–27.9 (overweight)	192 (83.1%)	92 (84.4%)	284 (83.5%)
≥ 28.0 (obese)	39 (16.9%)	17 (15.6%)	56 (16.5%)
HPF indicators			
Skeletal muscle mass (kg) [a]	33.07 ± 2.86	24.40 ± 2.49	30.29 ± 4.86
Skeletal muscle mass index (kg/m^2) [a]	11.00 ± 0.62	9.17 ± 0.68	10.43 ± 1.06
Body fat mass (kg) [b]	20.00 (5.80)	24.10 (5.00)	21.20 (6.40)
Body fat percentage (%) [b]	25.00 (5.06)	35.55 (4.34)	27.48 (9.64)
Grip strength (kg) [b]	36.50 (9.40)	25.60 (5.20)	33.60 (11.10)
Sit-and-reach (cm) [b]	4.10 (11.50)	9.15 (11.80)	5.90 (11.00)
Vital capacity (mL) [a]	3957.94 ± 844.10	2708.75 ± 624.92	3564.65 ± 979.17
Vital capacity index (mL/kg) [a]	50.66 ± 10.59	39.71 ± 9.54	47.40 ± 11.44
CVD risk factors			
UA (umol/L) [b]	384.00 (72.00)	301.50 (65.00)	363.00 (97.00)
TG (mmol/L) [b]	1.35 (0.79)	1.10 (0.65)	1.27 (0.79)
HDL-C (mmol/L) [a]	1.32 ± 0.24	1.54 ± 0.25	1.38 ± 0.42
LDL-C (mmol/L) [b]	2.96 (0.74)	2.65 (0.91)	2.92 (0.86)
TG/HDL-C ratio [b]	1.01 (0.70)	0.70 (0.53)	0.91 (0.72)
GLU (mmol/L) [a]	5.03 ± 0.43	5.07 ± 0.42	5.05 ± 0.51

Note: [a] Data are represented by mean ± SD; [b] Data are represented by median (IQR). Abbreviations: BMI: body mass index; UA: uric acid; TG: triglycerides; HDL-C: high-density lipoprotein cholesterol; LDL-C: low-density lipoprotein cholesterol; GLU: blood glucose.

Table 2 shows the associations between HPF indicators and CVD risk factors. BFP, SMI, and GS were positively associated with UA level (β = 0.239, β = 0.159, β = 0.139, $p < 0.05$). BFP was positively associated with TG and TG/HDL-C levels (β = 0.421, β = 0.259, $p < 0.05$). GS was positively associated with HDL-C level (β = 0.244, $p < 0.05$). SRT was negatively associated with GLU level (β = −0.130, $p < 0.05$).

Table 2. Associations between health-related physical fitness (HPF) indicators and cardiovascular disease (CVD) risk factors.

Dependent Variables [a]	Independent Variables [a]	β	β (95%CI)	SE	p	R^2
UA	SMI	0.159	(0.001, 0.318)	0.081	0.049 *	
	BFP	0.239	(0.076, 0.402)	0.083	0.004 *	
	GS	0.139	(0.018, 0.259)	0.061	0.024 *	0.363
	SRT	0.027	(−0.068, 0.122)	0.048	0.579	
	VCI	0.031	(−0.086, 0.147)	0.059	0.608	
TG	SMI	0.162	(−0.030, 0.353)	0.097	0.098	
	BFP	0.421	(0.226, 0.617)	0.099	0.000 *	
	GS	0.031	(−0.113, 0.175)	0.073	0.673	0.098
	SRT	−0.036	(−0.149, 0.078)	0.058	0.538	
	VCI	0.047	(−0.092, 0.187)	0.071	0.507	
HDL-C	SMI	−0.183	(−0.370, 0.003)	0.095	0.054	
	BFP	0.014	(−0.177, 0.205)	0.097	0.887	
	GS	0.244	(0.103, 0.385)	0.072	0.001 *	0.128
	SRT	−0.009	(−0.121, 0.103)	0.057	0.871	
	VCI	0.066	(−0.072, 0.203)	0.070	0.349	
LDL-C	SMI	0.045	(−0.148, 0.238)	0.054	0.646	
	BFP	0.131	(−0.068, 0.330)	0.010	0.197	
	GS	−0.009	(−0.155, 0.136)	0.005	0.900	0.063
	SRT	0.097	(−0.019, 0.212)	0.004	0.102	
	VCI	0.004	(−0.138, 0.147)	0.004	0.954	
TG/HDL-C	SMI	0.150	(−0.043, 0.344)	0.099	0.128	
	BFP	0.259	(0.061, 0.457)	0.101	0.011 *	
	GS	−0.054	(−0.201, 0.092)	0.074	0.465	0.070
	SRT	−0.029	(−0.145, 0.087)	0.059	0.622	
	VCI	−0.008	(−0.151, 0.134)	0.072	0.909	
GLU	SMI	0.181	(−0.007, 0.369)	0.096	0.059	
	BFP	0.128	(−0.065, 0.321)	0.098	0.192	
	GS	0.035	(−0.107, 0.177)	0.072	0.630	0.083
	SRT	−0.130	(−0.243, −0.017)	0.057	0.024 *	
	VCI	−0.052	(−0.190, 0.086)	0.070	0.461	

Note: the multiple linear regression model controlled for sex and age; [a] indicates the variable was z-standardized; * indicates statistical significance ($p < 0.05$); SE indicates standard error. Abbreviations: UA: uric acid; TG: triglycerides; HDL-C: high-density lipoprotein cholesterol; LDL-C: low-density lipoprotein cholesterol; GLU: blood glucose; SMI: skeletal muscle index; BFP: body fat percentage; GS: grip strength; SRT: sit-and-reach test; VCI: vital capacity index.

4. Discussion

This study evaluated the associations between HPF indicators and CVD risk factors in overweight and obese university staff. The main findings of this study were that reduced flexibility was associated with elevated GLU level, while high body fat percentage, muscle mass, and grip strength were associated with high UA level. We also observed that grip strength was positively associated with high-density lipoprotein cholesterol (HDL-C) level and that body fat percentage was positively associated with TG and TG/HDL-C levels. These results indicated that the HPF and CVD risk factors were related, and they provide a basis for nonmedical evaluations of CVD risk in overweight or obese university staff and the development of future exercise intervention strategies.

Our analysis of the association between HPF indicators and UA showed that body fat percentage was positively associated with UA level. This may be attributed to the fact that purine metabolism in adipose tissue is enhanced in obesity [27,28]. Furthermore, the distribution of body fat is closely related to UA level [29]. Huang et al. reported that visceral fat accumulation increased the risk of hyperuricemia in older Chinese adults [30]. This finding suggests that, in addition to the total body fat percentage, visceral fat is also an important indicator to consider in the prevention of hyperuricemia. We also observed that skeletal muscle index and grip strength were positively associated with UA level. This finding is consistent with those of previous cross-sectional studies in the elderly [31–33]. UA is the final product of purine metabolism. An excessive accumulation of UA in the body may cause not only gout but also heart failure [6,7]. In recent years, UA has been observed to slow age-related muscle decline [33,34]. In a longitudinal study, Macchi et al. [35] found that in people with an average age of 76 years, higher baseline serum UA levels were associated with better muscle function three years later. This muscular protection, however, was not observed in those under 60 years of age [36]. Furthermore, the possible physiological mechanisms by which UA protects muscles are not clear. Although studies have assumed that UA plays a protective role in the process of free radical damage to skeletal muscle protein [37], UA is also a pro-oxidant and may increase oxidative stress. Another study suggests that UA may be an indicator of dietary protein intake. High UA concentrations in patients with hyperuricemia are associated with better nutritional status [38]. Total protein intake, particularly those of meat and fish proteins, may be important for building and maintaining muscle mass [39]. Individuals with higher dietary protein intake, therefore, may maintain higher muscle mass as well as higher UA levels. Previous studies have shown that high body fat and muscle mass both place a burden on the cardiovascular system and increase the risk of cardiovascular disease [11], indicating that weight control and improvement to body composition are important for overweight and obese university staff.

Our study results revealed that flexibility was negatively associated with GLU level. Aparicio et al. [40] also reported a negative correlation between flexibility and GLU in menopausal women; however, their finding was not statistically significant, probably because flexibility was a self-reported scale score rather than an actual measured value. One possible explanation for the association between flexibility and GLU is disc degeneration. Hyperglycemia has a detrimental effect on disc cell viability, leading to disc degeneration and impaired lumbar flexibility [41]. Inflammatory cytokines, which mediate insulin resistance, also play a role in disc degeneration [42,43]. The relationship between flexibility and GLU metabolism, however, remains poorly understood, and as many factors affecting flexibility and blood glucose are not considered, the exact mechanism is not clear. Studies in recent years have begun to recognize the value of flexibility in evaluating and preventing chronic diseases. Gregorio et al. [44] reported that flexibility not only in the waist but also in the upper body is associated with cardiometabolic risk factors. Another study found that flexibility exercises reduced pro-inflammatory adipokines, such as PAI-1 and chemerin, and increased anti-inflammatory adipokines, such as adiponectin [45]. Future studies are needed to further confirm the effectiveness of flexibility training in reducing blood glucose and preventing CVD.

Our analysis of the relationship between HPF and blood lipids revealed that body fat percentage was positively associated with TG and TG/HDL-C levels. This finding is supported by previous studies using dual-energy X-rays and confirmed that body fat and its distribution are closely related to blood lipid levels [46,47]. Konieczna et al. [46] further compared regional and total body fat measurements, reporting that the ratio of visceral adipose tissue to total fat was a more effective evaluation indicator of TG. This may be because visceral fat mediates partial insulin resistance through the release of inflammatory adipokines [46]. As a result, lipolysis is intensified, and excess TGs enter the liver, causing an abnormally high TG level [48].

We observed that grip strength was positively associated with HDL-C level. Grip strength is an effective indicator of muscle strength and of potential health risks [49]. In a study of 8576 participants, Lee et al. found that participants with low grip strength had increased risks of CVD [50]. Another large sample study determined that higher relative grip strength was associated with healthier blood lipid levels in adults, such as lower TG and total cholesterol levels and higher HDL-C levels [19]. This may be related to the endocrine function of skeletal muscle and its metabolic benefits [51]. Cytokines secreted by the muscles may regulate the metabolic process through autocrine and paracrine mechanisms. Cytokines, such as myonectin and irisin, regulate lipid metabolism and improve insulin resistance [52,53].

One advantage of this study was that we first explored the associations between HPF and CVD risk factors in overweight or obese adults and provided new insight regarding CVD prevention and control strategies. Secondly, the HPF indicators included in this study were easy to measure and obtain. It is convenient, therefore, for the general population to conduct HPF self-assessments. Certainly, this study also has some limitations. Firstly, physical activity, nutritional status, and physiological indicators related to inflammation, such as blood pressure and CRP, were not included in the study. Secondly, our study cannot determine the causal relationship between HPF and CVD risk factors due to the cross-sectional design. Thirdly, the results of this study cannot be generalized for the overall population, as participants were overweight and obese adults. In the future, longitudinal or experimental studies should be considered to verify the causal relationship between HPF and CVD risk factors.

5. Conclusions

Among overweight and obese university staff, reduced flexibility was associated with high glucose level, while high body fat percentage, muscle mass, and grip strength were associated with high uric acid level. Additionally, grip strength was positively associated with HDL-C level, and body fat percentage was positively associated with TG and TG/HDL-C levels. The results of this study suggest that body composition, grip strength, and flexibility may be practical nonmedical markers for assessing cardiovascular disease risk. In the future, prospective studies should be conducted to investigate the extent to which exercise programs that improve body composition and increase muscle strength and flexibility may reduce the risk of cardiovascular disease.

Author Contributions: Conceptualization, J.Z.; methodology, J.C.; software, Y.Z.; formal analysis, J.C.; investigation, X.P., J.L., Y.Z., and H.Z.; data curation, X.L.; writing—original draft preparation, J.C.; writing—review and editing, J.Z. All authors have read and agreed to the published version of the manuscript.

Funding: This research was funded by the Project of Consultation of General Administration of Sport of China (YB20180419025), Special Fund for Innovation Guidance of Shaanxi Province (2020QFY01-03), and Special Fund for Basic Scientific Research Expenses of Central Colleges and Universities (18SZYB29).

Acknowledgments: The authors acknowledge the valuable contributions of all investigators and participants.

Conflicts of Interest: The authors declare no conflict of interest.

References

1. Zhou, M.; Wang, H.; Zhu, J.; Chen, W.; Wang, L.; Liu, S.; Li, Y.; Wang, L.; Liu, Y.; Yin, P.; et al. Cause-specific mortality for 240 causes in China during 1990-2013: A systematic subnational analysis for the Global Burden of Disease Study 2013. *Lancet* **2016**, *387*, 251–272. [CrossRef]
2. Liu, S.; Li, Y.; Zeng, X.; Wang, H.; Yin, P.; Wang, L.; Liu, Y.; Liu, J.; Qi, J.; Ran, S.; et al. Burden of Cardiovascular Diseases in China, 1990-2016: Findings From the 2016 Global Burden of Disease Study. *JAMA Cardiol.* **2019**, *4*, 342–352. [CrossRef]
3. Yu, Q.; Wang, B.; Wang, Y.; Dai, C.L. Level and trend of cardiovascular disease mortality in China from 2002 to 2016. *Zhonghua Xin Xue Guan Bing Za Zhi* **2019**, *47*, 479–485. [PubMed]
4. Shen, C.; Ge, J. Epidemic of Cardiovascular Disease in China: Current Perspective and Prospects for the Future. *Circulation* **2018**, *138*, 342–344. [CrossRef] [PubMed]
5. Joseph, P.; Leong, D.; McKee, M.; Anand, S.S.; Schwalm, J.D.; Teo, K.; Mente, A.; Yusuf, S. Reducing the Global Burden of Cardiovascular Disease, Part 1: The Epidemiology and Risk Factors. *Circ. Res.* **2017**, *121*, 677–694. [CrossRef] [PubMed]
6. Kleber, M.E.; Delgado, G.; Grammer, T.B.; Silbernagel, G.; Huang, J.; Kramer, B.K.; Ritz, E.; Marz, W. Uric Acid and Cardiovascular Events: A Mendelian Randomization Study. *J. Am. Soc. Nephrol.* **2015**, *26*, 2831–2838. [CrossRef] [PubMed]

7. Chiang, K.M.; Tsay, Y.C.; Vincent, N.T.; Yang, H.C.; Huang, Y.T.; Chen, C.H.; Pan, W.H. Is Hyperuricemia, an Early-Onset Metabolic Disorder, Causally Associated with Cardiovascular Disease Events in Han Chinese? *J. Clin. Med.* **2019**, *8*, 1202. [CrossRef]
8. Khan, S.S.; Ning, H.; Wilkins, J.T.; Allen, N.; Carnethon, M.; Berry, J.D.; Sweis, R.N.; Lloyd-Jones, D.M. Association of Body Mass Index With Lifetime Risk of Cardiovascular Disease and Compression of Morbidity. *JAMA Cardiol.* **2018**, *3*, 280–287. [CrossRef]
9. Barry, V.W.; Caputo, J.L.; Kang, M. The Joint Association of Fitness and Fatness on Cardiovascular Disease Mortality: A Meta-Analysis. *Prog. Cardiovasc. Dis.* **2018**, *61*, 136–141. [CrossRef]
10. Abdullah, A.; Wolfe, R.; Stoelwinder, J.U.; de Courten, M.; Stevenson, C.; Walls, H.L.; Peeters, A. The number of years lived with obesity and the risk of all-cause and cause-specific mortality. *Int. J. Epidemiol.* **2011**, *40*, 985–996. [CrossRef]
11. Ortega, F.B.; Lavie, C.J.; Blair, S.N. Obesity and Cardiovascular Disease. *Circ. Res.* **2016**, *118*, 1752–1770. [CrossRef] [PubMed]
12. Penha, J.; Gazolla, F.M.; Carvalho, C.; Madeira, I.R.; Rodrigues-Junior, F.; Machado, E.A.; Sicuro, F.L.; Farinatti, P.; Bouskela, E.; Collett-Solberg, P.F. Physical fitness and activity, metabolic profile, adipokines and endothelial function in children. *J. Pediatr.* **2019**, *95*, 531–537. [CrossRef] [PubMed]
13. Medrano, M.; Arenaza, L.; Migueles, J.H.; Rodriguez-Vigil, B.; Ruiz, J.R.; Labayen, I. Associations of physical activity and fitness with hepatic steatosis, liver enzymes, and insulin resistance in children with overweight/obesity. *Pediatr. Diabetes.* **2020**, *21*, 565–574. [CrossRef] [PubMed]
14. Lima, T.R.; Martins, P.C.; Guerra, P.H.; Silva, D. Muscular strength and cardiovascular risk factors in adults: Systematic review. *Phys. Sportsmed.* **2020**, *1*, 1–13. [CrossRef]
15. Chen, G.C.; Arthur, R.; Iyengar, N.M.; Kamensky, V.; Xue, X.; Wassertheil-Smoller, S.; Allison, M.A.; Shadyab, A.H.; Wild, R.A.; Sun, Y.; et al. Association between regional body fat and cardiovascular disease risk among postmenopausal women with normal body mass index. *Eur. Heart J.* **2019**, *40*, 2849–2855. [CrossRef]
16. Barry, V.W.; Baruth, M.; Beets, M.W.; Durstine, J.L.; Liu, J.; Blair, S.N. Fitness vs. fatness on all-cause mortality: A meta-analysis. *Prog. Cardiovasc. Dis.* **2014**, *56*, 382–390. [CrossRef]
17. Castro-Pinero, J.; Perez-Bey, A.; Segura-Jimenez, V.; Aparicio, V.A.; Gomez-Martinez, S.; Izquierdo-Gomez, R.; Marcos, A.; Ruiz, J.R. Cardiorespiratory Fitness Cutoff Points for Early Detection of Present and Future Cardiovascular Risk in Children: A 2-Year Follow-up Study. *Mayo Clin. Proc.* **2017**, *92*, 1753–1762. [CrossRef]
18. Simons, S.O.; Elliott, A.; Sastry, M.; Hendriks, J.M.; Arzt, M.; Rienstra, M.; Kalman, J.M.; Heidbuchel, H.; Nattel, S.; Wesseling, G.; et al. Chronic obstructive pulmonary disease and atrial fibrillation: An interdisciplinary perspective. *Eur. Heart J.* **2020**. [CrossRef]
19. Lawman, H.G.; Troiano, R.P.; Perna, F.M.; Wang, C.Y.; Fryar, C.D.; Ogden, C.L. Associations of Relative Handgrip Strength and Cardiovascular Disease Biomarkers in U.S. Adults, 2011-2012. *Am. J. Prev. Med.* **2016**, *50*, 677–683. [CrossRef]
20. Van der Palen, J.; Rea, T.D.; Manolio, T.A.; Lumley, T.; Newman, A.B.; Tracy, R.P.; Enright, P.L.; Psaty, B.M. Respiratory muscle strength and the risk of incident cardiovascular events. *Thorax* **2004**, *59*, 1063–1067. [CrossRef]
21. Garcia-Esquinas, E.; Rodriguez-Artalejo, F. Association between serum uric acid concentrations and grip strength: Is there effect modification by age? *Clin. Nutr.* **2018**, *37*, 566–572. [CrossRef] [PubMed]
22. Chang, K.V.; Hung, C.Y.; Li, C.M.; Lin, Y.H.; Wang, T.G.; Tsai, K.S.; Han, D.S. Reduced flexibility associated with metabolic syndrome in community-dwelling elders. *PLoS ONE* **2015**, *10*, e117167. [CrossRef] [PubMed]
23. Sita, C.; Sachita, S.; Mausumi, B.; Raghunath, M. A study on cardiovascular disease risk factors among faculty members of a tertiary care teaching institute of Kolkata. *J. Community Health Manag.* **2018**, *5*, 67–71. [CrossRef]
24. Cheong, S.M.; Kandiah, M.; Chinna, K.; Chan, Y.M.; Saad, H.A. Prevalence of obesity and factors associated with it in a worksite setting in Malaysia. *J. Community Health* **2010**, *35*, 698–705. [CrossRef] [PubMed]
25. Zhou, B.F. Predictive values of body mass index and waist circumference for risk factors of certain related diseases in Chinese adults–study on optimal cut-off points of body mass index and waist circumference in Chinese adults. *Biomed. Environ. Sci.* **2002**, *15*, 83–96.

26. Yeh, W.C.; Tsao, Y.C.; Li, W.C.; Tzeng, I.S.; Chen, L.S.; Chen, J.Y. Elevated triglyceride-to-HDL cholesterol ratio is an indicator for insulin resistance in middle-aged and elderly Taiwanese population: A cross-sectional study. *Lipids Health Dis.* **2019**, *18*, 176. [CrossRef]
27. Tsushima, Y.; Nishizawa, H.; Tochino, Y.; Nakatsuji, H.; Sekimoto, R.; Nagao, H.; Shirakura, T.; Kato, K.; Imaizumi, K.; Takahashi, H.; et al. Uric acid secretion from adipose tissue and its increase in obesity. *J. Biol. Chem.* **2013**, *288*, 27138–27149. [CrossRef]
28. Nagao, H.; Nishizawa, H.; Tanaka, Y.; Fukata, T.; Mizushima, T.; Furuno, M.; Bamba, T.; Tsushima, Y.; Fujishima, Y.; Kita, S.; et al. Hypoxanthine Secretion from Human Adipose Tissue and its Increase in Hypoxia. *Obesity* **2018**, *26*, 1168–1178. [CrossRef]
29. Yamada, A.; Sato, K.K.; Kinuhata, S.; Uehara, S.; Endo, G.; Hikita, Y.; Fujimoto, W.Y.; Boyko, E.J.; Hayashi, T. Association of Visceral Fat and Liver Fat With Hyperuricemia. *Arthritis Care Res.* **2016**, *68*, 553–561. [CrossRef]
30. Huang, X.; Jiang, X.; Wang, L.; Chen, L.; Wu, Y.; Gao, P.; Hua, F. Visceral adipose accumulation increased the risk of hyperuricemia among middle-aged and elderly adults: A population-based study. *J. Transl. Med.* **2019**, *17*, 341. [CrossRef]
31. Kawamoto, R.; Ninomiya, D.; Kasai, Y.; Kusunoki, T.; Ohtsuka, N.; Kumagi, T.; Abe, M. Serum Uric Acid Is Positively Associated with Handgrip Strength among Japanese Community-Dwelling Elderly Women. *PLoS ONE* **2016**, *11*, e151044. [CrossRef] [PubMed]
32. Xu, Z.R.; Zhang, Q.; Chen, L.F.; Xu, K.Y.; Xia, J.Y.; Li, S.M.; Yang, Y.M. Characteristics of hyperuricemia in older adults in China and possible associations with sarcopenia. *Aging Med.* **2018**, *1*, 23–34. [CrossRef] [PubMed]
33. Wu, Y.; Zhang, D.; Pang, Z.; Jiang, W.; Wang, S.; Tan, Q. Association of serum uric acid level with muscle strength and cognitive function among Chinese aged 50-74 years. *Geriatr. Gerontol. Int.* **2013**, *13*, 672–677. [CrossRef] [PubMed]
34. Dong, X.W.; Tian, H.Y.; He, J.; Wang, C.; Qiu, R.; Chen, Y.M. Elevated Serum Uric Acid Is Associated with Greater Bone Mineral Density and Skeletal Muscle Mass in Middle-Aged and Older Adults. *PLoS ONE* **2016**, *11*, e154692. [CrossRef]
35. Macchi, C.; Molino-Lova, R.; Polcaro, P.; Guarducci, L.; Lauretani, F.; Cecchi, F.; Bandinelli, S.; Guralnik, J.M.; Ferrucci, L. Higher circulating levels of uric acid are prospectively associated with better muscle function in older persons. *Mech. Ageing Dev.* **2008**, *129*, 522–527. [CrossRef]
36. Lee, J.; Hong, Y.S.; Park, S.H.; Kang, K.Y. High serum uric acid level is associated with greater handgrip strength in the aged population. *Arthritis Res. Ther.* **2019**, *21*, 73. [CrossRef]
37. Molino-Lova, R.; Sofi, F.; Pasquini, G.; Vannetti, F.; Del, R.S.; Vassale, C.; Clerici, M.; Sorbi, S.; Macchi, C. Higher uric acid serum levels are associated with better muscle function in the oldest old: Results from the Mugello Study. *Eur. J. Intern. Med.* **2017**, *41*, 39–43. [CrossRef]
38. Park, C.; Obi, Y.; Streja, E.; Rhee, C.M.; Catabay, C.J.; Vaziri, N.D.; Kovesdy, C.P.; Kalantar-Zadeh, K. Serum uric acid, protein intake and mortality in hemodialysis patients. *Nephrol Dial. Transpl.* **2017**, *32*, 1750–1757. [CrossRef]
39. Alexandrov, N.V.; Eelderink, C.; Singh-Povel, C.M.; Navis, G.J.; Bakker, S.; Corpeleijn, E. Dietary Protein Sources and Muscle Mass over the Life Course: The Lifelines Cohort Study. *Nutrients* **2018**, *10*, 1471. [CrossRef]
40. Aparicio, V.A.; Marin-Jimenez, N.; Coll-Risco, I.; de la Flor-Alemany, M.; Baena-Garcia, L.; Acosta-Manzano, P.; Aranda, P. Doctor, ask your perimenopausal patient about her physical fitness; association of self-reported physical fitness with cardiometabolic and mental health in perimenopausal women: The FLAMENCO project. *Menopause* **2019**, *26*, 1146–1153. [CrossRef]
41. Won, H.Y.; Park, J.B.; Park, E.Y.; Riew, K.D. Effect of hyperglycemia on apoptosis of notochordal cells and intervertebral disc degeneration in diabetic rats. *J. Neurosurg Spine* **2009**, *11*, 741–748. [CrossRef] [PubMed]
42. Wang, J.; Markova, D.; Anderson, D.G.; Zheng, Z.; Shapiro, I.M.; Risbud, M.V. TNF-alpha and IL-1beta promote a disintegrin-like and metalloprotease with thrombospondin type I motif-5-mediated aggrecan degradation through syndecan-4 in intervertebral disc. *J. Biol. Chem.* **2011**, *286*, 39738–39749. [CrossRef] [PubMed]
43. Dagistan, Y.; Cukur, S.; Dagistan, E.; Gezici, A.R. Importance of IL-6, MMP-1, IGF-1, and BAX Levels in Lumbar Herniated Disks and Posterior Longitudinal Ligament in Patients with Sciatic Pain. *World Neurosurg.* **2015**, *84*, 1739–1746. [CrossRef] [PubMed]

44. Gregorio-Arenas, E.; Ruiz-Cabello, P.; Camiletti-Moiron, D.; Moratalla-Cecilia, N.; Aranda, P.; Lopez-Jurado, M.; Llopis, J.; Aparicio, V.A. The associations between physical fitness and cardiometabolic risk and body-size phenotypes in perimenopausal women. *Maturitas* **2016**, *92*, 162–167. [CrossRef]
45. Supriya, R.; Yu, A.P.; Lee, P.H.; Lai, C.W.; Cheng, K.K.; Yau, S.Y.; Chan, L.W.; Yung, B.Y.; Siu, P.M. Yoga training modulates adipokines in adults with high-normal blood pressure and metabolic syndrome. *Scand. J. Med. Sci Sports* **2018**, *28*, 1130–1138. [CrossRef]
46. Konieczna, J.; Abete, I.; Galmes, A.M.; Babio, N.; Colom, A.; Zulet, M.A.; Estruch, R.; Vidal, J.; Toledo, E.; Diaz-Lopez, A.; et al. Body adiposity indicators and cardiometabolic risk: Cross-sectional analysis in participants from the PREDIMED-Plus trial. *Clin. Nutr.* **2019**, *38*, 1883–1891. [CrossRef]
47. Keswell, D.; Tootla, M.; Goedecke, J.H. Associations between body fat distribution, insulin resistance and dyslipidaemia in black and white South African women. *Cardiovasc. J. Afr.* **2016**, *27*, 177–183. [CrossRef]
48. Ormazabal, V.; Nair, S.; Elfeky, O.; Aguayo, C.; Salomon, C.; Zuniga, F.A. Association between insulin resistance and the development of cardiovascular disease. *Cardiovasc. Diabetol.* **2018**, *17*, 122. [CrossRef]
49. Lee, W.J.; Peng, L.N.; Chiou, S.T.; Chen, L.K. Relative Handgrip Strength Is a Simple Indicator of Cardiometabolic Risk among Middle-Aged and Older People: A Nationwide Population-Based Study in Taiwan. *PLoS ONE* **2016**, *11*, e160874. [CrossRef]
50. Lee, M.R.; Jung, S.M.; Kim, H.S.; Kim, Y.B. Association of muscle strength with cardiovascular risk in Korean adults: Findings from the Korea National Health and Nutrition Examination Survey (KNHANES) VI to VII (2014-2016). *Medicine* **2018**, *97*, e13240. [CrossRef]
51. Giudice, J.; Taylor, J.M. Muscle as a paracrine and endocrine organ. *Curr. Opin. Pharmacol.* **2017**, *34*, 49–55. [CrossRef] [PubMed]
52. Bostrom, P.; Wu, J.; Jedrychowski, M.P.; Korde, A.; Ye, L.; Lo, J.C.; Rasbach, K.A.; Bostrom, E.A.; Choi, J.H.; Long, J.Z.; et al. A PGC1-alpha-dependent myokine that drives brown-fat-like development of white fat and thermogenesis. *Nature* **2012**, *481*, 463–468. [CrossRef] [PubMed]
53. Seldin, M.M.; Peterson, J.M.; Byerly, M.S.; Wei, Z.; Wong, G.W. Myonectin (CTRP15), a novel myokine that links skeletal muscle to systemic lipid homeostasis. *J. Biol. Chem.* **2012**, *287*, 11968–11980. [CrossRef] [PubMed]

Publisher's Note: MDPI stays neutral with regard to jurisdictional claims in published maps and institutional affiliations.

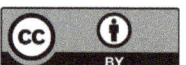

© 2020 by the authors. Licensee MDPI, Basel, Switzerland. This article is an open access article distributed under the terms and conditions of the Creative Commons Attribution (CC BY) license (http://creativecommons.org/licenses/by/4.0/).

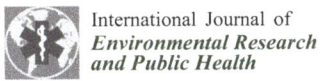 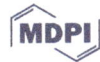

Article

Is Weight Gain Inevitable for Patients Trying to Quit Smoking as Part of Cardiac Rehabilitation?

Ahmad Salman * and Patrick Doherty

Department of Health Sciences, University of York, York YO10 5DD, UK; patrick.doherty@york.ac.uk
* Correspondence: as1816@york.ac.uk

Received: 21 September 2020; Accepted: 16 November 2020; Published: 18 November 2020

Abstract: The literature is uncertain about the extent to which those who attend cardiac rehabilitation (CR) gain weight while trying to quit smoking. This study aimed to determine the extent of CR-based smoking cessation provision and whether CR, as delivered in routine practice, is associated with helping patients quit smoking and avoid weight gain. Data from the UK National Audit of Cardiac Rehabilitation database, between April 2013 and March 2016, were used. Smoking status is categorised as smokers and quitters assessed by patient self-report. Outcomes included body weight, blood pressure, depression, and physical activity. A multiple linear regression model was constructed to understand the effect of continuing smoking or quitting smoking on CR outcomes. CR outcome scores were adjusted by the baseline CR score for each characteristic. An e-survey collected information about the smoking cessation support offered to patients attending CR. A total of 2052 smokers (58.59 ± 10.49 years, 73.6% male) and 1238 quitters (57.63 ± 10.36 years, 75.8% male) were analysed. Overall, 92.6% of CR programmes in the United Kingdom (UK) offer smoking cessation support for CR attenders. Quitting smoking during CR was associated with a mean increase in body weight of 0.4 kg, which is much less than seen in systematic reviews. Quitters who attended CR also had better improvements in physical activity status and psychosocial health measures than smokers. As delivered in routine practice, CR programmes in the UK adhere to the guideline recommendations for smoking cessation interventions, help patients quit smoking, and avoid weight gain on completion of CR.

Keywords: cardiac rehabilitation; cardiovascular diseases; smoking; weight gain

1. Introduction

Smoking is a risk factor for cardiovascular disease (CVD) and the cause of death for approximately 8 million people annually [1]. For developing non-communicable diseases such as cardiovascular, cancers, and respiratory diseases, smoking is considered a preventable risk factor [2].

A meta-analysis by Aubin et al. of 62 clinical trials that described weight gain in smokers who quit smoking for up to 12 months suggests that body weight increased on average by 1.12 kg, 2.26 kg, 2.85 kg, 4.23 kg, and 4.67 kg at one, two, three, six, and 12 months, respectively, after quitting [3]. Most of the weight gain occurs within three months of quitting, and estimates of weight gain were similar among smokers using different pharmacotherapies to support smoking cessation [3].

A large systematic review and meta-analysis of 35 prospective cohort studies with 63,403 quitters and 388,432 continuing smokers looking at the association between smoking cessation and weight gain found that quitting smoking was associated with a mean weight gain of 4.10 kg and mean body mass index (BMI) gain of 1.14 kg/m^2 over an average of 5 years [4]. The participants in this meta-analysis were similar to the general population in contrast to participants in the meta-analysis by Aubin et al. [3], making their findings more generalisable. In addition, the cohort studies in the meta-analysis by Tian et al. [4] had longer follow-up periods than those in the meta-analyses by

Aubin et al. [3], which allows for an assessment of the effects of quitting smoking on weight change beyond 12 months.

The cross-sectional studies of the four EUROASPIRE surveys, which took place between 1999 and 2013, investigated characteristics of successful quitters who had been pre-event smokers and reported a non-smoking status at the time of interview (median 1.2 years [range 0.5 to 3 years]) [5]. They also found that smoking cessation was associated with weight gain [5]. Numerous cohort studies have shown that people who stop smoking gain weight [6–12].

Gaining weight while stopping smoking can lead to anxiety and depression. Systematic reviews and meta-analyses found that overweight, obesity, and depression interacted reciprocally and that overweight and obesity increased the risk for anxiety and depression [13–15].

Cardiac rehabilitation (CR) is a structured, multi-disciplinary intervention that is offered to patients with CVD with the goal of reducing risk factors (smoking) and promoting psychosocial wellbeing [16–18]. Positive health outcomes, such as a reduction in cardiovascular mortality and hospital readmission, have been associated with CR participation [19,20]. In the United Kingdom (UK), patients with CVD have access to CR programmes. Programme uptake in the UK averages 50% and is considered one of the highest uptake figures compared to other countries [21]. CR programmes are delivered to the British Association for Cardiovascular Prevention and Rehabilitation (BACPR) standards with the goal of reducing cardiovascular risk and promoting quality of life through coordinated core components of CVD prevention and rehabilitation [17]. Recommendations include providing smoking cessation support and relapse prevention through lifestyle risk factor management as one of its core components [17]. On average, 94% of individuals who join CR programmes in the UK are classified as non-smokers [21]. The average increase in smoking cessation among individuals who participate in CR is approximately one percent (1.1%) [21].

A key aim of CR and a goal for most patients is to bring the body mass index (BMI) below <30 kg/m^2 [17]. On average, 30% of patients in the UK started CR with a BMI >30 kg/m^2 [21]. The contribution of CR to reducing BMI at a national level is low, with an average change of 0.2% in patients with BMI <30 kg/m^2 after CR [21]. This highlights the difficulty in addressing this risk factor. Additional factors need to be taken into account before drawing conclusions about how well CR programmes support weight management. Although smoking cessation results in considerable health improvements, it is often accompanied by weight gain, with patients who are trying to quit smoking more likely to put on 3–5 kg of weight in the first three months to a year [3]. Although weight gain does not offset the health benefits of smoking cessation, which far exceed any health risks that may result from smoking cessation-induced weight gain, it is frequently a source of concern for smokers planning to quit [7]. This substantial effect may inhibit the reporting of some successful weight loss programmes. The link between smoking and body weight is closely related and poses significant challenges for researchers investigating intervention effects in smokers. The most recent Cochrane review of 24 trials with a total of 7279 adult participants investigated the effectiveness of exercise-based interventions alone, or combined with a smoking cessation programmes and concluded no significant effect from adding exercise to smoking cessation [22]. The same authors do state and concludes that more studies are needed and that future trials may alter these conclusions [22]. Moreover, new research published in the British Journal of Pharmacology has confirmed that exercise can help smokers quit smoking and may aid smoking cessation by reducing the severity of smoking withdrawal symptoms [23]. As weight gain may be a barrier to quitting smoking or a reason to restart smoking, CR has not been evaluated in relation to weight gain after smoking cessation. As weight gain may be a barrier against quitting smoking, it is important to investigate smoking cessation support services provided in CR to help patients quit smoking while maintaining their weight status. Little is known about how routinely delivered CR programmes support smoking cessation.

This study determines the extent of CR-based smoking cessation provision and whether CR, as delivered in routine practice, is associated with helping patients quit smoking and avoid weight gain.

2. Materials and Methods

2.1. Data Source

Individual, patient-level data from the National Audit of Cardiac Rehabilitation (NACR) were used in the analyses of this study. The NACR, funded by the British Heart Foundation, is a web-based registry of CR in the UK. Data on patients who are eligible or referred to CR delivery are entered by practitioners into an electronic patient dataset according to a data dictionary (www.cardiacrehabilitation.org.uk/nacr/downloads.htm). The NACR team checks data quality from clinical teams who directly enters data into a secure online system (hosted by NHS Digital) who then provide NACR with anonymized local programme-level data. The NACR includes details of a patient's initiating event, treatment type, risk factors, drugs, patient demographics, and post-CR clinical outcomes. Anonymised data is collected for a range of clinical indicators for the purposes of audit and research under Section 251 of the NHS Act 2006 [21]. NHS Digital annually reviews data governance and approval for NACR projects that aim to improve service quality and patient outcomes. Separate approval for this study in addition to the e-survey project was not required, as it was considered part of the NACR quality and outcomes process. The Strengthening the Reporting of Observational Studies in Epidemiology (STROBE) guidelines were used for reporting this observational study [24].

2.2. Participants

Participants included in this study were from the research cohort added to the NACR database between 1 April 2013 and 31 March 2016. Data has been validated and extracted retrospectively and there were no exclusion criteria. Analyses included patient sociodemographic data and clinical characteristics of individuals who started a CR programme with both a baseline and follow-up smoking status assessments.

2.3. Smoking Outcome Measures

Smoking status is assessed via self-reported questionnaires in the NACR database [21]. Pre- and post-CR smoking status is categorised into one of the following: never smoked, ex-smoker, stopped smoking since the event, or current smoking. For the purposes of this study, patients were categorised as continued smokers (defined as current smokers in pre- and post-CR assessments) or quitters (defined as current smokers in pre- and no smoking status in post-CR assessment).

A range of patient-level variables collected by the NACR primary dataset were used for the present study. Variables included anthropometric data, physical, and psychosocial health measures. Anthropometric measures included weight (kg), height (m), body mass index (BMI) (kg/m^2), and waist circumference (cm). Alcohol consumption status was measured using self-reported questionnaires related to weekly alcohol consumption. Physical activity was self-reported and categorised into moderate physical activity (150 min/week; yes/no) or vigorous physical activity (75 min/week; yes/no)) using the Chief Medical Officer's Physical Activity Questionnaire [25]. Physical activity recommendations were based on the Department of Health guidelines for 19–64 and 65+ age groups. The Hospital Anxiety and Depression Scale (HADS), a reliable and well-validated scale, was used to assess psychosocial health status. Higher HADS scores represent worse symptoms.

2.4. e-Survey

With the knowledge that smoking cessation is a key part of secondary prevention and rehabilitation and is included in the BACPR core components of lifestyle risk factor management [17], a cross-sectional 11-item e-survey was sent to CR services to explore smoking cessation services provided by CR programmes in the UK. The sampling frame encompassed the 'coordinators' of the 224 CR programmes in the UK that electronically enter their data into the NACR. Several reminders were sent out via email over two months. Data collection took place in the summer of 2016 (May 2016–July 2016). The response rate was 78% (175/224 CR programmes registered in the NACR).

2.5. Statistical Analysis

All analyses were performed in the IBM Statistical Package for Social Sciences (SPSS) software statistics Version 24 (New York, NY, USA). A p-value < 0.05 was considered statistically significant.

Percentage or relative change was used to measure the difference in outcome (post-CR) from baseline (pre-CR) [26,27]. It was calculated by: (percentage change = pre-CR value − post-CR value/ pre-CR value) * 100

Outliers were detected by the median plus or minus 3 times the median absolute deviation (3 ± MAD) method [28]. Pre-and post-CR values with more than 3 ± MAD percentage change for each characteristic were eliminated from the analysis.

A multiple linear regression model was constructed to understand the effect of continuing smoking or quitting smoking on CR outcomes, with adjustments for the outcome CR score by the baseline CR score for each characteristic. Post-CR outcomes (with respect to baseline) were introduced into multiple linear regression models (as continuous dependent variables) and tested against smoking status (a score of 0 was categorised as a smoker, whereas a score of 1 was categorised as a quitter). We compared and described analyses of CR patients using the original data with analyses of all data after replacing missing values, which were handled through the expectation maximisation method [29]. Use of expectation maximisation to handle missing data gave similar results to the original analyses. Commonly used descriptive statistical parameters, including the number of programmes, percentages, means or medians, and standard deviations, were used to explore the data.

3. Results

3.1. Cohort Characteristics

A total of 49,725 patients had a pre- and post-CR smoking status recorded. Non-smokers comprised 93.4% of the sample (mean age 65.72 ± 11.08 years, 74.7% male), while 4.1% of the sample were classified as continued smokers (mean age 58.59 ± 10.49 years, 73.6% male) and 2.5% were quitters (mean age 57.63 ± 10.36 years, 75.8% male). The median duration of CR was 9 weeks. For the purposes of this research, patients were categorised as continued smokers or quitters (Table 1).

Table 1. Smoking categorisation groups.

Group	Frequency (n)	Percent (%)
Smokers	2052	62.4
Quitters	1238	37.6
Total	3290	100

n = Number of patients; % percentage of patients.

3.2. Smokers Versus Quitters (Outcomes)

The CR outcome results between smokers and quitters are summarised in Table 2.

Table 2. Baseline and outcome values for cardiac rehabilitation (CR) patients included in the analysis.

CR Outcome	Smokers			Quitters		
	Pre-CR	Post-CR	n	Pre-CR	Post-CR	n
Weight (Kg)	81.64	81.68	1499	83.83	84.28	881
BMI (kg/m2)	27.99	28.28	1442	28.01	28.47	833
Waist (cm)	98.47	98.09	657	97.39	97.11	272
Alcohol consumption	17.78	13.80	486	15.66	11.28	298
HADS anxiety score	7.89	7.39	1046	6.92	5.79	546
HADS depression score	6.53	5.68	1032	5.44	4.24	530

BMI, body mass index; CR, cardiac rehabilitation; HADS, hospital anxiety and depression scale; n = number of patients.

After controlling for baseline characteristics, predictions were made to determine outcome changes for patients who quit smoking while attending CR. Only CR patients with pre- and post-CR values were included in the analysis after excluding pre- and post-values with percentage change more than 3 ± MAD.

A multiple regression model was constructed to understand the effect of quitting smoking on CR outcomes with adjustments for the outcome CR score by the baseline CR score for each characteristic (Table 3). Moreover, post-CR outcomes (with respect to baseline) were introduced into multiple linear regression models (as continuous dependent variables) and tested against smoking status (score 0 for smokers; score 1 for quitters).

Table 3. Summary of multiple regression analysis.

Variable (n)		Unstandardised Coefficients		Standardised Coefficients		95% CI		Effect Size
		B	S.E.	Beta	Sig.	Lower	Upper	
Weight (n = 2380)	Constant	0.75	0.24		<0.001	0.28	1.23	
	Baseline weight	0.99	0.00	0.99	<0.001	0.99	1.00	0.01
	Smoking	0.43	0.11	0.01	<0.001 *	0.22	0.63	
BMI (n = 2275)	Constant	0.41	0.10		<0.001	0.22	0.61	
	Baseline BMI	0.99	0.00	0.99	<0.001	0.98	0.99	0.01
	Smoking	0.18	0.04	0.02	<0.001 *	0.10	0.25	
Waist (n = 929)	Constant	4.52	0.75		<0.001	3.05	5.99	
	Baseline waist	0.95	0.01	0.97	<0.001	0.94	0.97	0.00
	Smoking	0.05	0.23	0.00	0.83	−0.40	0.49	
Alcohol consumption (784)	Constant	3.86	0.54		<0.001	2.80	4.91	
	Baseline alcohol consumption	0.56	0.02	0.73	<0.001	0.52	0.60	0.01
	Smoking	−1.34	0.68	−0.05	0.05 *	−2.68	0.00	
HADS anxiety score (1592)	Constant	0.86	0.16		<0.001	0.56	1.17	
	Baseline HADS anxiety score	0.77	0.02	0.76	<0.001	0.74	0.80	0.02
	smoking	−0.75	0.15	−0.08	<0.001 *	−1.04	−0.45	
HADS depression score (1562)	Constant	0.64	0.14		<0.001	0.37	0.91	
	Baseline HADS depression score	0.74	0.02	0.74	<0.001	0.70	0.77	0.01
	smoking	−0.58	0.14	−0.07	<0.001*	−0.86	−0.30	

B = unstandardised regression coefficient; Beta = standardized coefficient; BMI, body mass index; CI = Confidence Interval for unstandardised regression coefficient; CR, cardiac rehabilitation; HADS, hospital anxiety and depression scale; n = Number of patients; S.E. = standard error of the coefficient. * $p < 0.05$.

A χ^2 test was conducted for the association between smokers and quitters and moderate physical activity (150 min/week) outcomes: improved (n = 679), no change (n = 1126), and worsened (n = 93). There was a statistically significant association between the smoking group and moderate physical activity outcomes: $\chi^2(2) = 23.50$, $p < 0.001$, and small association Cramér's V = 0.11 (Table 4). A χ^2 test was conducted for the association between smokers and quitters and vigorous physical activity (75 min/week) outcomes: improved (n = 338), no change (n = 1217), and worsened (n = 47). There was a statistically significant association between smoking status and vigorous physical activity outcomes: $\chi^2(2) = 17.88$, $p < 0.001$; small association Cramér's V = 0.11) (Table 4).

Table 4. Summary of multiple regression analysis.

Physical Activity Outcomes	Smokers (%)			Quitters (%)		
	Improve	No Change	Worsen	Improve	No Change	Worsen
Δ 150 min/week (moderate)	31.9	62.8	5.4	43	52.9	4.1
Δ 75 min/week (vigorous)	18.0	79.3	2.6	26.6	70.0	3.5

Δ, change; % percentage.

3.3. e-Survey

Overall, 175 CR programmes participated—a response rate of 78% (175/224 CR programmes registered in the NACR). The following results present an overview of the survey results (Figure 1).

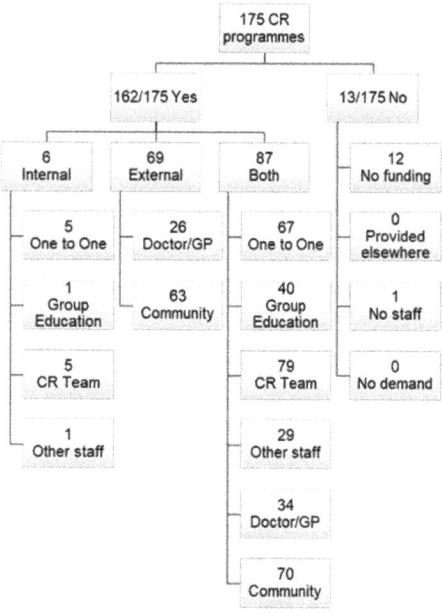

Figure 1. Number of cardiac rehabilitation programmes providing stopping smoking support. CR: cardiac rehabilitation; Internal: delivering the smoking cessation support services at the CR programme site; External: external referral.

Most CR programmes in the UK offered smoking cessation support for CR attenders: 162 (92.6%) programmes, while 13 (7.4%) of CR programmes did not provide patients with support to stop smoking.

About half of CR programmes (87 (49.7%) programmes) offered both internal and external smoking cessation support for CR attenders. Six CR programmes only offered internal support, by delivering smoking cessation support services at the CR programme sites, while 69 (39.4%) CR programmes only offered external referrals.

Notably, 72/93 (77.4%) CR programmes that delivered smoking cessation support at the CR programme sites (internal delivery: 6 only internal + 87 both = 93 internal) offered one-to-one sessions. On the other hand, 41 (44.1%) CR programmes offered group education support as a form of internal support.

Eighty four (90.3%) CR programmes that offered smoking cessation support delivered it internally through the CR team. On the other hand, 30 (32.3%) CR programmes delivered smoking cessation support through other qualified staff members.

Sixty (38.5%) CR programmes that offered external support for smoking cessation (external delivery: 69 only external + 87 both = 156 external) offered referrals to doctors or general practitioners and 133/156 (85.3%) CR programmes offered referrals to community-based cessation programmes.

For 73/162 (45.1%) CR programmes that offered smoking cessation support, patient preference was the most frequently cited factor for whether a patient attended an internal CR programme's smoking cessation service or was referred to external support (Table 5). However, eight (4.9%) CR programmes cited availability as a factor that influenced whether a patient would receive internal or external support; one (0.6%) reported funding constraints, and 36 (22.2%) CR programmes reported specific patient needs (e.g., hardened smoker).

Table 5. What might decide whether a patient would attend the CR Programme or be referred out?

Reason	n = 162	Percentage (%)
Availability	8	4.9
Patient preference	73	45.1
Service funding constraints	1	0.6
Specific patient needs	36	22.2

n = Number of programmes; % percentage of programmes.

Funding was the most common factor for not providing support for smoking cessation for CR attenders, given as the reason by 12/13 (92.3%) CR programmes that did not provide support for patients to stop smoking. The other factor reported by only one CR programme was lack of appropriate staff.

4. Discussion

Our research findings show that, after CR, quitters, on average, gain 0.43 kg more than those who continue to smoke ($p < 0.001$) and have a BMI of 0.18 kg/m^2 more than those who continue to smoke ($p < 0.001$). Although differences in weight and BMI scores after CR were statistically significantly different for quitters and continued smokers (driven by a large sample size of 49,725), the mean differences of 0.43 kg and 0.18 kg/m^2 were very small from a clinical perspective and much lower than previously cited reviews of smoking cessation where the mean weight gain was around 4 kg [3–5]. The lack of clinically relevant differences in this data are sufficient to make a strong clinical recommendation regarding the impact of CR to prevent weight gain when delivered alongside smoking cessation in patients with heart disease. Our study shows no clinically significant weight gain in the short term.

Evidence suggests that quitting smoking is associated with a mean increase in body weight of 3–5 kg, with most weight gain occurring within 3 months of quitting [3–5]; however, the research findings reported here show that smokers who quit smoking while attending CR do not gain weight, which aligns with the findings of Farley et al. that exercise could reduce post-cessation weight gain [30]. With regard to smoking and weight interactions, the extent of weight gain associated with smoking cessation in patients attending CR is much less than previous studies suggest. These research findings provide evidence that CR is positively associated with weight management during smoking cessation.

The confidence interval for mean difference in weight between continued smokers and quitters after CR was 0.22 to 0.63 kg and for mean difference in BMI, it was 0.1 to 0.25 kg/m^2. Because of the well-documented health benefits of quitting smoking, clinicians should inform smokers about the low likelihood of weight gain and encourage them to attend CR to avoid excess weight gain.

There is no clinical trial evidence for the effectiveness of smoking cessation interventions within CR; however, our research findings suggest CR as delivered in routine practice is associated with helping patients quit smoking and reduce the likelihood of weight gain beyond 1 kg. The NACR data regarding smoking status suggest that about 37.6% of patients who are smoking when recruited to CR successfully stop after CR. Quitting smoking is considered a core element in both primary and secondary prevention of cardiovascular disease [31].

Following CR, quitters on average drink 1.34 units of alcohol fewer than those who continue to smoke. Following CR, 43% and 26.6% of quitters improved to achieve the recommended UK moderate and vigorous physical activity guidelines, respectively, compared with 31.9% and 18% of continued smokers. An even stronger benefit was seen in both HADS anxiety and depression scores, which showed that quitters on average score 0.75 and 0.58 less anxious and less depressed than those who continue to smoke.

Our survey of smoking cessation support services, offered in routine practice to CR attenders, had a high response rate of 78%. Although one study has shown low levels of cessation support following hospital discharge [32], the e-survey showed that 92.6% of CR programmes in the UK offer smoking cessation support for patients attending CR. These results show that CR programmes in the UK adhere to guideline recommendations for smoking cessation interventions [17,33–35]. In addition, the research results suggest that CR programmes in the UK offer assistance for patients who smoke by delivering smoking cessation support at the CR programme site in the form of individualised one-to-one sessions or group educational sessions, as well as referral for external smoking cessation support. The internal support is provided by the CR team or another qualified member of staff. One-to-one sessions are the dominant service offered at the site of CR programmes, while external provision is predominantly through referral to community-based cessation programmes. Patient preference is the factor that most influences whether a patient would attend the CR programme (internal) or be referred out (external).

Provision of smoking cessation support in CR could have multiple benefits: the presence of such a programme could entice more smokers to attend CR, and the increased support for cessation they receive could encourage them to remain in the CR programme generally. Prior studies suggest that CR attendance improves smoking cessation rates, and Riley et al. found a strong relationship between smoking cessation and CR attendance [36].

Failure of adherence to guideline recommendations to provide support for smoking cessation for CR attenders was predominantly due to funding challenges. Cutting funds to CR services is a false economy, as evidence shows that smoking cessation services provide effective support for smokers who want to quit [37] and the lack of this provision leads to higher costs for the NHS to manage and treat diseases caused by smoking in the long term. The National Institute for Health and Care Excellence (NICE) estimates that for every pound invested in smoking cessation, £2.37 in benefits are generated [38]. Moreover, the lack of investment in CR programmes may impact on service provision. In Yorkshire, for example, a qualitative study found staff to be aware of limited service availability [39], which may influence which patients are invited. Finally, it should not have to be a choice that some smokers attending CR are supported to quit and others are not.

Comprehensive CR programmes seem to have a beneficial role in helping patients after a cardiac event or procedure, with significant improvements in smoking behaviour, weight management, physical activity levels, psychosocial health, and alcohol consumption. When a comprehensive CR includes exercise with smoking cessation and patient education, this research initiates evidence for improvements in cardiac risk factors, particularly increased smoking cessation and improvements in physical and psychosocial health.

Several limitations of our study must be noted. First, the retrospective observational study design is limited in capturing data and data quality from CR programmes. An 18% gap in data capture was identified due to some programmes not providing their data electronically. Approximately 31% of patients who began a CR programme did not have post-program data available, affecting data quality. Non-completion of the program leads to missingness in patient records that may affect the representativeness of our sample. Self-reported data poses a limitation in terms of determining smoking status and immediate post-CR analysis. Using self-reported data to determine smoking status might be subject to recall and social desirability biases. The self-reported smoking status was not validated with a biochemical marker. Some possible factors that influenced quitting smoking have been missed from the analysis due to high levels of missing data or may not have been collected in the NACR. Some smoking cessation drugs in addition to the intensity of the smoking cessation program (number and duration of the visits) may have affected the considered outcomes and they are not included as a confounder in the analyses for the outcomes related to smoking cessation and weight gain [40–42]. However, the strengths of our study include utilizing a prospective cohort design and an observational approach, and using data from a large-scale dataset that collects routine clinical information from CR programmes in the UK. This study also suggested that clinical and research efforts should be directed towards improving the rate of smoking cessation in patients with CVD by accounting for factors that predict quitting smoking among CR attendees [43].

5. Conclusions

Cardiac rehabilitation is an effective intervention to manage weight gain when quitting smoking. Quitting smoking during CR is associated with a mean increase of 0.4 kg in body weight following CR. Quitters who attended CR improved their physical activity status and psychosocial health measures compared with smokers.

This research is the first to evaluate smoking cessation support in CR services in the UK, with 92.6% of CR programmes in the UK offering smoking cessation support for CR attenders. These results demonstrate adherence of CR in the UK to the guideline recommendations for smoking cessation interventions.

Author Contributions: Conceptualization, A.S. and P.D.; Formal analysis, A.S.; Investigation, A.S.; Methodology, A.S. and P.D.; Validation, A.S. and P.D.; Visualization, A.S.; Writing—original draft, A.S.; Writing—review & editing, A.S. and P.D. All authors have read and agreed to the published version of the manuscript.

Funding: This research was funded by the British Heart Foundation, grant number (040/PSS/17/18/NACR).

Acknowledgments: The authors would like to acknowledge the support of NACR Team.

Conflicts of Interest: The authors declare no conflict of interest.

References

1. World Health Organisation. Tobacco: Fact Sheet. Available online: https://www.who.int/news-room/fact-sheets/detail/tobacco (accessed on 17 May 2020).
2. U.S. Department of Health and Human Services. *The Health Consequences of Smoking—50 years of Progress: A Report of the Surgeon General*; Department of Health and Human Services, Centers for Disease Control and Prevention, National Center for Chronic Disease Prevention and Health Promotion, Office on Smoking and Health: Atlanta, GA, USA, 2014.
3. Aubin, H.-J.; Farley, A.; Lycett, D.; Lahmek, P.; Aveyard, P. Weight gain in smokers after quitting cigarettes: Meta-analysis. *BMJ* **2012**, *345*. [CrossRef]
4. Tian, J.; Venn, A.; Otahal, P.; Gall, S. The association between quitting smoking and weight gain: A systemic review and meta-analysis of prospective cohort studies. *Obes. Rev.* **2015**, *16*, 883–901. [CrossRef]
5. Snaterse, M.; Deckers, J.W.; Lenzen, M.J.; Jorstad, H.T.; De Bacquer, D.; Peters, R.J.G.; Jennings, C.; Kotseva, K.; Scholte op Reimer, W.J.M. Smoking cessation in European patients with coronary heart disease. Results from the EUROASPIRE IV survey: A registry from the European Society of Cardiology. *Int. J. Cardiol.* **2018**, *258*, 1–6. [CrossRef]
6. Lycett, D.; Munafò, M.; Johnstone, E.; Murphy, M.; Aveyard, P. Associations between weight change over 8 years and baseline body mass index in a cohort of continuing and quitting smokers. *Addiction* **2011**, *106*, 188–196. [CrossRef] [PubMed]
7. Pistelli, F.; Aquilini, F.; Carrozzi, L. Weight gain after smoking cessation. *Monaldi Arch. Chest. Dis.* **2009**, *71*, 81–87. [CrossRef] [PubMed]
8. Eisenberg, D.; Quinn, B.C. Estimating the effect of smoking cessation on weight gain: An instrumental variable approach. *Health Serv. Res.* **2006**, *41*, 2255–2266. [CrossRef] [PubMed]
9. Filozof, C.; Fernández Pinilla, M.C.; Fernández-Cruz, A. Smoking cessation and weight gain. *Obes. Rev.* **2004**, *5*, 95–103. [CrossRef]
10. Froom, P.; Melamed, S.; Benbassat, J. Smoking cessation and weight gain. *J. Fam. Pract.* **1998**, *46*, 460–464.
11. Perkins, K.A. Weight gain following smoking cessation. *J. Consult. Clin. Psychol.* **1993**, *61*, 768–777. [CrossRef]
12. Klesges, R.C.; Meyers, A.W.; Klesges, L.M.; La Vasque, M.E. Smoking, body weight, and their effects on smoking behavior: A comprehensive review of the literature. *Psychol. Bull.* **1989**, *106*, 204–230. [CrossRef]
13. Gariepy, G.; Nitka, D.; Schmitz, N. The association between obesity and anxiety disorders in the population: A systematic review and meta-analysis. *Int. J. Obes.* **2010**, *34*, 407–419. [CrossRef] [PubMed]
14. Luppino, F.S.; de Wit, L.M.; Bouvy, P.F.; Stijnen, T.; Cuijpers, P.; Penninx, B.W.J.H.; Zitman, F.G. Overweight, Obesity, and Depression: A Systematic Review and Meta-analysis of Longitudinal Studies. *Arch. Gen. Psychiatry* **2010**, *67*, 220–229. [CrossRef] [PubMed]

15. Pereira-Miranda, E.; Costa, P.R.F.; Queiroz, V.A.O.; Pereira-Santos, M.; Santana, M.L.P. Overweight and Obesity Associated with Higher Depression Prevalence in Adults: A Systematic Review and Meta-Analysis. *J. Am. Coll. Nutr.* **2017**, *36*, 223–233. [CrossRef] [PubMed]
16. Piepoli, M.F.; Hoes, A.W.; Agewall, S.; Albus, C.; Brotons, C.; Catapano, A.L.; Cooney, M.T.; Corrà, U.; Cosyns, B.; Deaton, C.; et al. 2016 European Guidelines on cardiovascular disease prevention in clinical practice. The Sixth Joint Task Force of the European Society of Cardiology and Other Societies on Cardiovascular Disease Prevention in Clinical Practice. *Eur. Heart J.* **2016**, *37*, 2315–2381. [CrossRef] [PubMed]
17. BACPR. *The BACPR Standards and Core Components for Cardiovascular Disease Prevention and Rehabilitation 2017*, 3rd ed.; BACRP: London, UK, 2017.
18. Balady, G.J.; Ades, P.A.; Bittner, V.A.; Franklin, B.A.; Gordon, N.F.; Thomas, R.J.; Tomaselli, G.F.; Yancy, C.W. Referral, enrollment, and delivery of cardiac rehabilitation/secondary prevention programs at clinical centers and beyond: A presidential advisory from the American heart association. *Circulation* **2011**, *124*, 2951–2960. [CrossRef] [PubMed]
19. Anderson, L.; Oldridge, N.; Thompson, D.R.; Zwisler, A.-D.; Rees, K.; Martin, N.; Taylor, R.S. Exercise-Based Cardiac Rehabilitation for Coronary Heart Disease. *J. Am. Coll. Cardiol.* **2016**, *67*, 1–12. [CrossRef] [PubMed]
20. Rauch, B.; Davos, C.H.; Doherty, P.; Saure, D.; Metzendorf, M.-I.; Salzwedel, A.; Völler, H.; Jensen, K.; Schmid, J.-P. The prognostic effect of cardiac rehabilitation in the era of acute revascularisation and statin therapy: A systematic review and meta-analysis of randomized and non-randomized studies—The Cardiac Rehabilitation Outcome Study (CROS). *Eur. J. Prev. Cardiol.* **2016**, *23*, 1914–1939. [CrossRef]
21. NACR. *The National Audit of Cardiac Rehabilitation: Quality and Outcomes Report 2019*; British Heart Foundation: London, UK, 2019.
22. Ussher, M.H.; Faulkner, G.E.J.; Angus, K.; Hartmann-Boyce, J.; Taylor, A.H. Exercise interventions for smoking cessation. *Cochrane Database Syst. Rev.* **2019**, CD002295. [CrossRef]
23. Keyworth, H.; Georgiou, P.; Zanos, P.; Rueda, A.V.; Chen, Y.; Kitchen, I.; Camarini, R.; Cropley, M.; Bailey, A. Wheel running during chronic nicotine exposure is protective against mecamylamine-precipitated withdrawal and up-regulates hippocampal α7 nACh receptors in mice. *Br. J. Pharmacol.* **2018**, *175*, 1928–1943. [CrossRef]
24. Von Elm, E.; Altman, D.G.; Egger, M.; Pocock, S.J.; Gøtzsche, P.C.; Vandenbroucke, J.P. The Strengthening the Reporting of Observational Studies in Epidemiology (STROBE) statement: Guidelines for reporting observational studies. *J. Clin. Epidemiol.* **2008**, *61*, 344–349. [CrossRef]
25. Davies, D.S.C.; Atherton, F.; McBride, M.; Calderwood, C. *UK Chief Medical Officers' Physical Activity Guidelines*; Department of Health and Social Care: London, UK, 2019.
26. Zhang, L.; Han, K. *How to Analyze Change from Baseline: Absolute or Percentage Change?* Högskolan Dalarna: Borlänge, Sweden, 2009.
27. Törnqvist, L.; Vartia, P.; Vartia, Y.O. How should relative changes be measured? *Am. Stat.* **1985**, *39*, 43–46.
28. Leys, C.; Ley, C.; Klein, O.; Bernard, P.; Licata, L. Detecting outliers: Do not use standard deviation around the mean, use absolute deviation around the median. *J. Exp. Soc. Psychol.* **2013**, *49*, 764–766. [CrossRef]
29. Schafer, J.L. *Analysis of Incomplete Multivariate Data*; Chapman and Hall: London, UK, 1997; Volume 72, ISBN 0412040611.
30. Farley, A.; Hajek, P.; Lycett, D.; Aveyard, P. Interventions for preventing weight gain after smoking cessation (Review). *Cochrane Database Syst. Rev.* **2012**. [CrossRef] [PubMed]
31. Mons, U.; Muezzinler, A.; Gellert, C.; Schottker, B.; Abnet, C.C.; Bobak, M.; de Groot, L.; Freedman, N.D.; Jansen, E.; Kee, F.; et al. Impact of smoking and smoking cessation on cardiovascular events and mortality among older adults: Meta-analysis of individual participant data from prospective cohort studies of the CHANCES consortium. *BMJ* **2015**, *350*. [CrossRef] [PubMed]
32. Boggon, R.; Timmis, A.; Hemingway, H.; Raju, S.; Malvestiti, F.M.; Van Staa, T.P. Smoking cessation interventions following acute coronary syndrome: A missed opportunity? *Eur. J. Prev. Cardiol.* **2014**, *21*, 767–773. [CrossRef]
33. NICE. *Stop Smoking Interventions and Services*; NICE guideline 92; National Institute for Health and Care Excellence: London, UK, 2018.
34. SIGN. *SIGN 150 Cardiac Rehabilitation: A National Clinical Guideline*; Scottish Intercollegiate Guidelines Network: Edinburgh, UK, 2017.
35. NICE. *Myocardial Infarction: Cardiac Rehabilitation and Prevention of Further Cardiovascular Disease*; Clinical Guideline [CG172]; National Institute for Health and Care Excellence: London, UK, 2013.

36. Riley, H.; Headley, S.; Goff, S.; Lindenauer, P.; Szalai, H.; Pack, Q. Smoking cessation is strongly associated with attendance at cardiac rehab: But which comes first? *J. Am. Coll. Cardiol.* **2017**, *69*, 1844. [CrossRef]
37. Bauld, L.; Bell, K.; McCullough, L.; Richardson, L.; Greaves, L. The effectiveness of NHS smoking cessation services: A systematic review. *J. Public Health* **2009**, *32*, 71–82. [CrossRef]
38. Pokhrel, S.; Owen, L.; Coyle, K.; Lester-George, A.; Leng, G.; West, R.; Coyle, D. Costs of disinvesting from stop smoking services: An economic evaluation based on the NICE Tobacco Return on Investment model. *Lancet* **2016**, *388*, S95. [CrossRef]
39. Lindsay, S. How and why the motivation and skill to self-manage coronary heart disease are socially unequal. *Res. Sociol. Health Care* **2008**, *26*, 17–39.
40. Shang, C.; Chaloupka, F.J.; Kostova, D. Who Quits? An overview of quitters in low- and middle-income countries. *Nicotine Tob. Res.* **2014**, *16*, S44–S55. [CrossRef]
41. Li, L.; Borland, R.; Yong, H.H.; Fong, G.T.; Bansal-travers, M.; Quah, A.C.K.; Sirirassamee, B.; Omar, M.; Zanna, M.P.; Fotuhi, O. Predictors of smoking cessation among adult smokers in Malaysia and Thailand: Findings from the International Tobacco Control Southeast Asia survey. *Nicotine Tob. Res.* **2010**, *12*, S34–S44. [CrossRef] [PubMed]
42. Chandola, T.; Head, J.; Bartley, M. Socio-demographic predictors of quitting smoking: How important are household factors? *Addiction* **2004**, *99*, 770–777. [CrossRef] [PubMed]
43. Salman, A.; Doherty, P. Predictors of Quitting Smoking in Cardiac Rehabilitation. *J. Clin. Med.* **2020**, *9*, 2612. [CrossRef] [PubMed]

Publisher's Note: MDPI stays neutral with regard to jurisdictional claims in published maps and institutional affiliations.

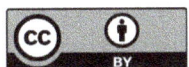

© 2020 by the authors. Licensee MDPI, Basel, Switzerland. This article is an open access article distributed under the terms and conditions of the Creative Commons Attribution (CC BY) license (http://creativecommons.org/licenses/by/4.0/).

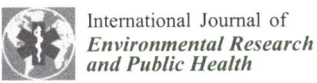

Review

Characteristics of Physical Exercise Programs for Older Adults in Latin America: A Systematic Review of Randomized Controlled Trials

Eduardo Vásquez-Araneda [1], Rodrigo Ignacio Solís-Vivanco [1], Sandra Mahecha-Matsudo [2], Rafael Zapata-Lamana [3] and Igor Cigarroa [4,*]

1. Programa de Magister en Fisiología Clínica del Ejercicio, Universidad Mayor, Santiago 8580000, Chile; vasquez.eduardo@hotmail.com (E.V.-A.); rsolivanko.10@gmail.com (R.I.S.-V.)
2. Facultad de Ciencias, Universidad Mayor, Santiago 8580000, Chile; sandra.mahecha@umayor.cl
3. Escuela de Educación, Universidad de Concepción, Los Ángeles 4440000, Chile; rafaelzapata@udec.cl
4. Escuela de Kinesiología, Facultad de Salud, Universidad Santo Tomás, Los Ángeles 4440000, Chile
* Correspondence: icigarroa@santotomas.cl; Tel.: +56-432536628

Abstract: Aim: To characterize physical exercise programs for older adults in Latin America. Methods: This review was conducted in accordance with the PRISMA statement. A search for randomized controlled trials (RCTs) published between the years 2015 and 2020 was performed in the Scopus, MedLine and SciELO databases. Results: A total of 101 RCTs were included. A large percentage of the studies had an unclear risk of bias in the items: selection, performance, detection and attribution. Furthermore, a heterogeneous level of compliance was observed in the CERT items. A total sample of 5013 older adults (79% women) was included. 97% of the studies included older adults between 60–70 years, presenting an adherence to the interventions of 86%. The studies were mainly carried out in older adults with cardiometabolic diseases. Only 44% of the studies detailed information regarding the place of intervention; of these studies, 61% developed their interventions in university facilities. The interventions were mainly based on therapeutic physical exercise (89% of the articles), with a duration of 2–6 months (95% of the articles) and a frequency of 2–3 times a week (95% of the articles) with sessions of 30–60 min (94% of the articles) led by sports science professionals (51% of the articles). The components of physical fitness that were exercised the most were muscular strength (77% of the articles) and cardiorespiratory fitness (47% of the articles). Furthermore, only 48% of the studies included a warm-up stage and 34% of the studies included a cool-down stage. Conclusions: This systematic review characterized the physical exercise programs in older adults in Latin America, as well the most frequently used outcome measures and instruments, by summarizing available evidence derived from RCTs. The results will be useful for prescribing future physical exercise programs in older adults.

Keywords: aging; physical aptitude; mental health; cognition; systematic review

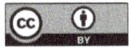

1. Introduction

The aging process of the population is advancing at an accelerated rate and is related to a longer life expectancy [1]. Thus, it is expected that the fraction of the world population over 65 years of age will increase from 9% to 16% by the year 2050 [2]. Latin America is in a similar situation, with a 156% increase in the population of older adults (OAs) [3].

Aging is characterized by physiological changes that, conditioned by extrinsic and intrinsic factors, translate into loss of health, conditioning a decline in the physical and mental skills of OAs [4]. Although current evidence supports the bio-psycho-social benefits of physical activity (PA) and physical exercise (PE), it is known that their practice decreases with age [5]. It is therefore a strong predictor of physical disability [6], associated with an increased risk of mortality. Along these lines, the World Health Organization (WHO) has reported that around 2.3 million deaths each year are due to physical inactivity [7]. The highest levels of physical inactivity in men and women (39%) are registered in Latin America and the Caribbean [8–10].

The practice of PA and PE through supervised programs contributes to improving physical fitness components such as cardiorespiratory fitness, muscular strength, gait and balance, and to avoid the risk of falls [11–13], being an effective intervention to delay the onset characteristic disorders of OA, such as sarcopenia and/or frailty syndrome, which cause a significant deterioration in functionality and quality of life [14–16]. On the other hand, PA and PE also generate positive effects associated with psychosocial and cognitive aspects in OAs, reducing symptoms of anxiety and depression [17].

Current PA and PE recommendations for aging suggest accumulating a minimum of 150 min of moderate aerobic PA or 75 min of vigorous aerobic PA and varied multicomponent physical activities three or more days a week, to improve functional capacity and prevent falls, in addition to perform activities that strengthen the main muscle groups two or more days a week [18–20].

At the Latin American level, different countries have proposed guidelines for PA recommendations (GPAR) for OAs [21–36]. Although the recommendations proposed by the WHO for the elaboration of GPAR have been considered as a reference, these are constantly being updated and differ in specific characteristics such as the type of exercise, frequency and duration, as well as the suggested age for their implementation. In relation to the age group to which these GPAR are directed, there are countries that classify those over 65 as elderly, while in Chile this category begins at 60 years. This allows us to infer that there could be a heterogeneity in the GPAR of the different Latin American countries. Along the same lines, it is of great interest to know if the current evidence that exists regarding the prescription of PA and PE in OAs has the same heterogeneity in characteristics such as the type of exercise, analysis variables, measurement instruments, effects on health outcomes, and risk of bias. In addition, knowing in depth the latest and updated research that is being done in the field of PA and PE and thus having a Latin American map of the programs developed in the last five years can serve as a basis for future guidelines, guides, recommendations or programs that wish to be guided by current evidence.

For this reason, the present systematic review aims to characterize the PE programs for OA in Latin America, focusing on the main characteristics of the interventions developed, participants, types of exercise, effects, variables and instruments used, risk of bias and level of compliance with the Consensus on Exercise Reporting Template (CERT) of the articles included. This will allow to start the discussion on the current state of research on PE for OA in the different Latin American countries.

2. Materials and Methods

The systematic review was carried out in accordance with the standards established by the PRISMA statement [36]. The PRISMA checklist can be found in the supplementary article files (Table S1). A systematic review protocol had previously been registered in the PROSPERO repository with the code: CRD42020208833.

2.1. Search Strategy for the Identification of Studies

The following databases were reviewed: MEDLINE by PubMed, SCOPUS by ELSEVIER and SciELO. The objective was to identify studies that developed PA and PE interventions for OAs in Latin America. The search covered the period between 2015 and 2020. For the development of the search, the MeSH terms used were: "Exercise", "Exercise Therapy" and "Aged", present in the MeSH Database. The search strategy followed the Peer Review of Electronic Search Strategies (PRESS) guidelines [37].

The general search syntax was: ("Exercise" OR "Exercise Therapy") AND ("Aged") and it was adapted to each database applying the following filters:

(a) PubMed: Type of article: randomized controlled trial, Date of publication: 5 years, Language: English, Spanish and Portuguese, Age: aged (65+ years) and 80 and over (80+ years).
(b) Scopus: Exclusion: Medline, Year of publication: 2015 to 2020, Status of publication: final, Type of document: article, Country: Latin American countries, Language: English, Spanish and Portuguese, Keyword: words that are related to the subject under study.
(c) SciELO: Country: Brazil, Colombia and Chile, Year of publication: 2015 to 2020, Type of literature: article.

Search strings for all databases are presented in the Supplementary Material (Table S2).

2.2. Selection of Studies and Inclusion Criteria

All those studies that met the search phrase were considered, and only those that met the following inclusion criteria were selected: (a) Country: interventions developed in countries belonging to Latin America; (b) Sample: people over 60 years of age; (c) Language: English, Spanish and Portuguese; (d) Methodological Design: Randomized controlled clinical trial. No reviews, editorial documents, protocols, or thesis were included. The articles selected by title and abstract had to meet the conditions indicated in Table 1.

Table 1. Inclusion criteria of the studies.

Criterion	Description
- Type of intervention - Single intervention - Duration	- Resistance, strength, multicomponent, concurrent, multidomain, HIIT or neuromotor, or other related to physical activity or exercise. - Only intervention based on physical activity or exercise (no other interventions). - Duration of at least four weeks.
- Age range	- Seniors, 60 years or older.
- Physical health - Mental health - Cognitive skills	- Physical fitness variables: balance, muscular strength, cardiorespiratory fitness, flexibility, proprioception, agility, other. - Psychological variables: depression, happiness, well-being, quality of life, anxiety, other. - Cognitive variables: memory, perception, language, attention, concentration, other.
- Article type	- Original article, with experimental design and random assignment.
- Country of origin of the population	- Latin American countries only.

2.3. Data Extraction

Duplicate articles were removed from the databases using Mendeley. Articles that met the inclusion criteria were selected, and when decisions could not be made considering only the title and abstract of the article, the full text was retrieved (Figure 1). A standardized questionnaire was used and applied by the authors to extract the data from the included articles, to synthesize the evidence. The information extracted included: (a) general characteristics of the studies and of the participants (author, year, initial and final sample, adherence, reasons for withdrawal, age range, sex, health condition, recruitment and place of intervention, (b) main characteristics of the interventions based on physical activity and exercise (duration of the intervention, number of sessions per week, time of the session, responsible professional, type of intervention and components of physical fitness addressed and the time allocated to each one of them); (c) main variables evaluated (physical health, mental health and cognitive abilities); (d) main assessment instruments used (physical health, mental health and cognitive abilities).

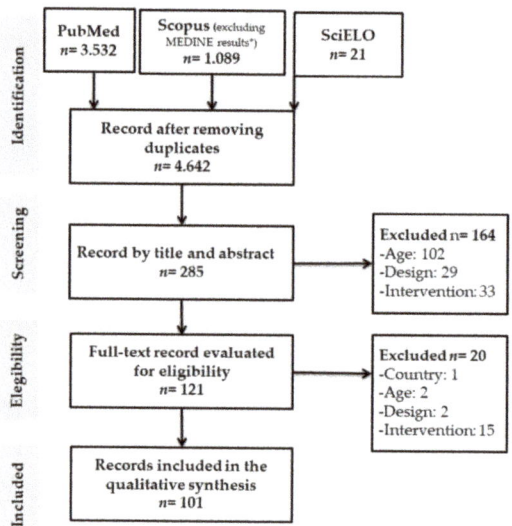

Figure 1. Literature search Flow chart. * Whole search strings for all databases are presented in the supplementary material (Table S2).

2.4. Risk of Bias Assessment Tool and Consensus on Exercise Reporting Template (CERT) Assessment Form

The Cochrane "Cochrane Manual of Systematic Reviews of Interventions" tool [38] was used to assess the methodological validity of the studies included in this review, evaluating the risk of bias in each of the items proposed by this manual, detailed as follows: (a) Selection bias, (b) Performance bias, (c) Detection bias, (d) Attrition bias and (e) Reporting bias. Only the item: "Other biases" was not considered. The results of this analysis are presented in Figure 2. In addition, the Consensus on Exercise Reporting Template (CERT) assessment form was added to know the proportion of articles that met the CERT items [39] (Table S3).

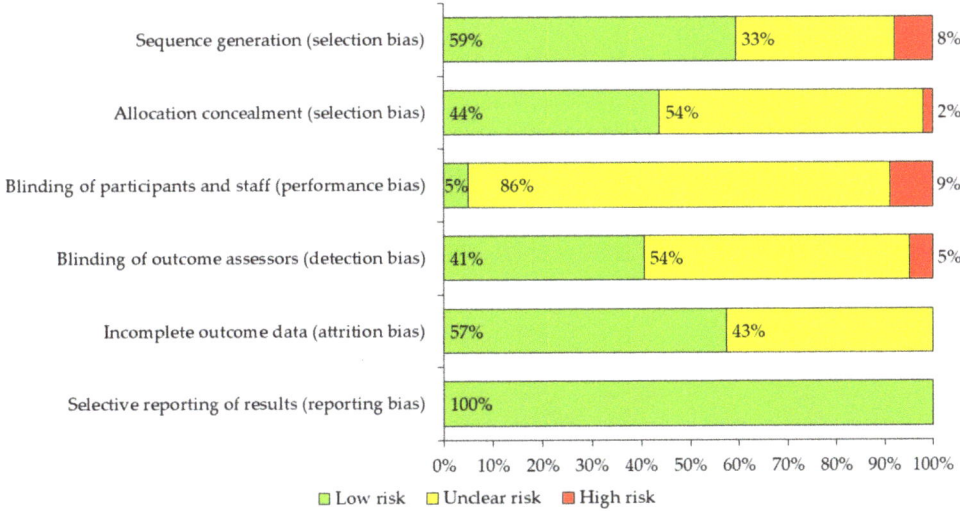

Figure 2. Evaluation of the methodological quality of the reviewed studies.

2.5. Strategy for Data Synthesis

A synthesis of the main findings of the included studies is provided, related to the interventions developed based on PE for OAs in Latin America. The main information is presented in summary tables. In addition, in the discussion, the most relevant methodological and applicability aspects are analyzed and some suggestions are given for future research, in order to standardize the application of this methodology.

3. Results

3.1. Literature Search

Figure 1 shows the flow chart of systematic reviews proposed by the PRISMA statement. 4.642 potential studies on PA and exercise in OAs in Latin America were identified. After the exclusion of the duplicates in the databases, the screening and eligibility criteria were applied. Finally, for data synthesis, 101 articles were included [40–140] (Figure 1).

3.2. General Characteristics of the Studies

A total of 101 articles were included, of these, 91 were from Brazil, five from Chile, two Colombia, two Mexico and one from Ecuador. The number of participants at the beginning of the studies was 5013 and 4334 at the end (79% women and 21% men), presenting a compliance with the interventions of 86%. Only 35% of the studies had 100% adherence. Three quarters of the studies suffered losses in their sample, the main reasons for withdrawal being categorized as follows: attendance, does not meet the criteria of the study and personal reasons, the latter being the one that was repeated the most (78%). Furthermore, in 15% of the cases the reason for withdrawal was not specified. Regarding the age range, 97% of the studies included participants between 60 and 70 years, 83% between 71 and 80 years, and only 16% included participants older than 80 years. The health condition with the highest prevalence was cardiometabolic diseases. Just over half (58%) of the OAs resided in the community and 44% of the studies detailed information regarding the place of intervention; of these studies, 61% of the interventions occurred at university facilities (Table 2).

Table 2. Characteristics of the articles.

Ref.	Authors (Year) Country	Initial/Final Sample	Percentage that Ended the Study (%)	Withdrawal Reason				Age Range (Years)				Sex		Health Condition				Recruitment				Place of Intervention		
				AT	PR	NMC	NS	60–70	71–80	80+	♀(%)	♂(%)	CD	NDD	CMD	CA	COM	HC	INST	HC	SC	UC
[ ]	Queiroz J. (2016) Brazil	62/62	100	1				1			0	100				-	1					
[ ]	Antunes A. (2015) Brazil	45/45	100					1			0	100				-	1					1
[ ]	Santos S. (2017) Brazil	40/26	65		1			1			31	69		1		-						1
[ ]	de Oliveira R. (2017) Brazil	24/23	96					1			56	44		1		-	1					
[ ]	Campos L. (2016) Brazil	32/32	100					1			100	0				-	1				1	
[ ]	Mazinmilho M. (2017) Brazil	79/79	100					1			100	0				-	1			1		
[ ]	Teodoro J. (2019) Brazil	36/36	100					1				100				-	1			1		
[ ]	Santos G. (2019) Brazil	34/18	53	1				1			100	0				-	1					
[ ]	Dueñas E. (2019) Colombia	125/105	84	1	1			1			84	16	1			-	1					
[ ]	Torres A. (2019) Brazil	64/56	88		1			1			91	9				-	1					
[ ]	Arantes P. (2015) Brazil	30/28	93					1			100	0				-	1					
[ ]	Lima L. (2015) Brazil	44/44	100					1			84	16				-	1			1		
[ ]	de Oliveira D. (2019) Brazil	24/19	79		1	1		1			100	0		1		-	1					
[ ]	da Silveira Ch. (2019) Brazil	60/52	87					1			77	23				-	1					
[ ]	do Nascimento M. (2019) Brazil	62/45	72		1	1		1			100	0				-	1					
[ ]	Oliveira F. (2016) Brazil	25/25	100					1			100	0		1		-	1					
[ ]	Galvão M. (2019) Brazil	30/24	80		1			1			100	0				-	1					
[ ]	Carvalo R. (2018) Brazil	22/21	95					1			75	25				-	1					
[ ]	Tiggemann C. (2016) Brazil	30/25	83					1			100	0				-	1					
[ ]	da Silva R. (2017) Brazil	30/30	100					1			100	0				-	1					
[ ]	Taglietti M. (2018) Brazil	60/49	81		1			1			68	32	1			-	1					
[ ]	Franco M. (2016) Brazil	82/71	87			1		1			93	7				-	1					
[ ]	Batisti C. (2018) Brazil	45/37	82					1			NS	NS				-	1					
[ ]	Lopez N. (2015) Chile	80/60	75				1	1			68	32		1		-	1					
[ ]	Shigoemitsu F. (2018) Brazil	37/31	84					1			60	40				-	1					
[ ]	Ortiz-Ortiz M. (2019) Mexico	50/50	100					1			100	0	1			-	1			1		
[ ]	Mansur J. (2016) Brazil	35/35	100					1			66	34				-	1					
[ ]	Clemente A. (2018) Brazil	41/35	86		1			1			100	0				-	1					
[ ]	Rodrigues-Krause J. (2018) Brazil	30/27	87		1	1		1			100	0				-	1					
[ ]	Ferrari R. (2016) Brazil	24/23	96					1								-						
[ ]	Ramírez-Campillo R. (2016) Chile	24/24	100					1			100	0				-	1					
[ ]	de Resende A. (2018) Brazil	32/32	100					1			100	0				-	1					
[ ]	Cavalcante E. (2018) Brazil	63/57	91					1			100	0				-		1				
[ ]	Pieta C. (2015) Brazil	26/19	73		1			1			55	45				-	1					
[ ]	Henrique P. (2019) Brazil	31/31	100	1				1			100	0	1			-	1					
[ ]	Ramirez-Villada J. (2019) Colombia	60/47	79					1			100	0				-	1					
[ ]	Gomes A. (2019) Brazil	47/47	100					1			100	0				-		1				
[ ]	Feitosa N. (2016) Brazil	30/23	77	1	1			1			100	0				-		1				
[ ]	Ribeiro J. (2018) Brazil	50/46	92					1			74	26				-	1					
[ ]	dos Santos L. (2018) Brazil	39/39	100					1			100	0				-	1					
[ ]	Gomenluka N. (2015) Brazil	33/26	79			1		1			73	27				-	1					
[ ]	Campos L. (2015) Brazil	32/32	100					1			NS	NS				-	1					
[ ]	de Souza R. (2018) Brazil	42/27	64		1			1			100	0				-		1				
[ ]	Macedo L. (2018) Brazil	23/19	83					1			100	0				-		1				
[ ]	Botton C. (2018) Brazil	44/26	59					1			41	59				-	1					
[ ]	Bonadias A. (2016) Brazil	133/133	100					1			100	0		1		-		1				
[ ]	Barbosa A. (2015) Brazil	30/30	100					1			100	0				-	1					
[ ]	Rodrigues W. (2015) Brazil	47/40	85					1			70	30		1		-	1					
[ ]	Gallo L. (2015) Brazil	31/26	84					1			100	0				-	1					
[ ]	Ruaro M. (2019) Brazil	40/33	83					1			100	0				-	1					
[ ]	Da silva C. (2018) Brazil	58/51	88					1			59	41				-		1				
[ ]	Mirando A. (2020) Chile	21/12	57				1	1			86	14				-	1					
[ ]	Cadore E. (2018) Brazil	65/52	80					1				100				-	1					
[ ]	de Resende A. (2018) Brazil	55/44	80					1			100	0				-	1					
[ ]	Silva I. (2018) Brazil	48/43	90					1			39	61		1		-			1			
[ ]	Rabelo M. (2019) Brazil	39/39	100					1			74	26				-	1					
[ ]	Ramirez-Campillo R. (2018) Chile	74/52	70					1			100	0				-	1					
[ ]	Brandão G. (2018) Brazil	131/125	95					1			88	12				-	1					
[ ]	Lopez J. (2017) Mexico	31/26	84					1								-					1	
[ ]	Medeiros L. (2018) Brazil	78/71	91	1				1			77	23				-	1					
[ ]	Vargas M. (2019) Ecuador	50/50	100					1			30	70				-	1					

Table 2. Cont.

Ref.	Authors (Year) Country	Initial/Final Sample	Percentage that Ended the Study (%)	Withdrawal Reason				Age Range (Years)				Sex		Health Condition					Recruitment				Place of Intervention	
				AT	PR	NMC	NS	60–70	71–80	80+		♀ (%)	♂ (%)	CD	NDD	CMD	CA	COM	HC	INST	HC	SC	UC
[ ]	Covolo-Scarabottolo C. (2017) Brazil	35/30	86	1								53	47										
[ ]	Damorim I. (2017) Brazil	64/55	86									71	29						1				
[ ]	Leal L. (2019) Brazil	54/54	100									50	50							1			
[ ]	Souza D. (2019) Brazil	25/21	84					1				100						1					1
[ ]	Santos G. (2015) Brazil	70/62	86					1				60	40										
[ ]	Moreira N. (2018) Brazil	46/45	98					1				100							1				
[ ]	Martínez A. (2018) Chile	33/33	100					1	1	1		39	61		–					1	1		1
[ ]	Santana M. (2016) Brazil	23/16	70	1					1			87	13		–					1	1		1
[ ]	Gomes/luka N. (2020) Brazil	33/26	79					1				72	28		–								
[ ]	Coelho-Junior H. (2019) Brazil	45/36	80					1	1			100						1					
[ ]	Silva M. (2016) Brazil	78/45	58		1			1	1			82	18		–			1					
[ ]	Gambassi B. (2015) Brazil	17/16	94	1								100			–			1					
[ ]	Tomeleri C. (2016) Brazil	38/35	92	1				1				100						1					
[ ]	Alex S. (2015) Brazil	30/30	100									100						1					1
[ ]	Cunha P. (2019) Brazil	48/48	100									100						1					1
[ ]	Ribeiro. S. (2017) Brazil	76/68	89						1			100			1			1					
[ ]	Alcantar T. (2019) Brazil	33/33	100		1				1			NS	NS		1			1					
[ ]	Tomeleri M. (2018) Brazil	53/45	85									100			–			1					
[ ]	Oliveira-Dantas F. (2020) Brazil	25/25	100									100			–			1					
[ ]	Lopez P. (2016) Brazil	55/37	67				1					100			–			1					
[ ]	da Silva P. (2015) Brazil	20/20	100									65	35					1					
[ ]	Alves W. (2019) Brazil	32/28	88		1							50	50			–			1				1
[ ]	Morales F. (2018) Brazil	35/35	100				1					NS	NS		–			1					
[ ]	Rosa C. (2017) Brazil	92/55	60				1					100						1					
[ ]	Rodacki A. (2017) Brazil	38/30	79	1								100						1					
[ ]	Aragao-Santos J. (2019) Brazil	44/44	100									40	60					1					
[ ]	Domínguez D. (2018) Brazil	72/62	86	1								100						1					
[ ]	Sbardelotto M. (2017) Brazil	55/55	100									100						1			1		
[ ]	Moreira H. (2015) Brazil	51/51	100									100				–							
[ ]	De Carvalho I. (2018) Brazil	20/20	100									100						1					
[ ]	Mendes M. (2017) Brazil	420/376	90	1								59	41					1					
[ ]	de Oliveira F. (2019) Brazil	56/46	82									43	57		–			1					
[ ]	Lixandrao M. (2016) Brazil	14/14	100		1						1	100						1					
[ ]	Ribeiro A. (2016) Brazil	29/25	86									100						1					
[ ]	Silveira Y. (2019) Brazil	83/40	48	1				1				33	67					1					
[ ]	Monteiro-junior R. (2017) Brazil	29/11	38									100							1				
[ ]	Chaves M. (2017) Brazil	36/36	100		1			1				100						1					
[ ]	Ribeiro S. (2018) Brazil	48/33	69		1							NS	NS					1					
[ ]	de Oliveira V. (2019) Brazil	52/43	83									100						1					
[ ]	Simao A. (2019) Brazil	15/15	100						1			100		1									

1: registered data, Withdrawal reasons: AT, Attendance; PR, Personal reasons; NMC, does not meet criteria; NS, Not specified, Blank space, Does not meet criterion. Age range: Blank space, does not meet criterion. Sex: NS, Not specified. Health condition: CD, Chronic disease; NDD, Neurodegenerative disease; CMD, cardio metabolic disease; CA, Cancer; -, Exclusion criterion of the study. Recruitment: COM, Community; HC, Health center; INST, Institutionalized. Place of intervention: HC, Health center; SC, Sports center; UC, University center.

3.3. Assessment of Risk of Bias and CERT Compliance Level

The risk of bias of the studies was assessed using the Cochrane 'Cochrane Handbook for Systematic Reviews of experimental study interventions' tool. The risk of bias was included for each of the items proposed by the manual, excluding the item "other biases". It was observed that the distribution of biases classified as unclear risk or high risk was similar between the items selection bias, detection bias and attrition bias (40–60% of the studies). However, it was observed that 95% of the studies had unclear risk and high risk of performance bias, and 100% of the studies had low risk of reporting bias (Figure 2).

Nine out of nineteen items compliant (rated "yes" on the CERT items) in at least 75% of the articles (C1 = 90%, C3 = 100%, C4 = 100%, C5 = 93%, C7b = 100%, C10 = 100%, C13 = 100%, C14a = 100%, C16a = 93%). The items categories with the highest level of compliance were those included in the materials (one item, C1 = 90%) and dosage (one item, C13 = 90%) categories. In contrast, the items categories with the lowest level of compliance were those related to the delivery (ten items, C6 = 5%, C7a = 50%, C8 = 21%, C9 = 0% and C11 = 41%) and location (one item, C12 = 40%) categories (Table S3).

3.4. Main Characteristics of the Interventions

95% of the articles had interventions with a duration of 2 to 6 months, 2% less than 2 months and 3% more than 9 months. 95% had a session frequency of 2 or 3 times a week. The sessions had a duration that varied between 30 and 60 min in 93.8% of the articles, taking into account that 20.8% of the studies did not specify this information. In 51% of the studies the sessions were led by physical activity qualified professionals, such as physical education teachers or personal trainers, while 14% of the studies presented interventions led by a health professional, most of whom were a physiotherapist. 35% of the studies did not specify this information. Regarding the training modality, 89% of the studies included interventions based on therapeutic PE, 11% of the studies included interventions based on non-traditional physical disciplines such as Tai Chi, Pilates and dance, 7% included interventions based in exercise with digital support, known as Exergames, 5% included interventions based on exercise complemented with other interventions such as vibration and auriculotherapy and 2% included interventions based on water training, known as hydrogymnastics. Regarding the components of physical fitness addressed during the interventions, 77% of the studies included muscular strength, 47% cardiorespiratory fitness, 27% balance, 14% coordination, 12% flexibility, 7% gait and 5% proprioception. Furthermore, 48% of the studies included a warm-up stage and 34% of the studies included a cool-down stage (Table 3).

Additionally, the characteristics of multicomponent exercise were analyzed according to the components of physical fitness. Muscle strength was commonly exercised with 1 to 3 sets (61%), 8–15 repetitions (71%), and one-minute rest (18%). The intensity of the exercise was controlled with scales of perception of effort (30%) and multifunctional machines were used to train (65%). In relation to cardiorespiratory fitness, this was developed mainly on a treadmill (39%), for 20 min or more (61%). The intensity of the exercise was controlled through the heart rate (52%). With regard to flexibility, this was exercised through static stretching (25%) and was controlled through the time performed (42%), With regard to gait, coordination, and proprioception, these components of fitness were trained primarily through circuits (56%, 50% and 40, respectively).

3.5. Outcome Variables Analyzed

Outcome variables were grouped and described in three broad categories: (a) physical health, (b) mental health and quality of life and (c) cognitive skills.

(a) Physical health: This category was considered in 100% of the studies and was divided into 10 outcome variables. Of these, the most evaluated was muscle strength (74 of the studies). The following most frequent were: nutritional status and diet, functionality, balance, gait and vital signs, blood tests and others (blood pressure, pain, dyspnea, heart rate variability and blood tests). The least evaluated was coordination (7 studies) (Figure 3a).

(b) Mental health and quality of life: The mental health and quality of life categories were considered only in 28% of the studies, and was grouped into nine outcome variables related to emotional, psychological and social well-being. The most evaluated was quality of life, included in 17 studies, followed by depression and fear of falling, evaluated in eight and six studies, respectively (Figure 3b).

(c) Cognitive Skills: the category of cognitive skills was considered only in 11% of the studies and 12 outcome variables were grouped. The most evaluated was language, included in six of the studies, followed by memory, attention and executive function, evaluated in five studies (Figure 3c).

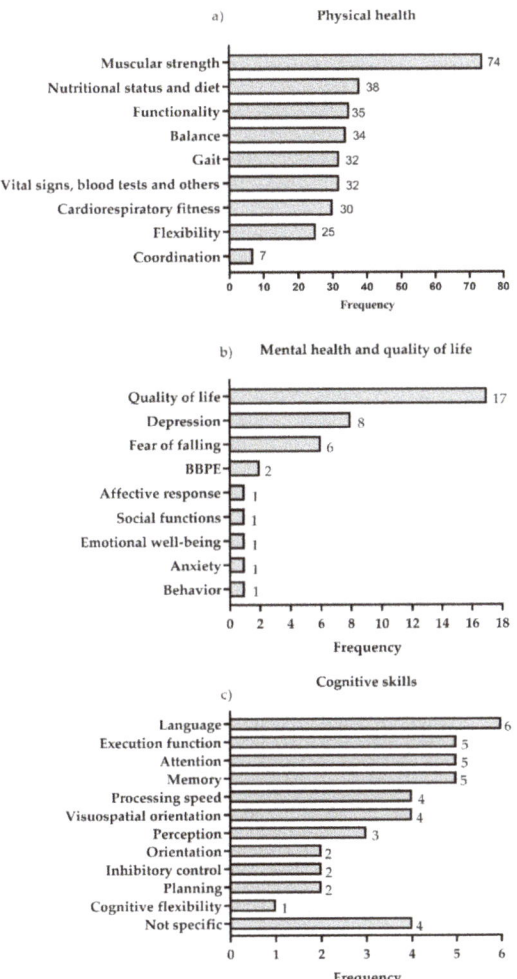

Figure 3. Variables of (**a**) physical health, (**b**) mental health and quality of life and (**c**) cognitive skills. The data are presented in absolute frequency. BBPE: Barriers and Benefits Perceived for the Execution of the Exercise.

Table 3. Characteristics of the interventions.

Ref.	Authors	Intervention Duration (Month)	Intervention Frequency (Sessions/Week)	Session Duration (min)	Professional in Charge				Type of Intervention (Experimental Group)								Components and Time of Each Intervention						
					HP	QP	NS	PEI	HI	NTI	DSI	IC	WS	CS	AER (min)	STR (min)	FLE (min)	GAI (min)	COO (min)	BAL (min)	PRO (min)
[40]	Queiroz J.	3	2	90			1						1	1	20–60						
[41]	Antunes A.	6	3	20–60			1	EG							60	NS					
[43]	Santos S.	2	2	60				EG1								NS		NS	NS	NS
								EG2								NS					
[43]	de Oliveira R.	6	2	60			1	EG1					1	1		NS	NS	NS	NS	NS	NS
								EG2					1	1	50						
[44]	Campos L.	3	2	60	1			EG2	EG1						15	15	60				
[45]	Mazirfilho M.	3	3	50/50		1		EG1					1	1	20	20					
								EG2					1	1	20–35	40					
[46]	Teodoro J.	5	2	65–85		1		EG1					1	1	20–35	40					
								EG2							20–35	40					
								EG3													
[47]	Santos G.	3	3	40		1		EG1					1	1	NS	20			NS	NS	
								EG2					1	1	10*	20				10*	
								EG3					1	1	10*	20				10*	
[48]	Dueñas E.	2	1	60		1		EG1					1	1	10*	NS			NS	NS	
[49]	Torres A.	6	3				1	EG1		EG2			1	1		NS					
								EG2					1	1		NS					
[50]	Arantes P.	3	2	60	1			EG					1	1	30	NS				60	
[51]	Lima L.	2.5	3	NS			1	EG1					1	1	30	NS					
[52]	de Oliveira D.	3.5	2	40	1			EG2					1	1	20–30	NS				NS	
[53]	da Silveira Ch.	6	2/3	60				EG							30	NS					
[54]	do Nascimento M.	3	2–3				1	EG1							30	NS					
[55]	Oliveira F.	2.5	2–3	60				EG							30	NS					
[56]	Galvao M.	2	3					EG1							30	NS					
								EG2							30	NS					
								EG3							NS	NS					
[57]	Carvalo R.	2	2	100		1		EG1			EG				30	NS				NS	
[58]	Tiggemann C.	3	2			1		EG1							30	NS					
[59]	da Silva R.	6	2/3			1		EG2								NS					
								EG1								NS					
[60]	Taglietti M.	2	2	60		1		EG		EG			1		20	15					
[61]	Franco M.	3	2	60		1		EG													
[62]	Batisti C.	3	3	40	1			EG							10,–20	15–30	10		10	10	10
[63]	Lopez N.	6	5	60				EG					1		40	NS				10	
[64]	Shiguemitsu F.	14	2	75			1	EG					1		NS	NS	NS			NS	
[65]	Ortiz-Ortiz M.	3	5	40–50		1		EG					1		NS	NS	NS		NS	NS	
[66]	Mansur J.	2	2	30			1	EG1					1		15–30	30					
								EG2													
								EG3													
[67]	Clemente A.	6	2	90		1		EG	EG1				1		45	30					
[68]	Rodrigues-Krause J.	2	3	60		1		EG					1		35	45					
[69]	Ferrari R.	2.5	2/3			1		EG1					1		50	50					
[70]	Ramirez-Campillo R.	3	2/3	60		1		EG1					1		40	NS				NS	NS
								EG2					1		30	NS					10
[71]	de Resende A.	2	3	60		1		EG2					1		30	NS					
[72]	Cavalcante E.	3	2/3	30		1		EG1					1	1	15	30	NS		NS	NS	
								EG2						1		NS	NS		15		
[73]	Pietta C.	3	2			1		EG1						1		NS					
[74]	Henrique P.	3	2	30		1		EG1			EG					NS					NS
[75]	Ramírez-Villada J.	8	3	60	1			EG					1		15	20			NE	NE	
[76]	Gomes A.	2–3	3	45				EG1					1		15	20			15	15	
								EG2													

112

Table 3. Cont.

Ref.	Authors	Intervention Duration (Month)	Intervention Frequency (Sessions/Week)	Session Duration (min)	Professional in Charge HP	QP	NS	Type of Intervention (Experimental Group) PEI	HI	NTI	DSI	IC	WS	CS	AER min	STR min	FLE min	GAI min	COO min	BAL min	PRO min
[ ]	Feitosa N. Ribeiro J.	3 1.75	3 2	50 60		1		EG EG2			EG1		1	1	NS 10	25 10	10		NS 10	NS 10	
[ ]	dos Santos L.	2	3	NS		1		EG1 EG2						1		NS NS					
[ ]	Gornefuka N.	3	3	30–60				EG2		EG1			1	1				30–50			
[ ]	Campos L.	3	2	60		1		EG		EG			1			40					
[ ]	de Souza R.	4	3	60		1		EG					1			NS					
[ ]	Macedo L.	3	3	50			1	EG					1			NS					
[ ]	Bottorn C.	3	3	NS				EG					1			NS					
[ ]	Bonadias A.	6	3	30				EG					1								
[ ]	Barbosa A.	2	3	NS		1		EG								NS					
[ ]	Rodrigues W.	2	2	40		1		EG								NS	40					
[ ]	Gallo L.	3	3	NS			1	EG					1			NS					
[ ]	Ruan M. F.	3.5	2	30–60				EG					1	1	25	5–15		30		NS	
[ ]	Da silva C. M.	2	3	60				EG					1	1	NS	NS					
[ ]	Mirando A. D.	1.5	2	NS				EG1 EG2							NS	NS					
[ ]	Cadore E.	3	2					EG3							NS	NS					
[ ]	de resende A.	3	3	60		1		EG1 EG2							25	25			15		
[ ]	Silva I.	3	3	60			1	EG1							15	25					
								EG2							NS	NS					
								EG3							NS	NS					
[ ]	Rabelo M.	3	3	50		1		EG1 EG2							25	20					
[ ]	Ramirez-Campillo R.	3	3	60				EG					1	1	NS	50	NS	NS	NS	NS	
[ ]	Brandao G.	3	3	40			1	EG					1	1	30	50					
[ ]	Lopez J.	3	5	50			1	EG					1	1	10	NS	10				
[ ]	Medeires L.	3	3	50				EG					1	1	15–						
[ ]	Vargas M.	6	2	30–60		1		EG							40						
[ ]	Covolo-Scarabottolo C.	3	2	40–50		1		EG						1	NS	NS		NS		NS	
[ ]	Damorim I.	4	3	30			1	EG2							30						
[ ]	Leal L.	6	2	30–40		1		EG								30–40					
[ ]	Souza D.	3.5	2	NS		1		EG1 EG2								NS NS					
[ ]	Santos G. D.	3	2	60			1	EG					1	1		50					
[ ]	Moreira N.	4	3	50			1	EG		EG			1	1		50	NS		NS	NS	
[ ]	Martinez A.	3	3	63				EG					1	1		NS					
[ ]	Santana M.	2	3	30				EG					1	1		NS					
[ ]	Gornefuka N.	2	3	NS		1		EG2		EG1				1	30	NS	NS	NS	NS	NS	
[ ]	Coelho-Junior H.	4.5	2	40				EG1 EG2					1		NS	NS					
[ ]	Silva M.	5	2	60			1	EG					1	1		NS					
[ ]	Gambassi B.	3	2	NS			1	EG					1	1		NS					
[ ]	Tomeleri C.	2	3	45				EG					1	1		45					
[ ]	Alex S.	4.2	6	45				EG1					1	1		NS	NS		NS		
[ ]	Cunha P.	3	3	20				EG2					1	1		NS					
[ ]	Ribeiro S.	2	3	60				EG					1	1		NS					
[ ]	Alcantar T.	5	2	40			1	EG					1	1		NS					
[ ]	Tomeleri M.	3	3	NS			1	EG1					1	1		NS					
[ ]	Oliveira-Dantas F.	2.5	2/3	60			1	EG2					1	1		NS					
[ ]	Lopez P.	3	3	60				G2					1	1		NS					
[ ]	da Silva P.	1.5	2	30		1								1		NS					

Table 3. Cont.

Ref.	Authors	Intervention Duration (Month)	Intervention Frequency (Sessions/Week)	Session Duration (min)	Professional in Charge HP	QP	NS	Type of Intervention (Experimental Group) PEI	HI	NTI	DSI	IC	WS	CS	Components and Time of Each Intervention AER (min)	STR (min)	FLE (min)	GAI (min)	COO (min)	BAL (min)	PRO (min)
[22]	Alves W.	4	2	30–40				EG					1			30– 35					
[23]	Morales F.	6	2	30–40			1	EG							40– 45	NS					
[24]	Rosa C.	6	2	60			1	G1 EG2					1	1	40– 45 40– 45	40– 45 45					
[25]	Rodacki A.	2	3	60				EG1	EG				1	1	NS	NS					
[26]	Aragao-Santos J.	3	3	50		1		EG2					1	1	15 15	25 25		15	15	NS 15	
[27]	Dominguez D.	2	3	50		1		EG1 EG2			EG1		1	1							
[28]	Sbardelotto M.	2	3	60			1	EG2 EG3					1	1	NS						
[29]	Moreira H.	6	3	60			1	EG2		EG1			1	1	30 15 35	30 30		NS	NS	NS	NS
[30]	De Carvalho I.	3	2	30			1	EG1			EG1 EG2		1		60					30 30	
[31]	Mendes M.	3	2	NE			1	EG1 EG2					1			NS NS					
[32]	de Oliveira F.	3	2	60		1		EG					1	1	20	20 NS					
[33]	Lixandrao M.	2.5	2	NS		1		G G1					1			NS NS					
[34]	Ribeiro A.	9	3	NS				G2					1			NS					
[35]	Silveira Y.	4	3	50					EG		EG		1	1	15	25					
[36]	Monteiro-junior R.	2	2	30–45		1			EG1				1		NS	NS					
[37]	Chaves M.	3	2	45			1	EG2 EG1													
[38]	Ribeiro S.	3	2	NS			1	EG2 EG1							NS NS	NS				NS NS	
[39]	de Oliveira V.	4	2	NS			1	EG2													
[40]	Simão A.	3	3	NS	1							EG1 EG2	1 1		NS NS	NS NS					

1: registered data, Professional in charge: HP, Health professional; QP, Physical activity qualified professional. Type of intervention: PEI, Therapeutic physical exercise-based intervention; HI, Hydrogymnastics-based intervention; NTI, Non-traditional physical disciplines-based intervention; DSI, Digitally supported exercise-based intervention; ICI, Exercise-based interventions complemented with other interventions. Components and time of each intervention: WS: warm-up stage; CS: cool down stage; AER, Aerobic; STR, Strength; FL, Flexibility; GAI: Gait; COO, Coordination; BAL, Balance; PRO, Proprioception.

3.6. Assessment Instruments Used

The evaluations were grouped and described in three broad categories: (a) physical health, (b) mental health and quality of life, and (c) cognitive skills.

(a) Physical health instruments: 63 instruments were used, which were grouped into ten categories (strength, flexibility, cardiorespiratory fitness, walk test, balance, chair test, step test, risk of falls, functionality and body composition), being the most used instruments the maximum repetition to measure muscle strength (33 studies), the sit-to-stand test in tests that use a chair (24 studies), the timed up and go in tests of risk of falling (20 studies) and the test of 6-min walk in walking tests (17 studies) (Figure 4a).

(b) Mental health and quality of life instruments: 18 instruments were used, which were grouped into four categories (quality of sleep, suspected depression, quality of life and others, which included instruments that evaluated affectivity, efficacy, mood, feelings, entertainment and perception barriers). The most widely used instruments were the Falls Efficacy Scale International (FES-I), the World Health Organization Quality of Life (WHOQoL), the Geriatric Depression Scale (GDS) and the Yesavage Geriatric Depression (YGDS) (Figure 4b).

(c) Cognitive skills instruments: 22 instruments were used that were grouped into two categories (cognitive skills and suspected dementia). Of all the instruments, the most used were the Mini Mental State Examination (MMSE) in five studies and the Montreal Cognitive Assessment (MoCA) (Figure 4c).

3.7. Effects by Sex and Type of Intervention

Regarding the effects of physical exercise interventions according to sex, in the physical health category, more than 50% of the articles with female-only samples presented significant effects in six of nine outcomes. More than 50% of the articles with male-only samples presented significant effects in four of seven outcomes, and more than 50% of the articles with mixed samples (both sexes) presented significant effects in three of nine outcome variables. In the mental health category, more than 50% of the articles with female-only samples presented significant effects in two of five outcomes. Articles with male-only samples did not include mental health outcome variables. More than 50% of the articles with mixed samples (both sexes) presented significant effects in four of six outcomes. Regarding the cognitive skills category, more than 50% of the articles with female-only samples presented significant effects in four of 10 outcomes. 100% of the articles with male-only samples presented significant effects in eight of eight outcome variables. More than 50% of the articles with mixed samples (both sexes) presented significant effects in five of 10 outcomes (Figure 5).

Regarding the effects according to the type of intervention, in the physical health category, more than 50% of the therapeutic physical exercise-based interventions presented significant effects in seven of nine outcomes. More than 50% of the hydrogymnastics-based interventions had significant effects in three of six outcomes. More than 50% of the non-traditional physical disciplines-based interventions had significant effects in two of nine outcomes. More than 50% of the digitally supported exercise-based interventions had significant effects in one of nine outcomes. More than 50% of the exercise-based interventions complemented with other interventions had significant effects in two of five outcomes. Regarding the mental health category, more than 50% of therapeutic physical exercise-based interventions presented significant effects in six of nine outcomes. There was no hydrogymnastics-based intervention that evaluated mental health outcomes. More than 50% of the non-traditional physical disciplines-based interventions had significant effects in one of three outcomes. More than 50% of the digitally supported exercise-based interventions had significant effects in one of three outcomes and 100% of the exercise-based interventions complemented with other interventions had significant effects on fear of falling. Regarding the category of cognitive skills, more than 50% of the therapeutic physical exercise-based interventions presented significant effects in 11 of 12 outcomes. There was no hydrogymnastics-based intervention that evaluated cognitive skills outcomes. More than 50% of the non-traditional physical disciplines-based interventions had significant effects in one of nine outcomes. 100% of the exercise-based interventions complemented with other interventions had significant effects in two of three outcomes (Figure 5).

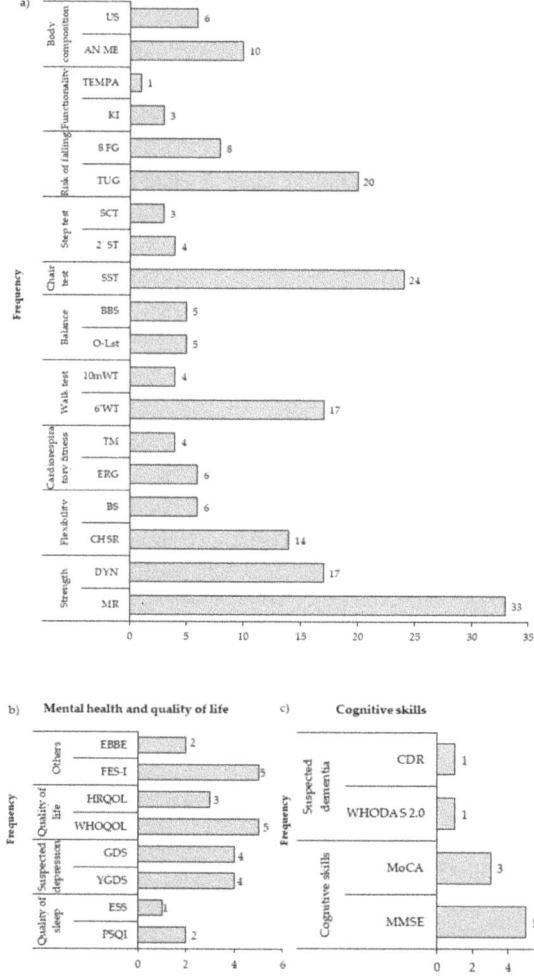

Figure 4. Instruments for measuring (**a**) Physical Health variables. Strength: MR, Maximum repetition; DYN, Dynamometer. Flexibility: CHSR, Chair sit and reach; BS, Back Scratch. cardiorespiratory fitness: ERG, Ergospirometry; TM, Treadmill. Walk test: 6'WT, 6-min walk test; 10 mWT, 10-m walk test. Balance: O-Lss, One-legged stand test; BBS, Berg Balance Scale. Chair test: SST, Sit to Stand Test. Step Test: 2'ST, 2 min Step Test, SCT, Stair Climb Test Risk of falling: TUG, Time up and go; 8FG, 8-fit and go. Functionality: KI, Katz index; TEMPA, Test d'Evaluation des Membres Supérieurs de Personnes Âgées. Body composition: ANT. ME., Anthropometric measures; US, Ultrasound. (**b**) Mental health and quality of life variables. Sleep quality: PSQI, Pittsburgh Sleep Quality Index; ESS, Epworth sleepiness scale. Suspected depression: YGDS, Yesavage Geriatric Depression Scale; GDS, Geriatric Depression Scale. Quality of life: WHOQOL, The World Health Organization Quality of Life; HRQOL, Health Related Quality of Life. Others: FES-I, Falls Efficacy Scale International; EBBE, Exercise Benefits Barriers Scale. (**c**) Cognitive skills variables. Cognitive skills: MMSE, Mini-Mental State Examination; MoCA, Montreal Cognitive Assessment. Suspected dementia: WHODAS 2.0, World Health Organization Disability Assessment Schedule; CDR, Clinical Dementia Rating. The data are presented in absolute frequency.

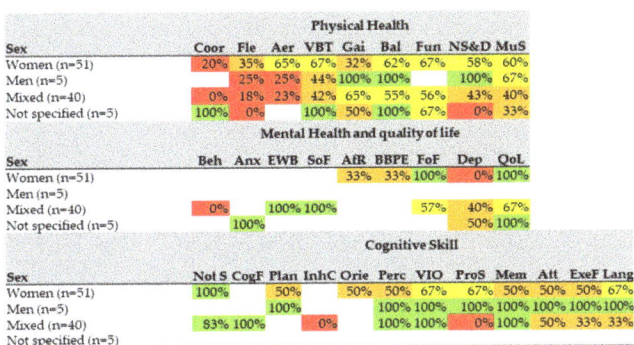

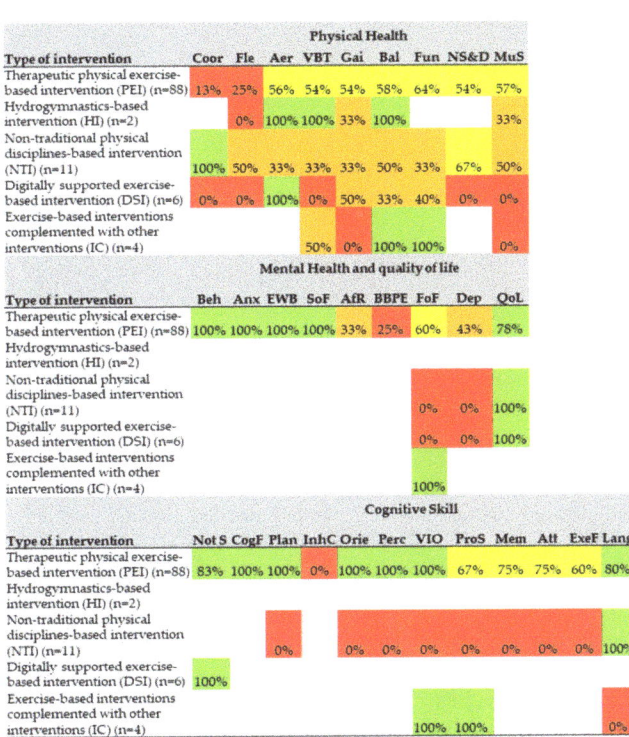

Figure 5. Effects by sex and by type of intervention on the outcomes of physical health and quality of life, mental health and cognitive skills. The percentage of articles that present significant effects on each health outcome measures is shown. 0–25% red, 26–50% orange, 51–75% yellow, 76–100% green and white: no studies. Physical health Coor: Coordination, Fle: Flexibility, Aer: cardiorespiratory fitness, VBT: Vital signs, blood tests and others, Gai: Gait; Bal: Balance, Fun: Functionality, NS&D: Nutritional status and diet, MuS: Muscular strength. Mental health and quality of life: Beh: Behavior, Anx: Anxiety, EWB: Emotional well-being, SoF: Social functions, AfR: Affective response, BBPE: Barriers and Benefits Perceived for the Execution of the Exercise, FoF: Fear of falling, Dep: Depression, QoL: Quality of life. Cognitive skills Not S: Not specific, CogF: Cognitive flexibility, Plan: Planning, InhC: Inhibitory control, Orie: Orientation, Perc: Perception, ViO: Visuospatial orientation, ProS: Processing speed, Mem: Memory, Att: Attention, ExeF: Execution Function, Lang: Language.

4. Discussion

The main results of this systematic review focused on five large areas: general characteristics, risk of bias and level of compliance with the CERT of the articles, characteristics of the interventions, outcome measures, and instruments used for their analysis. Its importance and possible implications are discussed below.

4.1. General Characteristics of the Articles Reviewed

Regarding the geographic location, the interventions occurred in only five Latin American countries, most of them in Brazil. This could be associated with the fact that Brazil is the country with the largest population in Latin America, and the sixth in the world [141], being also one of the Latin American countries that invests the most in developing and publishing research in the area of biological and medical sciences [142,143]. Regarding the characteristics of OA, female participants predominated (79%), which is striking considering that South American population surveys position women as more physically inactive than men [144]. Adherence was higher than 80% in 75% of the studies, which suggests a high degree of commitment to this type of intervention and contrasts with the evidence that indicates that the practice of AP decreases over the years [145]. In addition, OAs were mainly recruited from the community and most of the interventions were carried out in university facilities, suggesting that OA living in the community are willing to participate in PE-related activities. This could motivate researchers to develop interventions that include more OAs as study subjects in future research. Although the evidence is clear that the benefits of PA and PE are independent of age and health status [11], it is interesting that only 16% of the studies included people over 80 years of age, which could be associated with the higher prevalence of comorbidities at that age [146]. This would generate a higher risk of unwanted side effects related to exercise, although if the training program is prescribed properly, the risk of side effects should be like those that occur in OAs below 80 years [9,10]. Regarding the health condition of the OAs, the comorbidities with the highest prevalence were neurodegenerative and cardiometabolic diseases, which is related to the increase in NCDs worldwide [13].

4.2. Evaluation of the Methodological Quality of the Studies and CERT Compliance

From the results found, it stands out that 95% of the studies presented unclear risk and high risk in performance bias. This point is relevant as it is related to the blinding of the study participants and staff, and although the Cochrane manual states that simply blinding does not ensure successful blinding, it also states that the lack of blinding in this item could produce a bias by affecting the results of the participants [39]. In any case, the predominant classification in this item was unclear risk, which is associated with a lack of information on this bias by the authors, rather than a possible bias in the results. On the contrary, 100% of the studies presented a low-risk classification in the reporting bias item. This could be due to the fact that all the studies had an experimental and randomized methodological design (RCT), which corresponds to the best level of evidence in quantitative studies. Only nine out of nineteen items compliant in at least 75% of the RTC analyzed. Furthermore, the items categories with the highest level of compliance were those included in the materials and dosage categories. Conversely, the item categories with the lowest level of compliance were those related to the delivery and location categories. Similar results on the level of compliance had already been observed in another systematic review. This could be because the CERT was developed in 2016 with the goal of making exercise-based clinical trials transparent and replicable and have not yet been sufficiently assimilated by researchers [147].

4.3. Main Characteristics of the Interventions

Most of the interventions had a duration of 2 to 6 months, with a frequency of 2 to 3 times a week and a duration of 30 to 60 min per session, and were directed by qualified professionals, characteristics that are related to the WHO recommendations [19,20] and to the GPAR [21–35]. 89% of the interventions were based on traditional PE, while 11% of the studies included interventions based on non-traditional disciplines such as Tai Chi and Pilates, disciplines that in recent years have increased their adherence and level of evidence [44,81,111,125,148] being even included by some countries in their GPAR [21,27,29,32,33]. 7% of the studies included exercise-based interventions with digital support, known as Exergames [74,78,117,120,126] a modality not so well known today, which has been shown to be effective in improving balance and mobility function in OA [149,150]. On the other hand, some authors suggest that more research is lacking regarding this type of interventions and the effects they propose [151]. 2% of the studies included interventions based on hydro gymnastics [125,127], and although few studies have covered this type of exercise, it has shown positive effects on the physical functioning of OAs [152]. Finally, 5% included exercise interventions supplemented with other interventions such as vibration and auriculotherapy [48,57,82,140]. Regarding the vibration modality, benefits have been shown in physical performance [153] and in balance and gait of OAs [154], in addition to being an effective intervention to reduce the risk of falls [155]. However, some authors suggest that more evidence is needed to know which is the most effective vibration modality [156]. This indicates that although interventions based on traditional exercise predominate (mainly resistance training [157] and aerobic training [158]), whose effects have been widely supported, non-traditional interventions have been developed during the last decade that have shown to be as effective as traditional exercise interventions [48,57,82,140]. Regarding the components of the interventions, 77% considered the muscle strength component as the main training variable and 47% the aerobic exercise, the latter being the first recommendation by the WHO and the GPAR. This may be due to the fact that muscle strength training, associated with an improvement in muscle quality in OAs, is more closely related to improvements in functionality, decreased risk of falls, and health-related improvements in quality of life [159,160], variables in which aerobic training has a minor effect [160]. At the same time, the small number of studies that consider the training of balance, coordination and proprioception components within their interventions is striking, given that alteration of these components increases the risk of falls. This variable that is of great interest to OAs, because falls are associated with a decrease in functionality, a higher level of dependency and a higher risk of mortality [12–16]. Lastly, the flexibility component was considered only in 7% of the studies, a variable that is not specifically found within the WHO recommendations, and is only found in some of the GPAR. This contrasts with the fact that flexibility exercises have been shown to improve aspects of physical health and mental well-being in OAs [36,161].

A fifth of the studies included in this review developed combined PE interventions, modalities known as concurrent training and multicomponent training, which had positive effects on the variables studied. In particular, the multicomponent training modality, which has important scientific support in terms of its effectiveness [162,163], is being strongly recommended in the European continent for the development of PA in OA [164]. In addition, it could be that in the near future, the recommendations proposed by the WHO will undergo modifications, proposing multicomponent training as a more effective alternative than training each component of physical fitness in isolation in OA.

4.4. Outcome Variables Studied in the Articles and Instruments Used in Evaluations

The aging process is not only associated with deterioration in physical skills, but also with disorders of mental health and cognitive skills [165]. Along these lines, although the interventions were based on PE that considered physical health variables in 100% of the studies, 28% of the studies also considered the effects of these interventions on mental health variables and 11% on cognitive skills. Even though the percentage is low, this is related to understanding how exercise is a therapeutic agent with multiple benefits in the health of OA [17].

Sixty-three instruments were used to evaluate the physical health variables, 18 to evaluate the mental health variables, and 22 to evaluate the cognitive skills variables. This highlights the great diversity of instruments used to identify the effects of PE in OA, and although there are some instruments that are used more frequently, this highlights the lack of consensus that exists for the evaluation of the different variables.

4.5. Effects by Sex and by Type of Intervention

Regarding the effects of interventions by sex, positive effects were observed in a greater number of physical health outcome measures in male-only samples, in a greater number of mental health outcome measures in mixed samples, and in a greater number of cognitive function outcome measures in single samples of men. Older women are known to have lower levels of PA and fitness than older men [144]. Considering this baseline condition, a PE-based intervention could show greater benefits for women in the different physical health outcomes [166], Furthermore, it has been observed that mixed sample generates greater collaboration, motivation and challenge for OA of both genders [167].

In relation to the effects according to different types of exercise, positive effects were observed in a greater number of physical health, mental health and cognitive function outcome measures in therapeutic PE-based interventions. This could be related to the fact that this type of intervention is usually implemented as an intervention for OA with altered physical health status. In addition, this type of intervention is more structured, individualized and with specific objectives for each participant, allowing greater control of exercise dose such as intensity, frequency, length and training progression. Furthermore, therapeutic PE-based interventions commonly included in the same session a greater number of components of physical condition [45,100,103,131], than those interventions based on non-traditional disciplines. Hydro-gymnastics and with digital support, which although have shown positive effects in some interventions, some authors agree that evidence to support their effects is lacking [151,156]. In particular, therapeutic PE-based interventions seem to improve muscle strength in a greater number of RTC. This finding could be associated with the fact that other types of exercise such as hydro-gymnastics-based interventions and digitally supported exercise-based interventions consider very light workloads and are more focused on other fitness qualities, such as aerobic endurance, balance and coordination [151].

Additionally, the component of physical fitness with the most positive effects was balance, regardless of sex and type of intervention. The interventions were mainly with a duration of 3 months, a frequency of 3 times a week, with 30–60 min sessions. OAs often have problems with balance [168]. Thus, PE-based interventions could promote improvements in these components of physical fitness [169,170].

Particularly, quality of life improved regardless of the type of exercise trained, which reinforces the positive effect of PE on health-related quality of life of the elderly [171,172]. In cognitive skills, therapeutic PE-based interventions, presenting effectiveness greater than 60% of the articles in 11 of the 12 analyzed outcomes. It should be noted that few studies analyzed mental health and cognitive skills outcomes, most of which were therapeutic PE-based interventions. This finding suggests a lack of evidence on mental health and cognitive skills outcomes that should be explored in future research.

4.6. Limitations

Although articles from other countries such as Chile, Mexico, Ecuador and Colombia were considered, most of the included studies were developed in Brazil, which does not allow a complete overview in relation to PE interventions for OAs in all of Latin America. This in turn could be considered a challenge for researchers in the rest of the Latin American countries in terms of developing similar research in their respective countries. On the other hand, we restricted the search the last 5 years to find the latest and updated available evidence. We are aware that there may be high-quality evidence in previous years that was not included. Another limitation of this review was the quality of the RTCs included. Thus, a high percentage of RCTs had unclear risk of bias in selection bias, performance bias, detection bias, and attrition bias. In addition, 52.6% of the CERT items showed a low percentage of articles that complied with describing and detailing the CERT categories. Furthermore, this scoping review lacked meta-analysis due to the studies' heterogeneity, so there is only a qualitative analysis of the phenomenon studied.

4.7. How Does this Literature Review Contribute to the Existing One?

This systematic review provides a broad and updated view of the characteristics of the PA and PE interventions that are being developed in Latin America, thus allowing the generation of a profile, outcome variables, and evaluation instruments used. On the other hand, this review allowed to identify that, although there are certain similarities between the recommendations proposed by the WHO and the GPAR of the different Latin American countries, there are also differences, for example, in the type of exercise, its frequency and its duration. Therefore, this review could serve to determine the more and less frequent characteristics of the interventions used by Latin American researchers.

This review also provides updated information derived from RTC on the characteristics of PE based-interventions, as well as the most frequently used outcome measures and instruments that should serve to help exercise professionals prescribe exercise for older adults.

Additionally, it allowed the understanding of new PE modalities that are being implemented and their characteristics, being able to encourage the development of future studies that are based on non-traditional PE interventions, in little-explored age groups and health conditions.

5. Conclusions

A total of 101 articles were included (90% focused on Brazil), with a total sample of 5013 OA (79% women). 97% of the studies included participants between 60–70 years of age. The studies had an average adherence of 86%. The main cause of withdrawal was personal reasons (78% of cases). The studies were mainly carried out with OAs who lived in the community with the diagnosis of some disease, with cardiometabolic diseases being the most prevalent. A large percentage of studies had an unclear risk of bias in the items: selection, performance, detection and attrition. Furthermore, a heterogeneous level of compliance was observed in the CERT items. The interventions were mainly based on therapeutic PE, lasted between 2–6 months, with a frequency of 2–3 times a week, with a duration of sessions between 30–60 min and were led by professionals of PA sciences. For the most part, there was no warm-up stage before exercise and cool-down stage after exercise. As well as the components of physical fitness that were exercised the most were muscle strength and cardiorespiratory fitness.

This systematic review provides a broad and updated view of the characteristics of PE-based interventions that are being developed for OAs in Latin America. The findings will be useful for prescribing future PE programs for OAs, being able to encourage the development of future studies in this area of knowledge.

Supplementary Materials: The following are available online at https://www.mdpi.com/1660-4601/18/6/2812/s1, Table S1: PRISMA Checklist, Table S2: Search strings for all databases in the systematic review, Table S3: Proportions of "Yes" per CERT item for 101 included trials

Author Contributions: Conceptualization, E.V.-A., R.I.S.-V., S.M.-M., R.Z.-L. and I.C.; methodology, E.V.-A., R.I.S.-V., S.M.-M., R.Z.-L. and I.C.; validation, E.V.-A., R.I.S.-V., S.M.-M., R.Z.-L. and I.C.; formal analysis, E.V.-A., R.I.S.-V., S.M.-M., R.Z.-L. and I.C.; investigation, E.V.-A., R.I.S.-V., S.M.-M., R.Z.-L. and I.C.; data curation, E.V.-A., R.I.S.-V., S.M.-M., R.Z.-L. and I.C.; writing—original draft preparation, E.V.-A., R.I.S.-V., S.M.-M., R.Z.-L. and I.C.; writing—review and editing, E.V.-A., R.I.S.-V., S.M.-M., R.Z.-L. and I.C.; supervision, E.V.-A., R.I.S.-V., S.M.-M., R.Z.-L. and I.C.; project administration, E.V.-A., R.I.S.-V., S.M.-M., R.Z.-L. and I.C. All authors have read and agreed to the published version of the manuscript.

Funding: This research received no external funding.

Institutional Review Board Statement: Not applicable.

Informed Consent Statement: Not applicable.

Data Availability Statement: The systematic review protocol was registered in the PROSPERO repository with the code: CRD42020208833. This information was already provided in the methodology section of the systematic review.

Conflicts of Interest: The authors declare no conflict of interest.

References

1. WHO. Aging. WHO: Washington, DC, USA, 2015. Available online: http://www.who.int/topics/ageing/es/ (accessed on 24 July 2020).
2. World Population Prospects 2019: 2019 Revision | Multimedia Library—United Nations Department of Economics and Social Affairs Un.org. 2020. Available online: https://www.un.org/development/desa/publications/world-population-prospects-2019-highlights.html (accessed on 24 July 2020).
3. World Population Ageing 2019: 2019 Revision | Multimedia Library—United Nations Department of Economics and Social Affairs Un.org. 2020. Available online: https://www.un.org/en/development/desa/population/publications/pdf/ageing/WorldPopulationAgeing2019-Highlights.pdf (accessed on 24 July 2020).
4. Machado-Cuétara, R.L.; Bazán-Machado, M.A.; Izaguirre-Bordelois, M. Principales Factores de Riesgo Asociados a las Caídas en Ancianos del área de Salud Guanabo. *MEDISAN* **2014**, *18*, 158–164. Available online: http://scielo.sld.cu/scielo.php?script=sci_arttext&pid=S1029301920140000200003&lng=es (accessed on 21 July 2020).
5. Sun, F.; Norman, I.J.; While, A.E. Physical activity in older people: A systematic review. *BMC Public Health* **2013**, *13*, 449. [CrossRef]
6. Aguilar-Farías, N.; Martino-Fuentealba, P.; Infante-Grandon, G.; Cortinez-O'Ryan, A. Physical inactivity in Chile: we must answer to global call. *Rev. Méd. Chile* **2017**, *145*, 12.
7. World Health Organization. Diet and Physical Activity Factsheet. Secondary Diet and Physical Activity Factsheet. 2013. Available online: http://www.who.int/dietphysicalactivity/factsheet_inactivity/en/index.html (accessed on 21 July 2020).
8. Guthold, R.; Stevens, G.; Riley, L.; Bull, F.C. Worldwide trends in insufficient physical activity from 2001 to 2016: A pooled analysis of 358 population-based surveys with 1.9 million participants. *Lancet Glob. Health* **2018**, *6*, 1077–1086. [CrossRef]
9. Roca, R. Actividad Física y Salud en el adulto mayor de 6 países latinoamericanos: Review. *Rev. Cienc. Act. Física UCM* **2016**, *17*, 77–86.
10. Salinas, J.; Bello, M.; Flores, A.; Carbullanca, L.; Torres, M. Actividad física con adultos y adultos mayores en Chile: Resultados de un programa piloto. *Rev. Chil. Nutr.* **2005**, *32*, 215–224. [CrossRef]
11. Kruger-Gonçalves, A.; Ribeiro-Teixeira, A.; Cristina-Valentini, N.; Rodriguez de Varga, A.; Dias-Possamai, V.; Feijó-Martins, V. Multicomponent physical activity program: Study with faller and non-faller older adults. *J. Phys. Educ* **2019**, *30*. [CrossRef]
12. Ogawa, E.F.; You, T.; Leveille, S.G. Potential Benefits of Exergaming for Cognition and Dual-Task Function in Older Adults: A Systematic Review. *J. Aging. Phys. Act.* **2016**, *24*, 332–336. [CrossRef]
13. Costantino, S.; Paneni, F.; Cosentino, F. Ageing, metabolism and cardiovascular disease. *J. Physiol.* **2016**, *594*, 2061–2073. [CrossRef] [PubMed]
14. Cadore, E.L.; Rodríguez-Mañas, L.; Sinclair, A.; Izquierdo, M. Effects of different exercise interventions on risk of falls, gait agility, and balance in physical frail older adults: A sistematic review. *Rejuvenation Res.* **2013**, *16*, 105–114. [CrossRef]
15. Izquierdo, M.; Häkkinen, K.; Ibañez, J.; Garrues, M.; Antón, A.; Zúñiga, A.; Larrión, J.L.; Gorostiaga, E.M. Effects of strength training on muscle power and serum hormones in middle-aged and older men. *J. Appl. Physiol.* **2001**, *90*, 1497–1507. [CrossRef] [PubMed]
16. Izquierdo, M.; Ibañez, J.; Hakkinen, K.; Kraemer, W.J.; Larrión, J.L.; Gorostiaga, E.M. Once weekly combined resistance and cardiovascular training in healthy older men. *Med. Sci. Sports Exerc.* **2004**, *36*, 435–443. [CrossRef]
17. Cordero, A.; Solano, R. Impacto de la actividad física en salud mental de la persona mayor. *Rev. Médica Costa Rica Cent.* **2010**, *593*, 305310.
18. OMS. *Lucha contra las ENT: «Mejores Inversiones» y Otras Intervenciones Recomendadas Para la Prevención y el Control de las Enfermedades no Transmisibles*; Ginebra, Organización Mundial de la Salud: Geneva, Switzerland, 2017.
19. WHO Guidelines on Physical Activity and Sedentary Behaviour. World Health Organization: Geneva, Switzerland, 2020. Available online: https://www.who.int/publications/i/item/9789240015128 (accessed on 30 December 2020).
20. *ACTIVE: Paquete de Intervenciones Técnicas Para Acrecentar la Actividad Física [ACTIVE: A Technical Package for Increasing Physical Activity]*; Ginebra, Organización Mundial de la Salud: Geneva, Switzerland, 2019.
21. Fundación interamericana del corazón Argentina. *La Actividad Física en Personas Mayores: Guía Para Promover un Envejecimiento Activo*, 1st ed.; Fundación Navarro Viola: Buenos Aires, Argentina, 2018; pp. 17–26.
22. Ministerio de Salud, Secretaria Nacional del Deporte. Uruguay. 2004. Available online: http://www.codajic.org/ (accessed on 26 July 2020).
23. Rejas, N.; Ministerio de Salud. Documento Técnico: Gestión Para la Promoción de la Actividad Física Para la salud. Perú. 2015. Available online: http://docs.bvsalud.org/ (accessed on 26 July 2020).

24. Costa Rica. In *Ministerio de Salud y Ministerio del Deporte y Recreación. Plan Nacional de Actividad Física y Salud 2011–2021*, 1st ed.; El ministerio: San José, CA, USA, 2011. Available online: https://www.ministeriodesalud.org.cr (accessed on 27 July 2020).
25. Bukele, N. Deporte, Plan Cuscatlán. Un nuevo Gobierno Para el Salvador. El Salvador. 2019. Available online: https://www.plancuscatlan.com/ (accessed on 27 July 2020).
26. Guía para Actividad Física Para Adultos Mayores. Panamá. 2018. Available online: https://www.hospitalsantafepanama.com/ (accessed on 27 July 2020).
27. Paraguay; Ministerio de Salud Pública y Bienestar Social; Dirección General de Vigilancia de la Salud. *Dirección de Vigilancia de Enfermedades No Transmisibles*; Manual de Promoción de Actividad Física; MSP y BS: Asunción, Paraguay, 2014.
28. Comisión de Alimentación y Nutrición de Puerto Rico. Guía de Alimentación y Actividad Física Para Puerto Rico. Puerto Rico. 2015. Available online: http://www.salud.gov.pr/ (accessed on 27 July 2020).
29. Gobierno de Chile. *Recomendaciones Para la Práctica de Actividad Física Según Curso de la Vida*, 1st ed.; Gobierno de Chile: Santiago, Chile, 2017; pp. 48–51.
30. Honduras, Secretaria de Salud. *Guía de Actividad Física Para Facilitadores de Salud/Honduras*, 1st ed.; Línea Creative: Tegucigalpa, Honduras, 2016.
31. ACEMI. Se Activo Físicamente y Siéntete Bien. Colombia. 2011 [3 de agosto de 2020]. Available online: https://minsalud.gov.co/ (accessed on 27 July 2020).
32. Ministerio de Salud Pública del Ecuador Coordinación Nacional de Nutrición. Guía de Actividad Física Dirigida al Personal de Salud II. Ecuador. 2011. Available online: https://bibliotecapromocion.msp.gob.ec/ (accessed on 27 July 2020).
33. CONACYT, Consejo Nacional de Ciencia y Tecnología. Guías Alimentarias y de Actividad Física, en Contexto de Sobrepeso y Obesidad en la Población Mexicana. México. 2015. Available online: https://www.anmm.org.mx/ (accessed on 27 July 2020).
34. Matsudo, S.M.; Matsudo, V.R.; Araujo, T.L.; Andrade, D.R.; Andrade, E.L.; Oliveira, L.C.; Braggion, G.F. The agita São Paulo Program as a model for using physical activity to promote health. *Rev. Panam. Salud Publica* **2003**, *14*, 265–272. [CrossRef]
35. Matsudo, M.S.; Matsudo, R.V.; Araujo, T.L.; Andrade, D.R.; Oliveira, M.L. From diagnosis to action: The experience of Agita São Paulo program in promoting and active lifeestyle. *Rev. Bras. Ativ. Fís. Saúde* **2008**, *13*, 178–184. Available online: https://www.researchgate.net/publication/238744260_do_diagnostico_a_acao_a_experiencia_do_programa_agita_sao_paulo_na_promocao_do_estilo_de_vida_ativo (accessed on 24 July 2020).
36. Liberati, A.; Altman, D.; Tetzlaff, J.; Mulrow, C.; Gotzsche, P.; Ioannidis, J.; Clarke, M.; Devereaux, P.J.; Kleijnen, J.; Moher, D. The PRISMA statement for reporting systematic reviews and meta-analyses of studies that evaluate healthcare interventions: Explanation and elaboration. *BMJ* **2009**, *339*, b2700. [CrossRef] [PubMed]
37. McGowan, J.; Sampson, M.; Salzwedel, D.; Cogo, E.; Foerster, V.; Lefebvre, C. PRESS Peer Review of Electronic Search Strategies: 2015 Guideline Statement. *J. Clin. Epidemiol.* **2016**, *75*, 40–46. [CrossRef]
38. The Cochrane Collaboration; Higgins, J.P.T.; Green, S. (Eds.) Cochrane Handbook for Systematic Reviews of Interventions. Version 5.1.0 [updated March 2011]. 2011. Available online: www.cochrane-handbook.org (accessed on 20 February 2021).
39. Slade, S.C.; Dionne, C.E.; Underwood, M.; Buchbinder, R.; Beck, B.; Bennell, K. Consensus on Exercise Reporting Template (CERT): Modified Delphi Study. *Phys. Ther.* **2016**, *96*, 1514–1524. [CrossRef]
40. de Queiroz, J.L.; Sales, M.M.; Sousa, C.V.; Silva, S.; Asano, R.; Vila Nova-de Moraes, J.F. 12 weeks of Brazilian jiu-jitsu training improves functional fitness in elderly men. *Sport Sci. Health* **2016**, *12*, 291–295. [CrossRef]
41. Antunes, H.K.; De Mello, M.T.; de Aquino-Lemos, V.; Santos-Galduroz, R.F.; Camargo-Galdieri, L.; Amodeo-Bueno, O.F.; Tufik, S.; D'Almeida, V. Aerobic physical exercise improved the cognitive function of elderly males but did not modify their blood homocysteine levels. *Dement. Geriatr. Cogn. Dis. Extra* **2015**, *5*, 13–24. [CrossRef]
42. Santos, S.M.; da Silva, R.A.; Terra, M.B.; Almeida, I.A.; De Melo, L.B.; Ferraz, H.B. Balance versus resistance training on postural control in patients with Parkinson's disease: A randomized controlled trial. *Eur. J. Phys. Rehabil. Med.* **2017**, *53*, 173–183. [PubMed]
43. de Oliveira, R.T.; Felippe, L.A.; Bucken-Gobbi, L.T.; Barbieri, F.A.; Christofoletti, G. Benefits of Exercise on the Executive Functions in People with Parkinson Disease: A Controlled Clinical Trial. *Am. J. Phys. Med. Rehabil.* **2017**, *96*, 301–306. [CrossRef] [PubMed]
44. Oliveira, L.C.; Oliveira, R.G.; Pires-Oliveira, D.A. Comparison between static stretching and the Pilates method on the flexibility of older women. *J. Bodyw. Mov. Ther.* **2016**, *20*, 800–806. [CrossRef]
45. Mazini-Filho, M.L.; Aidar, F.J.; Costa-Moreira, O.; Gama de Matos, D.; Patrocínio de Oliveira, C.E.; Rezende de Oliveira-Venturini, G.; Paula-Costa, S.; Magalhaes-Curty, V.; Caputo-Ferreira, M.E. Comparison of the effect of two physical exercise programs on the functional autonomy, balance and flexibility of elderly women. *Med. Sport* **2017**, *70*, 288–298.
46. Teodoro, J.L.; da Silva, L.X.N.; Fritsch, C.G.; Baroni, B.M.; Grazioli, R.; Boeno, F.P.; Lopez, P.; Gentil, P.; Bottaro, M.; Pinto, R.S.; et al. Concurrent training performed with and without repetitions to failure in older men: A randomized clinical trial. *Scand J. Med. Sci. Sports* **2019**, *29*, 1141–1152. [CrossRef]
47. Santos, G.O.R.; Wolf, R.; Silva, M.M.; Rodacki, A.L.F.; Pereira, G. Does exercise intensity increment in exergame promote changes in strength, ¿functional capacity and perceptual parameters in pre-frail older women? A randomized controlled trial. *Exp. Gerontol.* **2019**, *116*, 25–30. [CrossRef]
48. Dueñas, E.P.; Ramírez, L.P.; Ponce, E.; Curcio, C.L. Efecto sobre el temor a caer y la funcionalidad de tres programas de intervención. Ensayo clínico aleatorizado [Effect on fear of falling and functionality of three intervention programs. A randomised clinical trial]. *Rev. Esp. Geriatr. Gerontol.* **2019**, *54*, 68–74. [CrossRef]

49. Pirauá, A.L.T.; Cavalcante, B.R.; de Oliveira, V.M.A.; Beltrao, N.B.; De Amorin Batista, G.; Pitangui, A.C.R.; Behm, D.; De Araújo, R.C. Effect of 24-week strength training on unstable surfaces on mobility, balance, and concern about falling in older adults. *Scand J. Med. Sci. Sports* **2019**, *29*, 1805–1812. [CrossRef]
50. Arantes, P.M.M.; Días, J.M.D.; Fonseca, F.F.; Oliveira, A.M.B.; Oliveira, M.C.; Pereira, L.S.M.; Dias, R.C. Effect of a Program Based on Balance Exercises on Gait, Functional Mobility, Fear of Falling, and Falls in Prefrail Older Women: A Randomized Clinical Trial. *Top. Geriatr. Rehabil.* **2015**, *31*, 113–120. [CrossRef]
51. Lima, L.G.; Bonardi, J.M.; Campos, G.O.; Bertani, R.F.; Scher, L.M.; Louzada-Junior, P.; Moriguti, J.C.; Ferrioli, E.; Lima, N.K. Effect of aerobic training and aerobic and resistance training on the inflammatory status of hypertensive older adults. *Aging Clin. Exp. Res.* **2015**, *27*, 483–489. [CrossRef]
52. De Oliveira, D.V.; Da Cunha, P.M.; Dos Santos-Campos, R.; Do-Nascimento, M.A.; Antunes, M.D.; Do Nascimento, J.R.A.; Mayhew, J.L.; Cavaglieri, C.R. Effect of circuit resistance training on blood biomarkers of cardiovascular disease risk in older women. *J. Phys. Educ.* **2019**, *30*. [CrossRef]
53. Langoni, C.D.S.; Resende, T.L.; Barcellos, A.B.; Cecchele, B.; Knob, M.S.; Silva, T.D.N.; da Rosa, J.N.; Diogo, T.S.; Filho, I.G.D.S.; Schwanke, C.H.A. Effect of Exercise on Cognition, Conditioning, Muscle Endurance, and Balance in Older Adults with Mild Cognitive Impairment: A Randomized Controlled Trial. *J. Geriatr. Phys. Ther.* **2019**, *42*, E15–E22. [CrossRef]
54. Nascimento, M.A.D.; Gerage, A.M.; Silva, D.R.P.D.; Ribeiro, A.S.; Machado, D.G.D.S.; Pina, F.L.C.; Tomeleri, C.M.; Venturini, D.; Barbosa, D.S.; Mayhew, J.L.; et al. Effect of resistance training with different frequencies and subsequent detraining on muscle mass and appendicular lean soft tissue, IGF-1, and testosterone in older women. *Eur. J. Sport Sci.* **2019**, *19*, 199–207. [CrossRef]
55. Dantas, F.F.; Brasileiro-Santos Mdo, S.; Batista, R.M.; do Nascimento, L.S.; Castellano, L.R.; Ritti-Dias, R.M.; Lima, K.C.; Santos-Ada, C. Effect of Strength Training on Oxidative Stress and the Correlation of the Same with Forearm Vasodilatation and Blood Pressure of Hypertensive Elderly Women: A Randomized Clinical Trial. *PLoS ONE* **2016**, *11*, e0161178. [CrossRef]
56. Leandro, M.P.G.; de Moura, J.L.S.; Barros, G.W.P.; da Silva-Filho, A.P.; Farias, A.C.O.; Carvalho, P.R.C. Effect of the aerobic component of combined training on the blood pressure of hypertensive elderly women. *Rev. Bras. Med. Esporte* **2019**, *25*, 469–473. [CrossRef]
57. de Carvalho-Fonseca, R.G.; Silva, A.M.; Teixeira, L.F.; Silva, V.R.; Dos Reis, L.M.; Silva-Santos, A.T. Effect of the Auricular Acupoint Associated with Physical Exercise in Elderly People: A Randomized Clinical Test. *J. Acupunct. Meridian Stud.* **2018**, *11*, 137–144. [CrossRef] [PubMed]
58. Tiggemann, C.L.; Días, C.P.; Radaelli, R.; Massa, J.C.; Bortoluzzi, R.; Schoenell, M.C.; Noll, M.; Alberton, C.L.; Kruel, L.F. Effect of traditional resistance and power training using rated perceived exertion for enhancement of muscle strength, power, and functional performance. *Age (Dordr)* **2016**, *38*, 42. [CrossRef]
59. da Silva, R.G.; da Silva, D.R.P.; Pina, F.L.C.; do Nascimento, M.A.; Ribeiro, A.S.; Cyrino, E.S. Effect of two different weekly resistance training frequencies on muscle strength and blood pressure in normotensive older women. *Rev. Bras. Cineantropometria Desempenho Hum.* **2017**, *19*, 118–127.
60. Taglietti, M.; Facci, L.M.; Trelha, C.S.; de Melo, F.C.; Da Silva, D.W.; Sawczuk, G.; Ruivo, T.M.; de Souza, T.B.; Sforza, C.; Cardoso, J.R. Effectiveness of aquatic exercises compared to patient-education on health status in individuals with knee osteoarthritis: A randomized controlled trial. *Clin. Rehabil.* **2018**, *32*, 766–776. [CrossRef]
61. Franco, M.R.; Sherrington, C.; Tiedemann, A.; Pereira, L.S.; Perracini, M.R.; Faria, C.R.; Pinto, R.Z.; Pastre, C.M. Effectiveness of Senior Dance on risk factors for falls in older adults (DanSE): A study protocol for a randomised controlled trial. *BMJ Open* **2016**, *30*, e013995. [CrossRef]
62. Ferreira, C.B.; Teixeira, P.D.S.; Alves Dos Santos, G.; Dantas Maya, A.T.; Americano Do Brasil, P.; Souza, V.C.; Córdova, C.; Ferreira, A.P.; Lima, R.M.; Nobrega, O.T. Effects of a 12-Week Exercise Training Program on Physical Function in Institutionalized Frail Elderly. *J. Aging Res.* **2018**, *2018*, 1–8. [CrossRef]
63. López, N.; Véliz, A.; Soto-Añari, M.; Ollari, J.; Chesta, S.; Allegri, R. Effects of a combined program of physical activity and cognitive training in Chilean patients with mild Alzheimer. *Neurol. Argent* **2015**, *7*, 131–139. [CrossRef]
64. Suzuki, F.S.; Evangelista, A.L.; Teixeira, C.V.L.S.; Paunksnis, M.R.R.; Rica, R.L.; de Toledo Evangelista, R.A.G.; Joao, G.A.; Doro, M.R.; Sita, D.M.; Serra, A.J.; et al. Effects of a multicomponent exercise program on the functional fitness in elderly women. *Rev. Bras. Med. Esporte* **2018**, *24*, 36–39. [CrossRef]
65. Ortiz-Ortiz, M.; Gómez-Miranda, L.M.; Chacón-Araya, Y.; Moncada-Jiménez, J. Effects of a physical activity program on depressive symptoms and functional capacity of institutionalized mexican older adults. *J. Phys. Educ. Sport* **2019**, *19*, 890–896.
66. Guedes, J.M.; Bortoluzzi, M.G.; Matte, L.P.; De Andrade, C.M.; Zulpo, N.C.; Sebben, V.; Filho, H.T. Effects of combined training on the strength, endurance and aerobic power in the elderly women. *Rev. Bras. Med. Esporte* **2016**, *22*, 480–484. [CrossRef]
67. Agner, V.F.C.; Garcia, M.C.; Taffarel, A.A.; Mourao, C.B.; da Silva, I.P.; da Silva, S.P.; Peccin, M.S.; Lombardi, I.J. Effects of concurrent training on muscle strength in older adults with metabolic syndrome: A randomized controlled clinical trial. *Arch. Gerontol. Geriatr.* **2018**, *75*, 158–164. [CrossRef]
68. Rodrigues-Krause, J.; Farinha, J.B.; Ramis, T.R.; Macedo, R.C.O.; Boeno, F.P.; Dos Santos, G.C.; Vargas, J.J.; Lopez, P.; Grazioli, R.; Costa, R.R.; et al. Effects of dancing compared to walking on cardiovascular risk and functional capacity of older women: A randomized controlled trial. *Exp. Gerontol.* **2018**, *114*, 67–77. [CrossRef] [PubMed]

69. Ferrari, R.; Fuchs, S.C.; Kruel, L.F.M.; Cadore, E.L.; Alberton, C.L.; Pinto, R.S.; Radaelli, R.; Schoenell, M.; Izquierdo, M.; Tanaka, H.; et al. Effects of different concurrent resistance and aerobic training frequencies on muscle power and muscle quality in trained elderly men: A randomized clinical trial. *Aging Dis.* **2016**, *7*, 697–704. [CrossRef]
70. Ramirez-Campillo, R.; Diaz, D.; Martinez-Salazar, C.; Valdés-Badilla, P.; Delgado-Floody, P.; Méndez-Rebolledo, G.; Cañas-Jamet, R.; Cristi-Moreno, C.; García-Moreno, A.; Celis-Morales, C.; et al. Effects of different doses of high-speed resistance training on physical performance and quality of life in older women: A randomized controlled trial. *Clin. Interv. Aging* **2016**, *11*, 1797–1804. [CrossRef] [PubMed]
71. Neto, A.G.R.; Santos, M.S.; Silva, R.J.S.; de Santana, J.M.; da Silva-Grigoletto, M.E. Effects of different neuromuscular training protocols on the functional capacity of elderly women. *Rev. Bras. Med. Esporte* **2018**, *24*, 140–144. [CrossRef]
72. Cavalcante, E.F.; Ribeiro, A.S.; do Nascimento, M.A.; Silva, A.M.; Tomeleri, C.M.; Nabuco, H.C.G.; Pina, F.L.C.; Mayhew, J.L.; Silva-Grigoletto, M.E.D.; da Silva, D.R.P.; et al. Effects of Different Resistance Training Frequencies on Fat in Overweight/Obese Older Women. *Int. J. Sports Med.* **2018**, *39*, 527–534. [CrossRef] [PubMed]
73. Días, C.P.; Toscan, R.; de Camargo, M.; Pereira, E.P.; Griebler, N.; Baroni, B.M.; Tiggeman, C.L. Effects of eccentric-focused and conventional resistance training on strength and functional capacity of older adults. *Age (Dordr)* **2015**, *37*, 99. [CrossRef]
74. Henrique, P.P.B.; Colussi, E.L.; De Marchi, A.C.B. Effects of Exergame on Patients' Balance and Upper Limb Motor Function after Stroke: A Randomized Controlled Trial. *J. Stroke Cerebrovasc. Dis.* **2019**, *28*, 2351–2357. [CrossRef]
75. Ramírez-Villada, J.F.; Cadena-Duarte, L.L.; Gutiérrez-Galvis, A.R.; Argothy-Bucheli, R.; Moreno-Ramírez, Y. Effects of explosive and impact exercises on gait parameters in elderly women. *Rev. Fac. Med.* **2019**, *67*, 493–501. [CrossRef]
76. de Resende-Neto, A.G.; Oliveira Andrade, B.C.; Cyrino, E.S.; Behm, D.G.; De-Santana, J.M.; Da Silva-Grigoletto, M.E. Effects of functional and traditional training in body composition and muscle strength components in older women: A randomized controlled trial. *Arch. Gerontol. Geriatr.* **2019**, *84*, 103902. [CrossRef]
77. De Lourdes Feitosa Neta, M.; De Resende-Neto, A.G.; Dantas, E.H.M.; De Almeida, M.B.; Wichi, R.B.; Da Silva Grigoletto, M.E. Effects of functional training on strength, muscle power and quality of life in pre-frail older women. *Motricidade* **2016**, *12*, 61–68.
78. Bacha, J.M.R.; Gomes, G.C.V.; de Freitas, T.B.; Viveiro, L.A.P.; da Silva, K.G.; Bueno, G.C.; Varise, E.M.; Torriani-Pasin, C.; Castilho-Alonso, A.; Silva-Luna, N.M.; et al. Effects of Kinect Adventures Games Versus Conventional Physical Therapy on Postural Control in Elderly People: A Randomized Controlled Trial. *Games Health* **2018**, *7*, 24–36. [CrossRef]
79. Dos Santos, L.; Ribeiro, A.S.; Cavalcante, E.F.; Nabuco, H.C.; Antunes, M.; Schoenfeld, B.J.; Cyrino, E.S. Effects of Modified Pyramid System on Muscular Strength and Hypertrophy in Older Women. *Int. J. Sports Med.* **2018**, *39*, 613–618. [CrossRef]
80. Gomeñuka, N.A.; Oliveira, H.B.; Silva, E.S.; Costa, R.R.; Kanitz, A.C.; Liedtke, G.V.; Schuch, F.B.; Peyré-Tartaruga, L.A. Effects of Nordic walking training on quality of life, balance and functional mobility in elderly: A randomized clinical trial. *PLoS ONE* **2019**, *14*, e0211472. [CrossRef]
81. De Oliveira, L.C.; De Oliveira, R.G.; De Almeida Pires-Oliveira, D.A. Effects of pilates on muscle strength, postural balance and quality of life of older adults: A randomized, controlled, clinical trial. *J. Phys. Ther. Sci.* **2015**, *27*, 871–876. [CrossRef]
82. Vale, R.G.D.S.; Da Gama, D.R.N.; Oliveira, F.B.D.; Almeida, D.S.D.M.; De Castro, J.B.P.; Meza, E.I.A.; Mattos, R.D.S.; Nunes, R.A.M. Effects of resistance training and chess playing on the quality of life and cognitive performance of elderly women: A randomized controlled trial. *J. Phys. Educ. Sport* **2018**, *18*, 1469–1477.
83. Santiago, L.Â.M.; Neto, L.G.L.; Pereira, G.B.; Leite, R.D.; Mostarda, C.T.; De Oliveira Brito Monzani, J.; Sousa, W.R.; Rodrigues Pinheiro, A.J.M.; Navarro, F. Effects of Resistance Training on Immunoinflammatory Response, TNF-alpha Gene Expression, and Body Composition in Elderly Women. *J. Aging Res.* **2018**. Available online: https://www.ncbi.nlm.nih.gov/pmc/articles/PMC6230406/ (accessed on 30 July 2020).
84. Botton, C.E.; Umpierre, D.; Rech Pfeifer, L.O.; Machado, C.L.F.; Teodoro, J.L.; Días, A.S.; Pinto, R.S. Effects of resistance training on neuromuscular parameters in elderly with type 2 diabetes mellitus: A randomized clinical trial. *Exp. Gerontol.* **2018**, *113*, 141–149. [CrossRef]
85. Gadelha, A.B.; Paiva, F.M.; Gauche, R.; de Oliveira, R.J.; Lima, R.M. Effects of resistance training on sarcopenic obesity index in older women: A randomized controlled trial. *Arch. Gerontol. Geriatr.* **2016**, *65*, 168–173. [CrossRef] [PubMed]
86. Barbosa Rezende, A.A.; Fernandes De Miranda, E.; Souza Ramalho, H.; Borges Da Silva, J.D.; Silva Carlotto Herrera, S.D.; Rossone Reis, G.; Dantas, E.H.M. Effects of sensory motor training of lower limb in sedentary elderly as part of functional autonomy. *Rev. Andaluza Med. Deporte* **2015**, *8*, 61–66. [CrossRef]
87. Martins, W.R.; Safons, M.P.; Bottaro, M.; Blasczyk, J.C.; Diniz, L.R.; Fonseca, M.C.F.; Bonini-Rocha, A.C.; Jacó de Oliveira, R. Effects of short term elastic resistance training on muscle mass and strength in untrained older adults: A randomized clinical trial. *BMC Geriatr.* **2015**, *15*, 99. [CrossRef]
88. Gallo, L.H.; Demantova Gurjão, A.L.; Gobbi, S.; Ceccato, M.; Garcia Prado, A.K.; Jambassi Filho, J.C.; Gomes, A. Effects of static stretching on functional capacity in older women: Randomized controlled trial. *J. Exerc. Physiol. Online* **2015**, *18*, 13–22.
89. Ruaro, M.F.; Santana, J.O.; Gusmão, N.; De Franca, E.; Carvalho, B.N.; Farinazo, K.B.; Bonorino, S.L.; Corralo, V.; Antonio De Sá, C.; Caperuto, E. Effects of strength training with and without blood flow restriction on quality of life in elderly women. *J. Phys. Educ. Sport* **2019**, *19*, 531–539.
90. Silva, C.M.D.S.E.; Gomes Neto, M.; Saquetto, M.B.; Conceição, C.S.D.; Souza-Machado, A. Effects of upper limb resistance exercise on aerobic capacity, muscle strength, and quality of life in COPD patients: A randomized controlled trial. *Clin. Rehabil.* **2018**, *32*, 1636–1644. [CrossRef]

91. Miranda-Aguilar, D.; Valdés-Badilla, P.; Herrera-Valenzuela, T.; Guzmán-Muñoz, E.; Magnani-Branco, B.H.; Méndez-Rebolledo, G.; Lopéz-Fuenzalida, A. ¿Bandas elásticas o equipos de gimnasio para el entrenamiento de adultos mayores? (¿Elastic bands or gym equipment for the training of older adults?). *Retos* **2019**, *37*, 370–378. [CrossRef]
92. Cadore, E.L.; Menger, E.; Teodoro, J.L.; Da Silva, L.X.N.; Boeno, F.P.; Umpierre, D.; Botton, C.E.; Ferrari, R.; Dos Santos-Cunha, G.; Izquierdo, M.; et al. Functional and physiological adaptations following concurrent training using sets with and without concentric failure in elderly men: A randomized clinical trial. *Exp. Gerontol.* **2018**, *110*, 182–190. [CrossRef]
93. De Resende Neto, A.G.; De Lourdes Feitosa Neta, M.; Santos, M.S.; La Scala Teixeira, C.V.; De Sá, C.A.; Da Silva-Grigoletto, M.E. Functional training versus traditional strength training: Effects on physical fitness indicators in pre-frail elderly women. *Motricidade* **2016**, *12*, 44–53.
94. Silva, I.G.; Silva, B.S.A.; Freire, A.P.C.F.; Santos, A.P.S.D.; Lima, F.F.; Ramos, D.; Ramos, E.M.C. Functionality of patients with Chronic Obstructive Pulmonary Disease at 3 months follow-up after elastic resistance training: A randomized clinical trial. *Pulmonology* **2018**, *24*, 354–357. [CrossRef]
95. Da Silva, M.A.R.; Baptista, L.C.; Neves, R.S.; De França, E.; Loureiro, H.; Rezende, M.A.C.; da Silva-Ferrerira, V.; Texeira-Veríssimo, M.; Martins, A. High intensity interval training improves health-related quality of life in adults and older adults with diagnosed cardiovascular risk. *J. Phys. Educ. Sport* **2019**, *19*, 611–618.
96. Ramirez-Campillo, R.; Alvarez, C.; Garcìa-Hermoso, A.; Celis-Morales, C.; Ramirez-Velez, R.; Gentil, P.; Izquierdo, M. High-speed resistance training in elderly women: Effects of cluster training sets on functional performance and quality of life. *Exp. Gerontol.* **2018**, *110*, 216–222. [CrossRef]
97. Brandão, G.S.; Gomes, G.S.B.F.; Brandão, G.S.; Callou-Sampaio, A.A.; Donner, C.F.; Oliveira, L.V.F.; Camelier, A.A. Home exercise improves the quality of sleep and daytime sleepiness of elderlies: A randomized controlled trial. *Multidiscip. Resp. Med.* **2018**, *13*, 1–9. [CrossRef]
98. Hall-López, J.A.; Ochoa-Martínez, P.Y.; Alarcón-Meza, E.I.; Moncada-Jiménez, J.A.; Garcia Bertruy, O.; Martin-Dantas, E.H. Hydrogymnastics training program on physical fitness in elderly women. *Rev. Int. Med. Cienc. Act. Fis. Deporte* **2017**, *17*, 283–298.
99. Medeiros, L.B.; Ansai, J.H.; De Souza-Buto, M.S.; Barroso, V.V.; Farche, A.C.S.; Rossi, P.G.; Andrade, L.P.; Takahashi, A.C. Impact of a dual task intervention on physical performance of older adults who practice physical exercise. *Rev. Bras. Cineantropometria Desempenho Hum.* **2018**, *20*, 10–19. [CrossRef]
100. Vargas, M.Á.; Rosas, M.E. Impact of an-aerobic physical activity program in hypertensive elderly adults. *Rev. Latinoam. Hipertens.* **2019**, *14*, 142–149.
101. Scarabottolo, C.C.; Garcia-Júnior, J.R.; Gobbo, L.A.; Alves, M.J.; Ferreira, A.D.; Zanuto, E.A.C.; Oliveira, W.; Destro-Christofaro, D.G. Influence of physical exercise on the functional capacity in institutionalized elderly. *Rev. Bras. Med. Esporte* **2017**, *23*, 200–203. [CrossRef]
102. Damorim, I.R.; Santos, T.M.; Barros, G.W.P.; Carvalho, P.R.C. Kinetics of Hypotension during 50 Sessions of Resistance and Aerobic Training in Hypertensive Patients: A Randomized Clinical Trial. *Arq. Bras. Cardiol.* **2017**, *108*, 323–330. [CrossRef] [PubMed]
103. Leal, L.C.; Abrahin, O.; Rodrigues, R.P.; Da Silva, M.C.; Araújo, P.M.; De Sousa, E.C.; Pimentel, C.P.; Cortinhas-Alves, E.A. Low-volume resistance training improves the functional capacity of older individuals with Parkinson's disease. *Geriatr. Gerontol. Int.* **2019**, *19*, 635–640. [CrossRef]
104. Souza, D.; Barbalho, M.; Vieira, C.A.; Martins, W.R.; Cadore, E.L.; Gentil, P. Minimal dose resistance training with elastic tubes promotes functional and cardiovascular benefits to older women. *Exp. Gerontol.* **2019**, *115*, 132–138. [CrossRef]
105. Santos, G.D.; Nunes, P.V.; Stella, F.; Brum, P.S.; Yassuda, M.S.; Ueno, L.M.; Gattaz, W.F.; Forlenza, O.V. Multidisciplinary rehabilitation program: Effects of a multimodal intervention for patients with Alzheimer's disease and cognitive impairment without dementia. *Rev. Psiquiatr. Clin.* **2015**, *42*, 153–156. [CrossRef]
106. Moreira, N.B.; Gonçalves, G.; da Silva, T.; Zanardini, F.E.H.; Bento, P.C.B. Multisensory exercise programme improves cognition and functionality in institutionalized older adults: A randomized control trial. *Physiother. Res. Int.* **2018**, *23*, e1708. [CrossRef] [PubMed]
107. Martinez, A.; Selaive, R.; Astorga, S.; Olivares, P. Neuromuscular training in institutionalized older adults: A functional approach to preventing fall. *Nutr. Clin. Diet. Hosp.* **2018**, *38*, 40–45.
108. Santana, M.; Pina, J.; Duarte, G.; Neto, M.; Machado, A.; Dominguez-Ferraz, D. Nintendo wii effects on cardiorespiratory fitness in older adults: A randomized clinical trial. a pilot trial. *Fisioterapia* **2016**, *38*, 71–77. [CrossRef]
109. Gomeñuka, N.A.; Oliveira, H.B.; da Silva, E.S.; Passos-Monteiro, E.; da Rosa, R.G.; Carvalho, A.R.; Costa, R.R.; Rodríguez, M.C.; Pellegrini, B.; Peyré-Tartaruga, L.A. Nordic walking training in elderly, a randomized clinical trial. Part II: Biomechanical and metabolic adaptations. *Sports Med. Open* **2020**, *6*. [CrossRef]
110. Coelho-Júnior, H.J.; de Oliveira-Gonçalvez, I.; Sampaio, R.A.C.; Sewo Sampaio, P.Y.; Cadore, E.L.; Izquierdo, M.; Marzetti, E.; Uchida, M.C. Periodized and non-periodized resistance training programs on body composition and physical function of older women. *Exp. Gerontol.* **2019**, *121*, 10–18.
111. Pestana, M.D.S.; Netto, E.M.; Pestana, M.C.S.; Pestana, V.S.; Schinoni, M.I. Pilates versus resistance exercise on the serum levels of hs-CRP, in the abdominal circumference and body mass index (BMI) in elderly individuals. *Motricidade* **2016**, *12*, 128. [CrossRef]

112. Gambassi, B.B.; Almeida, F.J.F.; Sauaia, B.A.; Novais, T.M.G.; Furtado, A.E.A.; Chaves, L.F.C. Resistance training contributes to variability in heart rate and quality of the sleep in elderly women without comorbidities. *J. Exerc. Physiol. Online* **2015**, *18*, 112–123.
113. Tomeleri, C.M.; Ribeiro, A.S.; Souza, M.F.; Schiavoni, D.; Schoenfeld, B.J.; Venturini, D.; Barbosa, D.S.; Landucci, K.; Sardinha, L.B.; Cyrino, E. Resistance training improves inflammatory level, lipid and glycemic profiles in obese older women: A randomized controlled trial. *Exp. Gerontol.* **2016**, *84*, 80–87. [CrossRef]
114. Ribeiro, A.S.; Schoenfeld, B.J.; Pina, F.L.C.; Souza, M.; Do Nascimento, M.A.; Santos, L.; Antunes, M.; Cyrino, E. Resistance Training in Older Women: Comparison of Single Vs. Multiple Sets on Muscle Strength and Body Composition. *Isokinet. Exerc. Sci.* **2015**, 53–60. [CrossRef]
115. Cunha, P.M.; Ribeiro, A.S.; Nunes, J.P.; Tomeleri, C.M.; Nascimiento, M.A.; Moraes, G.K.; Sugihara, P.; Barbosa, D.; Venturini, D.; Cyrino, E. Resistance training performed with single-set is sufficient to reduce cardiovascular risk factors in untrained older women: The randomized clinical trial. Active Aging Longitudinal Study. *Arch. Gerontol. Geriatr.* **2019**, *81*, 171–175. [CrossRef]
116. Ribeiro, A.S.; Schoenfeld, B.J.; Souza, M.F.; Tomeleri, C.M.; Silva, A.M.; Teixeira, D.C.; Sardinha, L.; Cyrino, E. Resistance training prescription with different load-management methods improves phase angle in older women. *Eur. J. Sport Sci.* **2017**, *17*, 913–921. [CrossRef]
117. de Lima, T.A.; Ferreira-Moraes, R.; Alves, W.M.G.D.C.; Alves, T.G.G.; Pimentel, C.P.; Sousa, E.C.; Abrahin, O.; Cortinhas-Alvees, E.A. Resistance training reduces depressive symptoms in elderly people with Parkinson disease: A controlled randomized study. *Scand J. Med. Sci. Sports* **2019**, *29*, 1957–1967. [CrossRef]
118. Tomeleri, C.M.; Souza, M.F.; Burini, R.C.; Cavaglieri, C.R.; Ribeiro, A.S.; Antunes, M.; Nunes, J.P.; Venturini, D.; Barbosa, D.S.; Sardinha, L.B.; et al. Resistance training reduces metabolic syndrome and inflammatory markers in older women: A randomized controlled trial. *J. Diabetes* **2018**, *10*, 328–337. [CrossRef]
119. Oliveira-Dantas, F.F.; Brasileiro-Santos, M.D.S.; Thomas, S.G.; Silva, A.S.; Silva, D.C.; Browne, R.A.V.; Farias-Junior, L.F.; Costa, E.; da Cruz, A. Short-Term Resistance Training Improves Cardiac Autonomic Modulation and Blood Pressure in Hypertensive Older Women: A Randomized Controlled Trial. *J. Strength Cond. Res.* **2020**, *34*, 37–45. [CrossRef]
120. Lopes, P.B.; Pereira, G.; Lodovico, A.; Bento, P.C.B.; Rodacki, A.L.F. Strength and Power Training Effects on Lower Limb Force, Functional Capacity, and Static and Dynamic Balance in Older Female Adults. *Rejuvenation Res.* **2016**, *19*, 385–393. [CrossRef]
121. Da Silva, P.B.; Antunes, F.N.; Graef, P.; Cechetti, F.; Pagnussat, A.D.S. Strength training associated with task-oriented training to enhance upper-limb motor function in elderly patients with mild impairment after stroke: A randomized controlled trial. *Am. J. Phys. Med. Rehabil.* **2015**, *94*, 11–19. [CrossRef]
122. Alves, W.M.; Alves, T.G.; Ferreira, R.M.; De Sousa, E.C.; Pimentel, C.P.; De Lima, T.A.; Abrahin, O.; Alves, E.A. Strength training improves the respiratory muscle strength and quality of life of elderly with Parkinson disease. *J. Sports Med. Phys. Fitness* **2019**, *59*, 1756–1762. [CrossRef]
123. Ferreira, R.M.; Alves, W.M.G.D.C.; de Lima, T.A.; Gibson-Alves, T.G.; Alves-Filho, P.A.; Pimentel, C.P.; Correa, E.; Cortinhas-Alves, E.A. The effect of resistance training on the anxiety symptoms and quality of life in elderly people with Parkinson's disease: A randomized controlled trial. *Arq. Neuropsiquiatr.* **2018**, *76*, 499–506. [CrossRef] [PubMed]
124. Rosa, C.; Vilaga-Alves, J.; Neves, E.B.; Saavedra, F.J.F.; Reckziegel, M.B.; Pohl, H.H.; Zanini, D.; Machado, V. The effect of weekly low frequency exercise on body composition and blood pressure of elderly women. *Arch. Med. Deporte* **2017**, *34*, 9–14.
125. Rodacki, A.L.F.; Cepeda, C.P.C.; Lodovico, A.; Ugrinowitsch, C. The Effects of a Dance-Based Program on the Postural Control in Older Women. *Top. Geriatr. Rehabil.* **2017**, *33*, 244–249. [CrossRef]
126. Aragão-Santos, J.C.; De Resende-Neto, A.G.; Nogueira, A.C.; Feitosa-Neta, M.L.; Brandao, L.H.; Chaves, L.M.; Da Silva-Grigoletto, M.E. The effects of functional and traditional strength training on different strength parameters of elderly women: A randomized and controlled trial. *J. Sports Med. Phys. Fitness* **2019**, *59*, 380–386. [CrossRef] [PubMed]
127. Ferraz, D.D.; Trippo, K.V.; Duarte, G.P.; Neto, M.G.; Bernardes-Santos, K.O.; Filho, J.O. The Effects of Functional Training, Bicycle Exercise, and Exergaming on Walking Capacity of Elderly Patients with Parkinson Disease: A Pilot Randomized Controlled Single-blinded Trial. *Arch. Phys. Med. Rehabil.* **2018**, *99*, 826–833. [CrossRef] [PubMed]
128. Sbardelotto, M.L.; Pedroso, G.S.; Pereira, F.T.; Soratto, H.R.; Brescianini, S.M.; Effting, P.S.; Thirupathi, A.; Nesi, R.T.; Silveira, P.CL.; Pinho, R.A. The effects of physical training are varied and occur in an exercise type-dependent manner in elderly men. *Aging Dis.* **2017**, *8*, 887–898. [CrossRef]
129. Antunes, H.K.; Santos-Galduroz, R.F.; De Aquino-Lemos, V.; Amodeu-Bueno, O.F.; Rzezak, P.; Goncalves-De Santana, M.; De Melo, M.T. The influence of physical exercise and leisure activity on neuropsychological functioning in older adults. *Age (Dordr)* **2015**, *37*, 9815. [CrossRef]
130. Carvalho, I.F.D.; Leme, G.L.M.; Scheicher, M.E. The Influence of Video Game Training with and without Subpatelar Bandage in Mobility and Gait Speed on Elderly Female Fallers. *J. Aging Res.* **2018**, *2018*, 1–9. [CrossRef]
131. Barbalho, M.S.M.; Gentil, P.; Izquierdo, M.; Fisher, J.; Steele, J.; Raiol, R.A. There are no no-responders to low or high resistance training volumes among older women. *Exp. Gerontol.* **2017**, *99*, 18–26. [CrossRef]
132. de Oliveira Silva, F.; Ferreira, J.V.; Plácido, J.; Sant'Anna, P.; Araújo, J.; Marinho, V.; Laks, J.; Deslandes, A.C. Three months of multimodal training contributes to mobility and executive function in elderly individuals with mild cognitive impairment, but not in those with Alzheimer's disease: A randomized controlled trial. *Maturitas* **2019**, *126*, 28–33. [CrossRef]

133. Lixandrão, M.E.; Damas, F.; Chacon-Mikahil, M.P.; Cavaglieri, C.R.; Ugrinowitsch, C.; Bottaro, M.; Vechin, F.C.; Conceicao, R.B.; Libardi, C.A. Time Course of Resistance Training-Induced Muscle Hypertrophy in the Elderly. *J. Strength Cond. Res.* **2016**, *30*, 159–163.
134. Ribeiro, A.S.; Schoenfeld, B.J.; Souza, M.F.; Tomeleri, C.M.; Venturini, D.; Barbosa, D.S.; Cyrino, E.S. Traditional and pyramidal resistance training systems improve muscle quality and metabolic biomarkers in older women: A randomized crossover study. *Exp. Gerontol.* **2016**, *79*, 8–15. [CrossRef] [PubMed]
135. Da Silveira Fontenele De Meneses, Y.P.; Cabral, P.U.L.; Orsano, F.E.; Da Silveira, C.M.L. Vascular function and nitrite levels in elderly women before and after hydrogymnastics exercises. *J. Phys. Educ.* **2019**, *30*. [CrossRef]
136. Monteiro-Junior, R.S.; Figueiredo, L.F.D.S.; Maciel-Pinheiro, P.T.; Abud, E.L.R.; Engedal, K.; Barca, M.L.; Nascimento, O.J.M.; Laks, J.; Deslandes, A.C. Virtual Reality-Based Physical Exercise With Exergames (PhysEx) Improves Mental and Physical Health of Institutionalized Older Adults. *J. Am. Med. Dir. Assoc.* **2017**, *18*, 454. [CrossRef]
137. Aveiro, M.C.; Avila, M.A.; Pereira-Baldon, V.S.; Ceccatto-Oliveira, A.S.B.; Gramani-Say, K.; Oishi, J.; Driusso, P. Water- versus land-based treatment for postural control in postmenopausal osteoporotic women: A randomized, controlled trial. *Climacteric* **2017**, *20*, 427–435. [CrossRef]
138. Silva, M.R.; Alberton, C.L.; Portella, E.G.; Nunes, G.N.; Martin, D.G.; Pinto, S.S. Water-based aerobic and combined training in elderly women: Effects on functional capacity and quality of life. *Exp. Gerontol.* **2018**, *106*, 54–60. [CrossRef]
139. De Oliveira, V.H.; Câmara, G.L.G.; Azevedo, K.P.M.; Neto, E.C.A.; Dos Santos, I.K.; Medeiros, H.J.; Knackfuss, M.I. Weight training program with imposed and self-selected intensity on body composition in elderly: A randomized clinical trial. *Rev. Andaluza. Med. Deporte* **2019**, *12*, 11–14.
140. Simao, A.P.; Mendonca, V.A.; Avelar, N.C.P.; Fonseca, S.F.D.; Santos, J.M.; Oliveira, A.C.C.; Tossige-Gomes, R.; Ribeiro, V.G.C.; Cunha, C.D.; Balthazar, C.E.; et al. Whole body vibration training on muscle strength and brain-derived neurotrophic factor levels in elderly woman with knee osteoarthritis: A randomized clinical trial study. *Front. Physiol.* **2019**, *10*, 756. [CrossRef] [PubMed]
141. Grupo Banco Mundial. Población Mundial Total. Washington, DC, USA. 2019 [04 de agosto de 2020]. Available online: https://www.bancomundial.org/ (accessed on 20 February 2021).
142. Carvajal-Tapia, A.; Carvajal-Rodríguez, E. Producción científica en ciencias de la salud en los países de América Latina, 2006 2015: Análisis a partir de SciELO. *Rev. Interam. Bibl.* **2019**, *42*, 15–21. [CrossRef]
143. Organización de las Naciones Unidas para la Educación, la Ciencia y la Cultura (UNESCO). *Informe de la UNESCO para la ciencia hacia 2030: Panorámica de América Latina y el Caribe*; Ediciones UNESCO: París, Francia, 2015.
144. Sallis, J.; Bull, F.; Guthold, R.; Heath, G.W.; Inoue, S.; Kelly, P.; Oyeyemi, A.L.; Perez, L.G.; Richards, J.; Hallal, P.C.; et al. Progress in physical activity over the Olympic quadrennium. *Lancet* **2016**, *388*, 1325–1336. [CrossRef]
145. Organización Mundial de la Salud. *Informe Mundial Sobre el Envejecimiento y la Salud*; Ginebra, OMS: Ginebra, Suiza, 2015.
146. Peranovich, A. Enfermedades crónicas y factores de riesgo en adultos mayores de Argentina: Años 2001–2009. *Saúde Debate* **2016**, *40*, 125–135. [CrossRef]
147. Hay–Smith, E.J.; Englas, K.; Dumoulin, Ch.; Ferreira, C.H.; Frawley, H.; Weatherall, M. The Consensus on Exercise Reporting Template (CERT) in a systematic review of exercise-based rehabilitation effectiveness: Completeness of reporting, rater agreement, and utility. *Eur. J. Phys. Rehabil. Med.* **2019**, *55*, 342–352. [CrossRef] [PubMed]
148. Roller, M.; Kachingwe, A.; Beling, J.; Ickes, D.M.; Cabot, A.; Shrier, G. Pilates Reformer exercises for fall risk reduction in older adults: A randomized controlled trial. *J. Bodyw. Mov. Ther.* **2018**, *22*, 983–998. [CrossRef] [PubMed]
149. Zheng, L.; Li, G.; Wang, X.; Huiru, Y.; Jia, Y.; Leng, M.; Li, H.; Chen, L. Effect of exergames on physical outcomes in frail elderly: A systematic review [published online ahead of print, 2019 Sep 13]. *Aging Clin. Exp. Res.* **2019**. [CrossRef]
150. Pacheco, T.B.F.; de Medeiros, C.S.P.; de Oliveira, V.H.B.; Vieira, E.R.; de Cavalcanti, F.A.C. Effectiveness of exergames for improving mobility and balance in older adults: A systematic review and meta-analysis. *Syst. Rev.* **2020**, *9*, 163. [CrossRef]
151. Waller, B.; Ogonowska-Słodownik, A.; Vitor, M.; Rodionova, K.; Lambeck, J.; Heinonen, A.; Daly, D. The effect of aquatic exercise on physical functioning in the older adult: A systematic review with meta-analysis. *Age Ageing* **2016**, *45*, 593–601. [CrossRef] [PubMed]
152. Lai, C.C.; Tu, Y.K.; Wang, T.G.; Huang, Y.T.; Chien, K.L. Effects of resistance training, endurance training and whole-body vibration on lean body mass, muscle strength and physical performance in older people: A systematic review and network meta-analysis. *Age Ageing* **2018**, *47*, 367–373. [CrossRef] [PubMed]
153. Aboutorabi, A.; Arazpour, M.; Bahramizadeh, M.; Farahmand, F.; Fadayevatan, R. Effect of vibration on postural control and gait of elderly subjects: A systematic review. *Aging Clin. Exp. Res.* **2018**, *30*, 713–726. [CrossRef]
154. Jepsen, D.B.; Thomsen, K.; Hansen, S.; Jørgensen, N.R.; Masud, T.; Ryg, J. Effect of whole-body vibration exercise in preventing falls and fractures: A systematic review and meta-analysis. *BMJ Open* **2017**, *7*, e018342. [CrossRef]
155. Rogan, S.; de Bruin, E.D.; Radlinger, L.; Joehr, C.; Wyss, C.; Stuck, N.J.; Bruelhart, Y.; de Bie, R.A.; Hilfiker, R. Effects of whole-body vibration on proxies of muscle strength in old adults: A systematic review and meta-analysis on the role of physical capacity level. *Eur. Rev. Aging Phys. Act* **2015**, *12*, 12. [CrossRef]
156. Hart, P.D.; Buck, D.J. The effect of resistance training on health-related quality of life in older adults: Systematic review and meta-analysis. *Health Promot. Perspect.* **2019**, *9*, 1–12. [CrossRef]
157. Bouaziz, W.; Vogel, T.; Schmitt, E.; Kaltenbach, G.; Geny, B.; Lang, P.O. Health benefits of aerobic training programs in adults aged 70 and over: A systematic review. *Arch. Gerontol. Geriatr.* **2017**, *69*, 110–127. [CrossRef]

158. Lopez, P.; Pinto, R.S.; Radaelli, R.; Rech, A.; Grazioli, R.; Izquierdo, M.; Cadore, E.L. Benefits of resistance training in physically frail elderly: A systematic review. *Aging Clin. Exp. Res.* **2018**, *30*, 889–899. [CrossRef]
159. Guizelini, P.C.; de Aguiar, R.A.; Denadai, B.S.; Caputo, F.; Greco, C.C. Effect of resistance training on muscle strength and rate of force development in healthy older adults: A systematic review and meta-analysis. *Exp. Gerontol.* **2018**, *102*, 51–58. [CrossRef]
160. Hollings, M.; Mavros, Y.; Freeston, J.; Fiatarone-Singh, M. The effect of progressive resistance training on aerobic fitness and strength in adults with coronary heart disease: A systematic review and meta-analysis of randomised controlled trials. *Eur. J. Prev. Cardiol.* **2017**, *24*, 1242–1259. [CrossRef]
161. Galloza, J.; Castillo, B.; Micheo, W. Benefits of Exercise in the Older Population. *Phys. Med. Rehabil. Clin. N. Am.* **2017**, *28*, 659–669. [CrossRef]
162. Jadczak, A.D.; Makwana, N.; Luscombe-Marsh, N.; Visvanathan, R.; Schultz, T.J. Effectiveness of exercise interventions on physical function in community-dwelling frail older people: An umbrella review of systematic reviews. *JBI Database Syst. Rev. Implement Rep.* **2018**, *16*, 752–775. [CrossRef]
163. Abdullah-Alfadhel, S.A.; Vennu, V.; Alotaibi, A.D.; Algarni, A.M.; Saad-Bindawas, S.M. The effect of a multicomponent exercise programme onelderly adults' risk of falling in nursing homes: A systematic review. *J. Pak. Med. Assoc.* **2020**, *70*, 699–704.
164. Izquierdo, M.; Casas, A.; Zambom, F.; Martínez, N.; Alonso, C.; Rodriguez, L.; VIVIFRAIL. Guía Práctica Para la Prescripción de un Programa de Entrenamiento Físico Multicomponente Para la Prevención de la Fragilidad y Caídas en Mayores de 70 años. Navarra, España. 2017. Available online: http://vivifrail.com/es/inicio/ (accessed on 24 July 2020).
165. Li, S.Y.H.; Bressington, D. The effects of mindfulness-based stress reduction on depression, anxiety, and stress in older adults: A systematic review and meta-analysis. *Int. J. Ment. Health Nurs.* **2019**, *28*, 635–656. [CrossRef] [PubMed]
166. Gómez-Cabello, A.; Vila-Maldonado, S.; Pedrero-Chamizo, R.; Villa-Vicente, J.G.; Gusi, G.; Espino, L.; González, M.; Casajus, J.; Ara, I. La actividad física organizada en las personas mayores, una herramienta para mejorar la condición física en la senectud. *Rev. Esp. Salud Pública* **2018**, *92*, e201803013.
167. Kruisselbrink, L.D.; Dodge, A.M.; Swanburg, S.L.; & MacLeod, A.L. Influence of Same-Sex and Mixed-Sex Exercise Settings on the Social Physique Anxiety and Exercise Intentions of Males and Females. *J. Sport Exerc. Psychol.* **2004**, *26*, 616–622. [CrossRef]
168. Rodríguez, E.; Ara, I.; Mata, E.A.; Aguado, X. Jump and balance performance in an active young and elderly Spanish population. *Apunts Med. Esport* **2012**, *47*.
169. Claros, J.; Cruz, M.V.; Beltrán, Y. Effects of physical exercise on functional fitness and stability in older adults. *Rev. Hacia. Promoción Salud* **2012**, *17*, 79–90.
170. Zech, A.; Hübscher, M.; Vogt, L.; Banzer, W.; Hänsel, F.; Pfeifer, K. Balance Trainning for Neuromuscular Control and Performance Enhancement: A systematic Review. *J. Athl. Train.* **2010**, *45*, 392–403. [CrossRef] [PubMed]
171. Bize, R.; Johnson, J.A.; Plotnikoff, R.C. Physical activity level and health-related quality of life in the general adult population: A systematic review. *Prev. Med.* **2007**, *45*, 401–415. [CrossRef]
172. Anokye, N.K.; Trueman, P.; Green, C.; Pavey, T.G.; Taylor, R.S. Physical activity and health related quality of life. *BMC Public Health* **2012**, *12*, 624. [CrossRef]

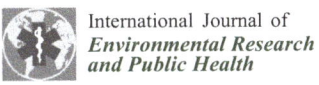

Review

Isokinetic Trunk Strength in Acute Low Back Pain Patients Compared to Healthy Subjects: A Systematic Review

Waleska Reyes-Ferrada [1,2], Luis Chirosa-Rios [1], Angela Rodriguez-Perea [1], Daniel Jerez-Mayorga [3,*] and Ignacio Chirosa-Rios [1]

1. Department Physical Education and Sports, Faculty of Sport Sciences, University of Granada, 18011 Granada, Spain; waleska.reyes@unab.cl (W.R.-F.); lchirosa@ugr.es (L.C.-R.); angrp91@gmail.com (A.R.-P.); ichirosa@ugr.es (I.C.-R.)
2. Faculty of Rehabilitation Sciences, Universidad Andres Bello, Viña del Mar 2531015, Chile
3. Faculty of Rehabilitation Sciences, Universidad Andres Bello, Santiago 7591538, Chile
* Correspondence: daniel.jerez@unab.cl; Tel.: +56-9-77697643

Abstract: Background: The purpose of this systematic review was to: (I) determine the quality of evidence from studies assessing trunk isokinetic strength in subjects with acute low back pain (ALBP) compared to healthy subjects and (II) establish reference values of isokinetic trunk strength in subjects with ALBP. Methodology: Preferred Reporting Items for Systematic Review and Meta-Analyses (PRISMA) statements were followed using keywords associated with trunk, strength and low back pain. Four databases were used: PubMed, Web of Science, Scopus and SPORTDiscus. Methodological quality was assessed using the Quality Assessment of Diagnostic Accuracy Studies (QUADAS). Results: A total of 1604 articles were retrieved, four included in this review. All were evaluated as high risk of bias (Rob). Due to the high Rob and the diversity of protocols, instruments and variables used, it was not possible to determine reference values for subjects with ALBP, we can only establish a range of flexion peak torque (PT) between 175.1 and 89.7 Nm at 60°/s and between 185 and 81.5 Nm at 120°/s, and for extension PT between 240.0 and 91.5 Nm at 60°/s and between 217.5 and 69.2 Nm at 120°/s in subjects with ALBP. Conclusions: Due to the low quality of the evidence and the diversity of protocols used when measuring trunk isokinetic strength, it is necessary to carry out new high-quality research to establish reference values of trunk strength in subjects with ALBP.

Keywords: dynamometer; core muscles; trunk strength testing; reference data; peak torque

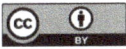

1. Introduction

Low back pain (LBP) is among the three leading causes of years lived with disability [1], only in 2017 577 million people suffered from LBP [2]. LBP refers to pain, muscle tension or stiffness below the costal border and over the lower gluteal fold, with or without sciatia. It can be classified according to its duration in acute low back pain (ALBP), less than six weeks, or chronic low back pain (CLBP) when the pain persists for more than three months [3]. It is estimated that 80% of the population will suffer from LBP at least once in their lives [4,5], but these symptoms should disappear within six weeks. Although a significant number of patients will have recurrences or persistent pain and disability [6,7], even in the follow-up to one year, some patients will still show mild to moderate levels of pain and disability [8]. Da Silva et al. [9] reports a pain episode recurrence in 70% of the patients within 12 months after recovery from the first ALBP episode, of which 40% will suffer a moderate functional limitation or will need to use the health system, suggesting that the good prognosis of ALBP has been overestimated.

Regarding the cause of the LBP, it is not often possible to determine an anatomical source of pain (e.g., epidural abscess, compression fracture, spondyloarthropathy, malignancy or cauda equina syndrome) [10]. Most of the times, in 90% of cases, no specific cause is identified for which it is denominated non-specific LBP (NSLBP) [10]. However, multiple factors have been associated with the occurrence of NSLBP, among them the alteration of the neuromuscular response of the trunk [11,12], the deconditioning (or decrease in the function) of the lumbar musculature [13,14], the reduction in the muscular mass of the trunk [15], and the reduction in the muscular strength of the trunk [13,16,17].

The spine needs to be mechanically stable at all times to avoid injuries that can eventually lead to pain [18]. Maintaining this stability is role of the active neuromuscular system [19], and thus the trunk strength plays an important role in different aspects related to health and sport [20–23]. The trunk is the center of the kinematic chains, transferring forces and acting as a bridge between the upper and lower extremities [24]. Arms and legs can be compared with their contralateral to define deficits or imbalances but, unlike the extremities, the trunk does not have this possibility, which makes it difficult to find parameters of normality or reference. Trunk strength has been related to injury prevention [25,26], which is why it plays an important role in the functional evaluation of people or athletes [27,28].

To evaluate trunk strength, several methods have been developed. The gold standard is the isokinetic dynamometry, which consists of measuring muscle strength capacity under linear or rotational movements at constant velocities [29]. This method allows a quick quantification of several muscle function parameters at different positions and angular velocities, and its use has been recommended for clinical and research purposes [30].

Prospective studies have shown that trunk strength imbalance [17] and decreased trunk muscle strength could be considered risk factors for developing NSLBP, specifically isometric and isokinetic strength of trunk flexors and lumbar extensors muscles [16]. To the best of our knowledge, there are no reference values in the development of the first episode of ALBP; instead, the evidence shows that, when comparing healthy subjects with CLBP patients, the lumbar extensor peak torque is lower, but the flexor peak torque does not decrease in the same way, so the ratio flexors/extensors (F/E) do not decrease [31]. These data are important since the parameters of isokinetic strength could be used for the early detection of people at risk for developing NSLBP. However, these reference data correspond to subjects with CLBP, and were obtained from reviews in which no assessment of the quality of the evidence was carried out. This could limit our confidence in the reported data [31,32]. Furthermore, in CLBP, the evidence shows that pain and disability do have physical causes and have multifactorial etiology [33], with psychological factors [34], central sensitization [35] and kinesiophobia [36] playing a role in this type of patient. De Souza et al. [37] demonstrated that the peak torque of lumbar extensors in women with CLBP who have fear or negative beliefs related to the activity could be modified merely by using kinesiotape. This suggests that probably the strength values obtained in this type of patient may be influenced by other processes related to chronic pain and may not be an appropriate measurement on their own.

This allows us to question whether we estimate the ability to exert maximum trunk strength in subjects with chronic pain. Establishing whether an alteration in trunk muscle strength is present in those subjects who suffer from ALBP compared to healthy subjects is paramount in order to be able to develop training programs for preventing ALBP in the general population, and to manage this type of patient, avoiding its progression to CLBP. It is necessary to have data on the trunk's isokinetic strength in patients with ALBP that will allow determination of which people are at risk for developing ALBP and thus prevent its appearance in healthy people. Moreover, this is necessary to manage it and avoid its progression to CLBP. Thus, the objective of this systematic review was (I) to determine the quality of evidence from studies assessing trunk isokinetic strength in subjects with ALBP compared to healthy subjects and (II) establish reference values of isokinetic trunk strength in subjects with ALBP.

2. Materials and Methods

The Preferred Reporting Items for Systematic Review and Meta-Analyses guidelines (PRISMA) were used [38] (Supplementary Table S1). The protocol of this review was registered in PROSPERO (CRD42020193458).

2.1. Study Search

Two authors (WR-F and DJ-M) conducted the search. The databases used were PubMed, Web of Science, Scopus and SPORTDiscus. The search was carried out from their inception to October 2020, the following keywords were included: "isokinetic", "muscle strength", "dynamometer", "CORE", "abdominal muscles", "abdominal wall", "torso", "trunk", "low back pain", "low back ache" y "lumbago". Search strategies are presented in Supplementary Table S2.

2.2. Eligibility Criteria

Articles that met the following criteria were included in this review. For aim (I): adult participants (age $\geq$18 years old), measures of isokinetic trunk flexors and extensors strength comparing a group of individuals with ALBP with a healthy control group, full-text available, and articles in English. For aim (II), the criteria for aim (I) were applied, but all the studies assessing isokinetic trunk flexors and extensors strength in individuals with ALBP, regardless of having a healthy control group or not, were included. Studies that only included either healthy people or subjects with chronic low-back pain were excluded.

2.3. Study Selection

Articles that were found eligible for inclusion in this review were entered into the Rayyan QCRI application, an app that assists in the article selection process, optimizing the screening time and allowing collaborative tasks (available for free at http://rayyan.qcri.org (accessed on 19 June 2020)) [39]. Duplicate references were removed, and two independent researchers (WR-F and DJ-M) reviewed titles and abstracts to identify articles met the eligibility criteria. The selected articles were then read in full, and the reference list was checked for relevant articles that could be included.

2.4. Assessment of the Risk of Bias and Quality of Evidence

Each article included in this systematic review was independently assessed for methodological quality and risk of bias by two researchers (WR-F and DJ-M). To the best of our knowledge, there is no scale for methodological evaluation adequate for the purpose of this review; therefore, we used the checklist proposed by Castro et al. [40], which combines some items from QUADAS [41] and a checklist to evaluate the methodological quality of both randomized and non-randomized studies of health care interventions [42]. This scale has 15 items divided into three sections (study sample, test procedures and data analysis, and results presentation). Each item was scored as "yes," "no," "unclear," or "not applied". A study was considered high risk of bias (low quality) when it received five or more "no" or "unclear" scores; in contrast, a study was considered low risk of bias (high quality) when it received less than five "no" or "unclear" scores. This cut-off score was determined on the basis of previous reviews that determined that 30% of negative results discriminate between studies of low or high methodological quality [43]. In case of disagreement among researchers, the consensus approach was used; for the case in which consensus could not be reached, a third researcher was consulted (LC-R).

2.5. Data Extraction and Analysis

The data extraction was performed by each researcher independently; the information extracted was related to the identification of the article (authors, year of publication, design and objective), the characteristics of the participants (total sample, gender, age, weight and height) and the isokinetic evaluation protocol (movement, position, range of movement, angular velocity, repetitions and contraction mode), in addition to results and main conclusions.

3. Results

3.1. Article Selection

No systematic reviews with a similar objective as the present study were found. From the initial search, a total of 1603 articles were retrieved (Figure 1), of which 610 were eliminated because they were duplicates. One additional article was identified from other sources. All the articles that assessed isokinetic trunk strength in individuals with ALBP presented a control group. Therefore, the number of articles included for aim (I) and aim (II) were the same. After evaluating titles and abstracts, 977 articles were excluded because they did not meet the inclusion criteria, leaving 17 articles for full-text analysis.

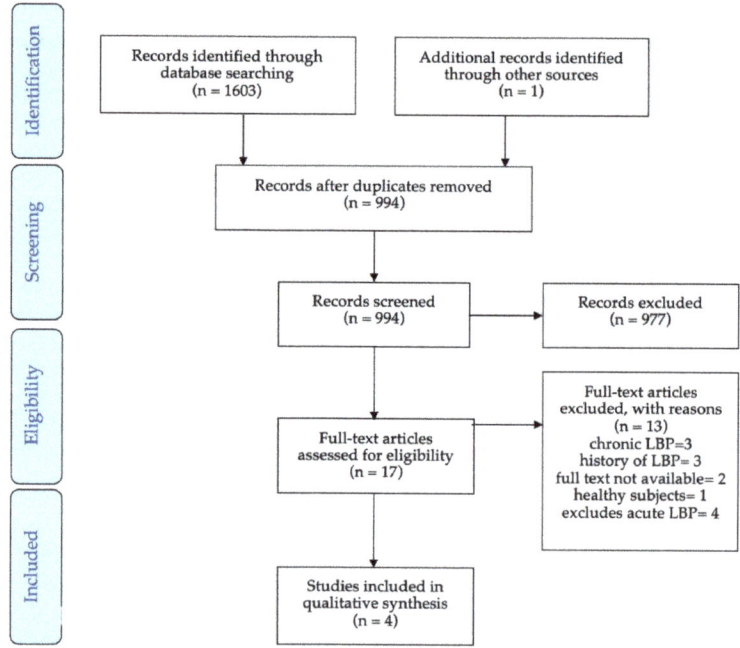

Figure 1. Flow chart for the systematic review.

Of the 17 articles, two could not be retrieved because when contacting the authors, they did not have a digital copy to share due to the age of the publication (1982 and 1994). Of the remaining 15, after reading the full text, 11 articles were eliminated because they did not include the evaluation of subjects with ALBP. Thus, four articles were selected, and their reference lists were checked, and there were no new articles found.

3.2. Characteristics of the Studies

Table 1 presents the main characteristics of the included studies. One study [44] divided patients according to the duration of symptoms as acute and chronic, two [45,46] did so in acute, subacute and chronic, and only one [47] considered only subjects with acute pain. The number of participants with ALBP ranged from 21 to 46 subjects; Gabr et al. [46] do not indicate the exact number of ALBP subjects enrolled in their study. Age was not specified in the ALBP group in three of four studies, with only Hupli et al. [47] reporting an average age of 40.1 ± 8.9 years for men and 43.5 ± 9.2 for women. The physical activity profile was reported in only one study [47], but it does not specify which tool is measured.

Table 1. Characteristics of individual studies.

Study	Objective	Participants	Age, Weight and Height (Mean ± SD)	Movement, Position and ROM	Velocity and Repetitions	Contraction Mode	Measured Outcomes
Suzuki et al. [44]	To measure the muscle strength and fatigability of the trunk flexors and extensors in normal pain-free subjects and in patients with LBP and to determine the role of the trunk muscles in LBP syndrome.	LBP group: 90 men. Acute pain: 38 Control group: 50 healthy men.	LBP group: 29.7 ± 5.4 yrs., 61.1 ± 8.5 kg, 167.8 ± 4.6 cm. Control group: 28.3 ± 4.3 yrs., 59.8 ± 7.5 kg, 167.8 ± 5.2 cm.	Flexion 1: Supine with hands behind the neck, with hips and knees extended. Flexion 2: supine, hands behind the head, hips and knees bent. Extension: prone arms at the sides. ROM: 30° flexion and extension.	30°/s 1 rep of 90 s	Isometric: no distinction according to duration of symptoms. Isokinetic: concentric, according to duration of symptoms (ALBP and CLBP).	Torque isometric (J); Trunk flexion (Joule), Trunk extension (J), abdominal strength (J)
Akebi et al. [45]	To examine the difference in coefficient of variance (CV) of isokinetic trunk strength between healthy subjects and LBP patients.	LBP group: 143 (93 men and 50 women) Acute pain: 46, men 29 and women 17. Subacute pain: 38 Chronic pain: 59 Control group: 200 healthy subjects (112 men and 88 women)	LBP group: Men 51 ± 15.7 yrs., women: 50 ± 14.7 yrs. Control group: Men 49 ± 15.5 yrs., women 51 ± 15.3 yrs. Weight and height not described.	Standing with knees in semi-flexion. ROM: 0°–60° flexion and extension.	60°/s 3 rep 120°/s 5 rep	Isokinetic: concentric.	Coefficient of variance (%)
Hupli et al. [47]	To compare of trunk strength measurements between two different isokinetic devices used in clinical settings	LBP group: 21 (11 men and 10 women). Control group: 20 healthy subjects (10 men and 10 women)	LBP group: Men 40.1 ± 8.9 yrs., 79.5 ± 9.4 kg, 177.6 ± 4.9 cm. Women: 43.5 ± 9.2 yrs., 66.0 ± 13.3 kg, 164.9 ± 6.4 cm. Control group: Men: 39.7 ± 7.6 yrs., 78.9 ± 5.6 kg, 180.5 ± 6.8 cm. Women: 43.2 ± 7.2 yrs., 65.5 ± 6.8 kg, 168.6 ± 5.2 cm.	Standing with knees in semi-flexion. ROM: natural movement from vertical to flexion that each subject could perform.	60°/s and 120°/s 5 rep.	Isokinetic: concentric.	Average peak torque (Nm)
Gabr et al. [46]	To check and compare the muscle torque and power velocity of the trunk muscles in healthy men and male patients with low back pain to detect the relationship between low back pain and trunk muscles strength in the absence of structural neurological lesions.	LBP group: 50 men. Does not specify number per acute, subacute and chronic group. Control group: 50 healthy men.	LBP group: 22.9 ± 3.4 yrs., 77.7 ± 21.1 kg, 170.6 ± 6.4 cm. Control group: 23.4 ± 3.9 yrs., 76.1 ± 15.5 kg, 170.6 ± 7.9 cm.	Semi standing position. ROM: adjusted to each subject for maximum flexion and extension.	60°/s and 120°/s	Isokinetic: concentric.	Peak torque, flexors/extensor ratio, average power of trunk flexor and extensor.

SD: standard deviation; ROM: Range of motion; LBP: Low back pain; yrs.: years; rep: repetitions; s: seconds; ALBP: acute low back pain; CLBP: chronic low back pain.

Regarding the isokinetic dynamometer used, Suzuki et al. [44] used Cybex II, Akebi et al. [45] did not specify it, Hupli et al. [47] compared two dynamometers: Ariel 5000 (Ariel dynamics Inc., Trabuco Canyon, CA, USA) and Lido Multi-Joint II (loredan Biomedical, Inc., West Sacramento, CA, USA), while Gabr et al. [46] used biodex system 4 pro. Regarding the position in which the trunk strength was measured, three studies were performed in the standing position with knees in semi-flexion [45–47] and one study [44] used the supine position. In relation to the range of movement used, there was no concordance among the studies. One study used natural movement [47], another one 30° of flexion–extension [44], another one [45] a range of 0°–60° and another one the movement of maximum flexion and extension [46]. Three studies measured at velocities of 60°/s and 120°/s [45–47], while Suzuki et al. [44] used 30°/s.

The strength variables calculated were: (I) average peak torque (Nm), (II) trunk flexion (J), (III) trunk extension (J), (IV) abdominal strength (J), (V) average power, (VI) flexion-extension ratio (%) (flexion strength/extensor strength), (VII) fatigue (%) calculated as: (initial muscle strength–final muscle strength/initial muscle strength) x 100, and (VIII) Coefficient of Torque Variation (%).

3.3. Methodological Quality and Risk of Bias

In this review, 57 items (95%) were evaluated in the agreement between the two reviewers, the remaining three were decided by agreement (Table 2).

Table 2. Methodological quality of the studies included.

Studies	\multicolumn{15}{c}{Items}	Total of N/UC	Total RoB
	1	2	3	4	5	6	7	8	9	10	11	12	13	14	15		
Suzuki et al. [44]	Y	N	N	N	UC	UC	NA	Y	UC	UC	UC	UC	N	Y	UC	11	High RoB
Akebi et al. [45]	N	N	N	Y	UC	UC	NA	Y	UC	UC	UC	UC	N	UC	Y	11	High RoB
Hupli et al. [47]	Y	N	N	Y	UC	Y	NA	Y	UC	Y	Y	UC	N	Y	UC	7	High RoB
Gabr et al. [46]	Y	Y	N	UC	UC	UC	NA	Y	UC	UC	Y	UC	N	Y	Y	8	High RoB

Items considered for rating: 1. Was the study population adequately described (i.e., sex, age, body mass, body height, kind of physical activity/lifestyle (sedentary, athlete, level of physical activity))?; 2. Was the description of selection criteria presented?; 3. Was there justification of appropriate sample size (through calculation or guidelines)?; 4. Were warm-ups and a familiarization protocol performed?; 5. Were type of muscle action (i.e., concentric and eccentric), sequence of action (i.e., concentric–concentric, concentric–eccentric, eccentric–eccentric), and velocity of movement described?; 6. Was the order of tests (velocities and trunk) randomized or counterbalanced?; 7. Was the lower limb dominance considered?; 8. Was the standardization of positions, movements and stabilization performed and properly described?; 9. Did participants receive the same encouragement during the test?; 10. Was gravity correction considered?; 11. Were the outcome measures clearly described?; 12. Were data extracted from the isokinetic load range?; 13. Were measures of reliability (e.g., Intraclass correlation coefficients (ICC), Standard error of the mean (SEM)) presented?; 14. Were results clearly described?; 15. Were appropriate inferential statistics presented?. N: no; Y: yes; UC: unclear; NA: not applied; RoB: risk of bias.

3.3.1. Sample

Regarding the sample, three studies [44,46,47] describe the sample properly (item 1), however, only Gabr et al. [46] specified the inclusion criteria (item 2), none of the included articles explained how the sample size was calculated (item 3).

3.3.2. Procedure

In relation to the trunk isokinetic evaluation procedure, two studies [45,47] report a familiarization process prior to measurement (item 4), none of them properly report the type or sequence of contraction only reporting the angular velocity used (item 5), only one study [47] reports a randomized order in the evaluations (item 6), and none of the four inform of the dominance of the extremities (item 7) which was evaluated as "not applied" because it is the trunk. All four studies [44–47] correctly describe the assessment position, the movements, and the form of stabilization used (item 8). None of the studies specify whether or not the same encouragement was given to each participant during the assessment (item 9). Considering the data analysis, only Hupli et al. [47] report that the

Lido dynamometer software compensates for gravity, while Ariel does not (item 10); it is not clear if the other three studies performed gravity correction. Regarding the dependent variable, two studies clearly describe how the data extraction was performed [46,47], while, in the other two studies [44,45], it is not clear how data such as fatigue or the coefficient of variation were determined. None of the studies clarify whether the data were extracted from the isokinetic load range (item 12), and none report reliability measures, such as the intra-class correlation coefficient or standard error measurement (item 13).

3.3.3. Presentation of Results

Regarding the presentation of results, three studies [44,46,47] adequately presented the results (item 14) and two [45,46] properly presented the inferential statistics (item 15). In summary, the four studies showed a high risk of bias [44–47].

3.4. Trunk Strength Parameters

Only two studies [46,47] measured peak torque in a similar way (Table 3).

3.4.1. Average Peak Torque in Flexion and Extension

Two studies [46,47] determined the average peak torque in flexion and extension in healthy subjects and those with ALBP, measuring in standing, concentric mode, at velocities of 60°/s and 120°/s. Hupli et al. [47] compared men and women with ALBP and healthy subjects using two dynamometers, finding small, non-statistically significant differences between groups. Gabr et al, [46] when comparing men with ALBP and healthy controls, found significant differences in the peak torque of flexors ($p = 0.004$) and extensors ($p = 0.003$) at 60°/s and flexors ($p < 0.001$) and extensors ($p < 0.001$) at 120°/s, with an inverse F/E ratio at speeds of 120°/s in the ALBP group (Table 3).

3.4.2. Coefficient of Variation

Akebi et al. [45] evaluated the relationship of the variability of the torque curves (CV) between subjects with ALBP and healthy controls finding CV values lower than the evaluation at 60°/s compared to 120°/s and, in addition, in both men and women the CV was lower in the control subjects compared to ALBP (Table 3).

3.4.3. Average Power

Gabr et al. [46] found significant differences between average power in flexion ($p = 0.004$) and extension ($p = 0.014$) at 60°/s and between average power in flexion ($p = 0.001$) and extension ($p = 0.045$) at 120°/s between men with ALBP and a control group (Table 3).

3.5. Adverse Outcome from Trunk Isokinetic Assessment

From all the articles reviewed, none report adverse effects during trunk strength measurement using an isokinetic dynamometer in patients with ALBP. Suzuki et al. [44] and Gabr et al. [46] report that the assessment was performed without any complaints, Akebi et al. [45] do not report any undesirable effects during the assessment, and only Hupli et al. [47] reports a pain measured with visual analogue scale (VAS) (0–100) of 26.3 using the Ariel dynamometer and 15.2 with the Lido dynamometer in subjects with ALBP.

Table 3. Isokinetic trunk strength in acute low back pain patients (ALBP) and healthy adults for trunk extension and flexion.

Movement	Position	Acute LBP Group (Mean ± SD)	Control Group (Mean ± SD)	Unit	Study
Flexion	Supine	71.20 ± 22.85 (J)	86.69 ± 27.66 (J)	Trunk flexion (J)	Suzuki et al. [44]
		49.7 ± 21.7	42.0 ± 21.7	Fatigue (%)	Suzuki et al. [44]
	Standing	Ariel: 60°/s: 175.1 ± 61.4 Nm 120°/s: 155.7 ± 58.3 Nm Lido: 60°/s: 165.2 ± 47.7 Nm 120°/s: 185.0 ± 54.0 Nm	Ariel: 60°/s: 171.3 ± 45.2 Nm 120°/s: 165.2 ± 47.2 Nm Lido: 60°/s: 168.4 ± 48.8 Nm 120°/s: 187.0 ± 61.7 Nm	Average peak torque (Nm)	Hupli et al. [47]
		60°/s: Men: 89.7 ± 34.5 Nm 120°/s: Men: 81.5 ± 34.9 Nm	60°/s: Men: 118.7 ± 37.1 Nm 120°/s: Men: 121.1 ± 39.7 Nm	Average Peak torque	Gabr et al. [46]
		60°/s: Men: 38.9 ± 19.7 120°/s: Men: 32.0 ± 24.9	60°/s: Men 56.0 ± 25.2 120°/s: Men: 57.7 ± 36.5	Average Power	Gabr et al. [46]
		60°/s: Men: 12.2 ± 5.4 Women: 12.2 ± 7.1. 120°/s: Men: 20.4 ± 9.2 Women: 29.7 ± 15.5	60°/s: Men: 8.9 ± 6.5 Women: 9.5 ± 4.9. 120°/s: Men: 17.3 ± 6.2 Women: 21.1 ± 8.0	Coefficient of variance (%)	Akebi et al. [45]
Extension	Supine	132.98 ± 29.91	156.72 ± 37.66	Trunk extension (J)	Suzuki et al. [44]
		19.3 ± 13.2	17.2 ± 10.8	Fatigue (%)	Suzuki et al. [44]
	Standing	Ariel: 60°/s: 178.9 ± 55.2 Nm 120°/s: 165.6 ± 52.6 Nm Lido: 60°/s: 240.0 ± 85.4 Nm 120°/s: 217.5 ± 89.5 Nm	Ariel: 60°/s: 189.3 ± 49.4 Nm 120°/s: 182.4 ± 52.6 Nm Lido: 60°/s: 264.0 ± 73.1 Nm 120°/s: 249.5 ± 68.3 Nm	Average peak torque (Nm)	Hupli et al. [47]
		60°/s: Men: 91.5 ± 57.1 Nm 120°/s: Men: 69.2 ± 49.6 Nm	60°/s: Men: 141.0 ± 64.5 Nm 120°/s: Men: 125.5 ± 68.1 Nm	Average Peak torque [46]	Gabr et al. [46]
		60°/s: Men: 41.8 ± 35.2 120°/s: Men: 37.6 ± 37.1	60°/s: Men: 68.4 ± 47.6 120°/s: Men: 61.7 ± 59.0	Average Power [46]	Gabr et al. [46]
		60°/s: Men: 11.4 ± 6.9 Women: 11.6 ± 5.9 120°/s: Men: 21.9 ± 9.0 Women: 24.5 ± 14.1.	60°/s: Men: 8.0 ± 5.8 Women: 9.2 ± 5.3. 120°/s: Men: 16.6 ± 6.6 Women: 22.2 ± 9.0.	Coefficient of variance (%)	Akebi et al. [45]
Flexion–Extension ratio (%)	Supine	55.9 ± 18.8	57.2 ± 16.0	% Trunk flexion/extension (J)	Suzuki et al. [44]
Abdominal Strength	Supine	69.73 ± 24.13	79.04 ± 29.22	Joule	Suzuki et al. [44]

SD: standard deviation; s: seconds.

4. Discussion

The present systematic review was designed to (I) determine the quality of evidence from studies assessing trunk isokinetic strength in subjects with ALBP compared to healthy subjects and (II) establish reference values of isokinetic trunk strength in subjects with ALBP. The main findings of this study were (I) the articles included in this review present a high risk of bias; therefore, this indicates low quality of evidence, and (II) it was not possible to determine reference values, neither was it possible to determine whether trunk strength can distinguish between patients with ALBP and healthy subjects. However, based on data provided in the articles reviewed, we can report a range of peak flexion torque between 175. 1 Nm and 89.7 Nm at 60°/s and between 185 Nm and 81.5 Nm at 120°/s, and for peak torque in extension between 240.0 Nm and 91.5 Nm at 60°/s and between 217.5 Nm and 69.2 Nm at 120°/s in subjects with ALBP.

In addition to considering research with a low risk of bias, we should also consider studies with similar evaluation protocols to suggest reference values. Estrázulas et al. [48] after reviewing the literature, recommend reliable protocols for the evaluation of trunk flexors and extensors, carried out in a sitting position at velocities of 30°/s and 60°/s with a range of 30° (10° of flexion and 20° of extension) and/or in a standing position at velocities of 60°/s and 90°/s with a range between 90° and 95° of flexion and 15° of extension, both protocols in concentric mode with the axis in the anterior superior iliac spine. In the four studies reviewed, none included evaluation in sitting position; three of them [45–47] used the standing position but in a different range to the suggested and with velocities of 60°/s and 120°/s, which are commonly used in the measurement of trunk strength [48].

Concerning the variable analyzed, we know that the peak torque is widely used as a reference, allowing a direct comparison between studies. It has been previously used by Mueller et al. [31,49] to analyze subjects with low back pain, to determine deficits and to assess the effectiveness of training or therapy. In this review, two of the four included studies used peak torque in their analysis; however, Hupli et al. [47] found differences between the dynamometers used and therefore conclude and recommend that these data should not be compared among themselves. Analyzing this same variable, Gabr et al. [46] found that, unlike patients with CLBP, patients with ALBP have a significant reduction in the strength of trunk flexors and extensors, with an inverse F/E ratio at 120°/s, that is, greater than one, which indicates that the extensor muscles were mostly affected by the weakness. Mueller et al. [31] had previously reported the same, but with data from CLBP subjects, where a greater decrease in extensors' strength was observed than in flexors, so the F/E ratio was higher than in healthy subjects. It is important to note that only the 60°/s flexor values obtained by Gabr et al. [46] are similar to those described by Mueller et al. [31] for the CLBP group, and those of 60°/s flexors in healthy subjects by Hupli et al. [47] with the control group by Mueller et al. [31]. On the other hand, Suzuki et al. [44] report differences in the strength of flexors and trunk extensors between ALBP and asymptomatic subjects, however, this variable was measured in Joules, which does not allow comparison, and also only indicates the existence of statistical differences, but does not report the p-value.

It is important to consider that none of the studies included in this review performed an isometric strength assessment of trunk flexors and extensors in subjects with ALBP using an isokinetic dynamometer. Among the studies reviewed, only Suzuki et al [44] evaluated isometric strength; however, they considered as a single group patients with acute and chronic pain (who had an average of eleven years of pain); so, unfortunately, it was not possible to distinguish isometric strength values in subjects with ALBP. Isometric evaluation is reliable in subjects with CLBP [50], and lower values of trunk strength have been observed in athletes and non-athletes with CLBP compared to healthy individuals. Cho et al. [16] propose that the risk for LBP and its severity would be associated with isokinetic weakness and the isometric weakness of trunk flexors and extensors.

From this, it is necessary to consider the importance of measuring these parameters in patients with ALBP, which could be used as an indicator of functionality or prognosis in these subjects, since isokinetic dynamometry has been widely used to evaluate the trunk strength but in patients with CLBP [50–53]; however, few studies have evaluated patients with ALBP.

Based on this systematic review, we cannot recommend reference values for the strength of trunk flexors and extensors in subjects with ALBP due to the high risk of bias of the articles included and the diversity of protocols, instruments and variables used in each article. Although three [44–46] of the four studies reviewed report differences in some strength parameters between individuals with ALBP and healthy subjects, these data are not confident given the limited quality of the evidence. Thus, it was also not possible to determine whether strength levels can help us distinguish between patients with ALBP and healthy subjects. On the other hand, we did not identify any studies that compared eccentric strength among these people. The eccentric contraction occurs when the external force is greater than the muscle strength, therefore, it plays an important role in the activities of daily life and sports, in the deceleration of the body during movements [54], so it would be interesting to investigate different types of contraction and eccentric/concentric ratio in subjects with ALBP compared to healthy subjects to understand the muscle dynamics of the trunk in different contexts or activities.

We can consider this review's strength as having considered research with no prior date limit until 2020. However, that presents us with an associated difficulty since the studies we include have a range of 36 years of difference, time in which the standards of scientific publication have changed, and new guidelines have been developed [55,56], which could explain the high risk of bias found in this review.

In this context, it is necessary to conduct rigorous longitudinal studies, based on current methodological guidelines, that allow us to detect people at risk for developing ALBP and that consider the multiple aspects involved in LBP, both physical and psychological. For this reason, we can suggest the formation of working groups to determine consensus on the best way to approach the evaluation of this type of patient. For the reasons mentioned earlier, we consider it necessary to carry out new studies of high methodological quality that allow us to clarify if there are levels of strength associated with ALBP and to be able to prevent its appearance. In addition, given the questions regarding the evaluation of unnatural movements or those that do not necessarily represent the physiology or velocity of the movement performed on the isokinetic dynamometer [57], it is necessary to develop new technologies [28,58] that allow the evaluation of trunk strength related to a functional or athletic context that mimics the functional demands of the athlete or patient.

5. Conclusions

The findings of this systematic review indicate that the quality of studies assessing isokinetic trunk strength in subjects with ALBP compared to healthy controls was weak. Moreover, the available data did not allow presentation of reference values in patients with ALBP. Future research of high methodological quality is needed to establish reference values of trunk isokinetic strength in subjects with ALBP and to determine the ability of trunk strength to discriminate ALBP patients from healthy individuals.

Supplementary Materials: The following are available online at https://www.mdpi.com/1660-4601/18/5/2576/s1, Table S1: PRISMA 2009 check list, Table S2: Search strategy for each database and number of articles found.

Author Contributions: Conceptualization, W.R.-F. and D.J.-M.; methodology, W.R.-F. and D.J.-M.; formal analysis, W.R.-F., D.J.-M., A.R.-P., L.C.-R.; writing—original draft preparation W.R.-F. and D.J.-M.; writing—review and editing, W.R.-F., D.J.-M., A.R.-P., L.C.-R., I.C.-R.; visualization, W.R.-F., D.J.-M., A.R.-P., L.C.-R., I.C.-R.; supervision, W.R.-F., L.C.-R. and D.J.-M. All authors have read and agreed to the published version of the manuscript.

Funding: This study has been partially supported by FEDER/ Ministry of Science, Innovation and Universities-State Research Agency (Dossier number: RTI2018-099723-B-I00).

Institutional Review Board Statement: Not applicable.

Informed Consent Statement: Not applicable.

Acknowledgments: This paper will be part of Waleska Reyes-Ferrada's Doctoral Thesis performed in the Biomedicine Doctorate Program of the University of Granada, Spain.

Conflicts of Interest: The authors declare no conflict of interest.

References

1. James, S.L.; Abate, D.; Abate, K.H.; Abay, S.M.; Abbafati, C.; Abbasi, N.; Abbastabar, H.; Abd-Allah, F.; Abdela, J.; Abdelalim, A.; et al. Global, regional, and national incidence, prevalence, and years lived with disability for 354 Diseases and Injuries for 195 countries and territories, 1990–2017: A systematic analysis for the Global Burden of Disease Study 2017. *Lancet* **2018**, *392*, 1789–1858. [CrossRef]
2. Wu, A.; March, L.; Zheng, X.; Huang, J.; Wang, X.; Zhao, J.; Blyth, F.M.; Smith, E.; Buchbinder, R.; Hoy, D. Global low back pain prevalence and years lived with disability from 1990 to 2017: Estimates from the Global Burden of Disease Study 2017. *Ann. Transl. Med.* **2020**, *8*, 299. [CrossRef]
3. Vlaeyen, J.W.S.; Maher, C.G.; Wiech, K.; Van Zundert, J.; Meloto, C.B.; Diatchenko, L.; Battié, M.C.; Goossens, M.; Koes, B.; Linton, S.J. Low back pain. *Nat. Rev. Dis. Prim.* **2018**, *4*, 52. [CrossRef] [PubMed]
4. Cassidy, J.D.; Carroll, L.J.; Côté, P. The Saskatchewan Health and Back Pain Survey. *Spine* **1998**, *23*, 1860–1866. [CrossRef] [PubMed]
5. Freburger, J.K.; Holmes, G.M.; Agans, R.P.; Jackman, A.M.; Darter, J.D.; Wallace, A.S.; Castel, L.D.; Kalsbeek, W.D.; Carey, T.S. The rising prevalence of chronic low back pain. *Arch. Intern. Med.* **2009**, *169*, 251–258. [CrossRef] [PubMed]
6. Pengel, L.H.M.; Herbert, R.D.; Maher, C.G.; Refshauge, K.M. Acute low back pain: Systematic review of its prognosis. *Br. Med. J.* **2003**, *327*, 323–325. [CrossRef] [PubMed]
7. Hoy, D.; Brooks, P.; Blyth, F.; Buchbinder, R. The Epidemiology of low back pain. *Best Pract. Res. Clin. Rheumatol.* **2010**, *24*, 769–781. [CrossRef]
8. Menezes Costa, L.D.C.; Maher, C.G.; Hancock, M.J.; McAuley, J.H.; Herbert, R.D.; Costa, L.O.P.P. The prognosis of acute and persistent low-back pain: A meta-analysis. *Can. Med. Assoc. J.* **2012**, *184*, E613–E624. [CrossRef] [PubMed]
9. da Silva, T.; Mills, K.; Brown, B.T.; Pocovi, N.; de Campos, T.; Maher, C.; Hancock, M.J. Recurrence of low back pain is common: A prospective inception cohort study. *J. Physiother.* **2019**, *65*, 159–165. [CrossRef]
10. Maher, C.; Underwood, M.; Buchbinder, R. Non-specific low back pain. *Lancet* **2017**, *389*, 736–747. [CrossRef]
11. Cholewicki, J.; Greene, H.; Polzhofer, G.; Galloway, M.; Shah, R.; Radebold, A. Neuromuscular Function in Athletes. *J. Orthop. Sport. Phys. Ther.* **2002**, *32*, 568–575. [CrossRef]
12. Radebold, A.; Cholewicki, J.; Panjabi, M.M.; Patel, T.C. Muscle Response Pattern to Sudden Trunk Loading in Healthy Individuals and in Patients with Chronic Low Back Pain. *Spine* **2000**, *25*, 947–954. [CrossRef] [PubMed]
13. Catalá, M.M.; Schroll, A.; Laube, G.; Arampatzis, A.; Catala, M.M.; Schrollia, A.; Laube, G.; Ararnpatzis, A.; Moreno Catalá, M.; Schroll, A.; et al. Muscle Strength and Neuromuscular Control in Low-Back Pain: Elite Athletes Versus General Population. *Front. Neurosci.* **2018**, *12*, 436. [CrossRef] [PubMed]
14. Steele, J.; Bruce-Low, S.; Smith, D. A reappraisal of the deconditioning hypothesis in low back pain: Review of evidence from a triumvirate of research methods on specific lumbar extensor deconditioning. *Curr. Med. Res. Opin.* **2014**, *30*, 865–911. [CrossRef] [PubMed]
15. Hori, Y.; Hoshino, M.; Inage, K.; Miyagi, M.; Takahashi, S.; Ohyama, S.; Suzuki, A.; Tsujio, T.; Terai, H.; Dohzono, S.; et al. ISSLS PRIZE IN CLINICAL SCIENCE 2019: Clinical importance of trunk muscle mass for low back pain, spinal balance, and quality of life—A multicenter cross-sectional study. *Eur. Spine J.* **2019**, *28*, 914–921. [CrossRef]
16. Cho, K.H.; Beom, J.W.; Lee, T.S.; Lim, J.H.; Lee, T.H.; Yuk, J.H. Trunk muscles strength as a risk factor for nonspecific low back pain: A pilot study. *Ann. Rehabil. Med.* **2014**, *38*, 234–240. [CrossRef] [PubMed]
17. Lee, J.H.; Hoshino, Y.; Nakamura, K.; Kariya, Y.; Saita, K.; Ito, K. Trunk muscle weakness as a risk factor for low back pain. A 5-year prospective study. *Spine* **1999**, *24*, 54–57. [CrossRef] [PubMed]
18. Oxland, T.R. Fundamental biomechanics of the spine-What we have learned in the past 25 years and future directions. *J. Biomech.* **2016**, *49*, 817–832. [CrossRef]
19. Panjabi, M.M. The stabilizing system of the spine: Part I. function, dysfunction, adaptation, and enhancement. *J. Spinal Disord.* **1992**, *5*, 383–389. [CrossRef]
20. Barbado, D.; Lopez-Valenciano, A.; Juan-Recio, C.; Montero-Carretero, C.; Van Dieën, J.H.; Vera-Garcia, F.J. Trunk stability, trunk strength and sport performance level in judo. *PLoS ONE* **2016**, *11*, 1–12.
21. Golubić, A.; Šarabon, N.; Marković, G. Association between trunk muscle strength and static balance in older women. *J. Women Aging* **2019**, 1–10. [CrossRef]
22. Granacher, U.; Gollhofer, A.; Hortobágyi, T.; Kressig, R.W.; Muehlbauer, T. The importance of trunk muscle strength for balance, functional performance, and fall prevention in seniors: A systematic review. *Sport. Med.* **2013**, *43*, 627–641. [CrossRef] [PubMed]
23. Zouita, A.B.M.; Salah, F.Z.B.; Dziri, C.; Beardsley, C.; Ben Moussa Zouita, A.; Ben Salah, F.Z.; Dziri, C.; Beardsley, C. Comparison of isokinetic trunk flexion and extension torques and powers between athletes and nonathletes. *J. Exerc. Rehabil.* **2018**, *14*, 72–77. [CrossRef]
24. Kibler, W.B.; Press, J.; Sciascia, A. The Role of Core Stability in Athletic Function. *Sport. Med.* **2006**, *36*, 189–198. [CrossRef]
25. Cronström, A.; Creaby, M.W.; Nae, J.; Ageberg, E. Modifiable Factors Associated with Knee Abduction During Weight-Bearing Activities: A Systematic Review and Meta-Analysis. *Sport. Med.* **2016**, *46*, 1647–1662. [CrossRef] [PubMed]
26. Heebner, N.R.; Abt, J.P.; Lovalekar, M.; Beals, K.; Sell, T.C.; Morgan, J.; Kane, S.; Lephart, S. Physical and performance characteristics related to unintentional musculoskeletal injury in special forces operators: A prospective analysis. *J. Athl. Train.* **2017**, *52*, 1153–1160. [CrossRef] [PubMed]

27. Juan-Recio, C.; Lopez-Plaza, D.; Barbado Murillo, D.; Pilar Garcia-Vaquero, M.; Vera-Garcia, F.J. Reliability assessment and correlation analysis of 3 protocols to measure trunk muscle strength and endurance. *J. Sports Sci.* **2018**, *36*, 357–364. [CrossRef]
28. Rodriguez-Perea, A.; Chirosa Ríos, L.J.; Martinez-Garcia, D.; Ulloa-Díaz, D.; Guede Rojas, F.; Jerez-Mayorga, D.; Chirosa Rios, I.J. Reliability of isometric and isokinetic trunk flexor strength using a functional electromechanical dynamometer. *PeerJ* **2019**, *7*, e7883. [CrossRef]
29. Stark, T.; Walker, B.; Phillips, J.K.; Fejer, R.; Beck, R. Hand-held dynamometry correlation with the gold standard isokinetic dynamometry: A systematic review. *PM R* **2011**, *3*, 472–479. [CrossRef]
30. Kannus, P. Isokinetic Evaluation of Muscular Performance. *Int. J. Sports Med.* **1994**, *15*, S11–S18. [CrossRef]
31. Mueller, S.; Stoll, J.; Mueller, J.; Mayer, F. Validity of isokinetic trunk measurements with respect to healthy adults, athletes and low back pain patients. *Isokinet. Exerc. Sci.* **2012**, *20*, 255–266. [CrossRef]
32. Zouita Ben Moussa, A.; Zouita, S.; Ben Salah, F.; Behm, D.; Chaouachi, A. Isokinetic Trunk Strength, Validity, Reliability, Normative data and Relation to Physical Performance and Low back pain: A Review of the Literature. *Int. J. Sports Phys. Ther.* **2020**, *15*, 160–174. [CrossRef]
33. Cholewicki, J.; Breen, A.; Popovich, J.M.; Reeves, N.P.; Sahrmann, S.A.; van Dillen, L.R.; Vleeming, A.; Hodges, P.W. Can Biomechanics Research Lead to More Effective Treatment of Low Back Pain? A Point-Counterpoint Debate. *J. Orthop. Sport. Phys. Ther.* **2019**, *49*, 425–436. [CrossRef] [PubMed]
34. Nicholas, M.K.; Linton, S.J.; Watson, P.J.; Main, C.J. Early identification and management of psychological risk factors ("yellow flags") in patients with low back pain: A reappraisal. *Phys. Ther.* **2011**, *91*, 737–753. [CrossRef] [PubMed]
35. Sanzarello, I.; Merlini, L.; Rosa, M.A.; Perrone, M.; Frugiuele, J.; Borghi, R.; Faldini, C. Central sensitization in chronic low back pain: A narrative review. *J. Back Musculoskelet. Rehabil.* **2016**, *29*, 625–633. [CrossRef] [PubMed]
36. Comachio, J.; Magalhães, M.O.; Campos Carvalho E Silva, A.P.D.M.; Marques, A.P. A cross-sectional study of associations between kinesiophobia, pain, disability, and quality of life in patients with chronic low back pain. *Adv. Rheumatol.* **2018**, *58*, 8. [CrossRef] [PubMed]
37. de Souza Júnior, J.R.; Lemos, T.V.; Hamu, T.C.D.D.S.; Calaça, F.I.R.; dos Santos, M.G.R.; Faria, A.M.; Silva, A.T.; Matheus, J.P.C. Effects of Kinesio Taping on peak torque and muscle activity in women with low back pain presenting fears and beliefs related to physical activity. *J. Bodyw. Mov. Ther.* **2020**, *24*, 361–366. [CrossRef]
38. Moher, D.; Liberati, A.; Tetzlaff, J.; Altman, D.G.; Altman, D.; Antes, G.; Atkins, D.; Barbour, V.; Barrowman, N.; Berlin, J.A.; et al. Preferred reporting items for systematic reviews and meta-analyses: The PRISMA statement. *PLoS Med.* **2009**, *6*, e1000097. [CrossRef]
39. Ouzzani, M.; Hammady, H.; Fedorowicz, Z.; Elmagarmid, A. Rayyan-a web and mobile app for systematic reviews. *Syst. Rev.* **2016**, *5*, 1–10. [CrossRef]
40. Castro, M.P.D.; Ruschel, C.; Santos, G.M.; Ferreira, T.; Pierri, C.A.A.; Roesler, H. Isokinetic hip muscle strength: A systematic review of normative data. *Sport. Biomech.* **2018**, *19*, 26–54. [CrossRef]
41. Whiting, P.; Rutjes, A.W.S.; Reitsma, J.B.; Bossuyt, P.M.M.; Kleijnen, J. The development of QUADAS: A tool for the quality assessment of studies of diagnostic accuracy included in systematic reviews. *BMC Med. Res. Methodol.* **2003**, *3*, 1–13. [CrossRef]
42. Downs, S.H.; Black, N. The feasibility of creating a checklist for the assessment of the methodological quality both of randomised and non-randomised studies of health care interventions. *J. Epidemiol. Community Health* **1998**, *52*, 377–384. [CrossRef]
43. Cook, C.; Mabry, L.; Reiman, M.P.; Hegedus, E.J. Best tests/clinical findings for screening and diagnosis of patellofemoral pain syndrome: A systematic review. *Physiotherapy* **2012**, *98*, 93–100. [CrossRef] [PubMed]
44. Suzuki, N.; Endo, S. A quantitative study of trunk muscle strength and fatigability in the low-back-pain syndrome. *Spine* **1983**, *8*, 69–74. [CrossRef]
45. Akebi, T.; Saeki, S.; Hieda, H.; Goto, H. Factors affecting the variability of the torque curves at isokinetic trunk strength testing. *Arch. Phys. Med. Rehabil.* **1998**, *79*, 33–35. [CrossRef]
46. Gabr, W.; Eweda, R.S. Isokinetic Strength of Trunk Flexors and Extensors Muscles in Adult Men with and without Nonspecific Back Pain: A Comparative Study. *J. Behav. Brain Sci.* **2019**, *9*, 340–350. [CrossRef]
47. Hupli, M.; Sainio, P.; Hurri, H.; Alaranta, H. Comparison of trunk strength measurements between two different isokinetic devices used at clinical settings. *J. Spinal Disord. Tech.* **1997**, *10*, 391–397. [CrossRef]
48. Estrázulas, J.A.; Estrázulas, J.A.; de Jesus, K.; de Jesus, K.; da Silva, R.A.; Libardoni dos Santos, J.O. Evaluation isometric and isokinetic of trunk flexor and extensor muscles with isokinetic dynamometer: A systematic review. *Phys. Ther. Sport* **2020**, *45*, 93–102. [CrossRef]
49. Mueller, S.; Stoll, J.; Cassel, M.; Engel, T.; Mueller, J.; Mayer, F. Trunk peak torque, muscle activation pattern and sudden loading compensation in adolescent athletes with back pain. *J. Back Musculoskelet. Rehabil.* **2019**, *32*, 379–388. [CrossRef]
50. Verbrugghe, J.; Agten, A.; Eijnde, B.O.; Vandenabeele, F.; De Baets, L.; Huybrechts, X.; Timmermans, A. Reliability and agreement of isometric functional trunk and isolated lumbar strength assessment in healthy persons and persons with chronic nonspecific low back pain. *Phys. Ther. Sport* **2019**, *38*, 1–7. [CrossRef]
51. Dvir, Z.; Keating, J.L. Trunk extension effort in patients with chronic low back dysfunction. *Spine* **2003**, *28*, 685–692. [CrossRef] [PubMed]
52. Ripamonti, M.; Colin, D.; Rahmani, A. Maximal power of trunk flexor and extensor muscles as a quantitative factor of low back pain. *Isokinet. Exerc. Sci.* **2011**, *19*, 83–89. [CrossRef]

53. Yahia, A.; Jribi, S.; Ghroubi, S.; Elleuch, M.; Baklouti, S.; Habib Elleuch, M. Evaluation of the posture and muscular strength of the trunk and inferior members of patients with chronic lumbar pain. *Jt. Bone Spine* **2011**, *78*, 291–297. [CrossRef]
54. Shirado, O.; Ito, T.; Kaneda, K.; Strax, T.E. Concentric and eccentric strength of trunk muscles: Influence of test postures on strength and characteristics of patients with chronic low-back pain. *Arch. Phys. Med. Rehabil.* **1995**, *76*, 604–611. [CrossRef]
55. Schulz, K.F.; Altman, D.G.; Moher, D. CONSORT 2010 Statement: Updated guidelines for reporting parallel group randomised trials. *BMJ* **2010**, *340*, 698–702. [CrossRef] [PubMed]
56. von Elm, E.; Altman, D.G.; Egger, M.; Pocock, S.J.; Gøtzsche, P.C.; Vandenbroucke, J.P. The Strengthening the Reporting of Observational Studies in Epidemiology (STROBE) statement: Guidelines for reporting observational studies. *Lancet* **2007**, *370*, 1453–1457. [CrossRef]
57. Bouilland, S.; Loslever, P.; Lepoutre, F.X. Biomechanical comparison of isokinetic lifting and free lifting when applied to chronic low back pain rehabilitation. *Med. Biol. Eng. Comput.* **2002**, *40*, 183–192. [CrossRef] [PubMed]
58. Martinez-Garcia, D.; Rodriguez-Perea, A.; Barboza, P.; Ulloa-Díaz, D.; Jerez-Mayorga, D.; Chirosa, I.; Ríos, L.J.C. Reliability of a standing isokinetic shoulder rotators strength test using a functional electromechanical dynamometer: Effects of velocity. *PeerJ* **2020**, *8*, 1–15. [CrossRef]

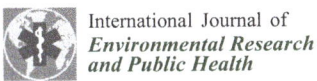

Systematic Review

The Effects of Martial Arts on Cancer-Related Fatigue and Quality of Life in Cancer Patients: An Up-to-Date Systematic Review and Meta-Analysis of Randomized Controlled Clinical Trials

Daniel Sur [1,2,*], Shanthi Sabarimurugan [3] and Shailesh Advani [4]

1. 11th Department of Medical Oncology, University of Medicine and Pharmacy "Iuliu Hatieganu", 400015 Cluj-Napoca, Romania
2. Department of Medical Oncology, Oncology Institute "Prof. Dr. Ion Chiricuta", 400015 Cluj-Napoca, Romania
3. School of Biomedical Sciences, Faculty of Health and Medical Sciences, University of Western Australia, Nedlands, WA 6009, Australia; shanthi.sabarimurugan@uwa.edu.au
4. Terasaki Institute of Biomedical Innovation, Los Angeles, CA 90024, USA; shailesh.advani735@gmail.com
* Correspondence: dr.geni@yahoo.co.uk; Tel.: +40-009840745778434

Citation: Sur, D.; Sabarimurugan, S.; Advani, S. The Effects of Martial Arts on Cancer-Related Fatigue and Quality of Life in Cancer Patients: An Up-to-Date Systematic Review and Meta-Analysis of Randomized Controlled Clinical Trials. *Int. J. Environ. Res. Public Health* **2021**, *18*, 6116. https://doi.org/10.3390/ijerph18116116

Academic Editor: Alberto Soriano-Maldonado

Received: 19 March 2021
Accepted: 2 June 2021
Published: 6 June 2021

Publisher's Note: MDPI stays neutral with regard to jurisdictional claims in published maps and institutional affiliations.

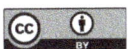

Copyright: © 2021 by the authors. Licensee MDPI, Basel, Switzerland. This article is an open access article distributed under the terms and conditions of the Creative Commons Attribution (CC BY) license (https://creativecommons.org/licenses/by/4.0/).

Abstract: Background: To evaluate and synthesize the existing evidence of the effects of practicing martial arts by cancer patients and cancer survivors in relation to overall quality of life (QoL) and cancer-related fatigue (CRF). Methods: Randomized controlled trials (RCTs) from 1 January 2000 to 5 November 2020 investigating the impact of martial arts were compared with any control intervention for overall QoL and CRF among cancer patients and survivors. Publication quality and risk of bias were assessed using the Cochrane handbook of systematic reviews. Results: According to the electronic search, 17 RCTs were retrieved including 1103 cancer patients. Martial arts significantly improved social function, compared to that in the control group (SMD = -0.88, 95% CI: -1.36, -0.39; $p = 0.0004$). Moreover, martial arts significantly improved functioning, compared to the control group (SMD = 0.68, 95% CI: 0.39–0.96; $p < 0.00001$). Martial arts significantly reduced CRF, compared to that in the control group (SMD = -0.51, 95% CI: -0.80, -0.22; $p = 0.0005$, I2 > 95%). Conclusions: The results of our systematic review and meta-analysis reveal that the effects of practicing martial arts on CRF and QoL in cancer patients and survivors are inconclusive. Some potential effects were seen for social function and CRF, although the results were inconsistent across different measurement methods. There is a need for larger and more homogeneous clinical trials encompassing different cancer types and specific martial arts disciplines to make more extensive and definitive cancer- and symptom-specific recommendations.

Keywords: cancer; QOL; fatigue; martial arts; clinical trial; meta-analysis

1. Introduction

In 2020, 19.3 million new cancer cases were diagnosed globally, where breast, lung, and prostate were the most frequent type of malignancies [1]. Cancer is the second cause of mortality worldwide after ischemic heart disease, with 8.97 million deaths, and it is predicted to become the leading cause of death by 2060 with approximately 18.63 million deaths [2]. Improvements in diagnostics and treatments have increased the survival rate of the most prevalent cancers in developed countries [3]. As of January 2019, there were an estimated 16.9 million cancer survivors in the United States. The number of cancer survivors is projected to increase to 22.2 million by 2030 [4]. Furthermore, the burden of cancer incidence and survivors continues to increase in low- and middle-income countries as well [5].

The physical, emotional, and financial impacts of cancer diagnosis and its management, along with the side effects of treatments, normally have long-term consequences on the patient's overall quality of life (QoL) that can interfere in their activities of daily living [6,7]. The World Health Organization (WHO) defines QoL as an individual's perception of their position in life in the context of the culture, as well as the value systems in which they live and in relation to their goals, expectations, standards, and concerns [8]. Cancer-specific QoL encompasses all stages of the disease [9].

Cancer standard treatment (surgery, radiation, chemotherapy, hormone therapy, targeted therapy, and immunotherapy) can cause a series of side effects, including nausea, vomiting, diarrhea, constipation, fatigue, depression, and weight loss, which affects physical and psychological functioning, as well as overall QoL [10–12]. Fatigue remains one of the most important components of QoL that can vary in intensity and impact based on the stage of disease, treatment received, and patients' functional status [13]. Cancer-related fatigue (CRF) seems to be due mainly to alterations promoted by cancer in patient homeostasis, such as proinflammatory cytokine upregulations, hydroxytryptophan dysregulation, hypothalamic–pituitary–adrenal axis dysfunction, circadian rhythm disturbances, and increased vagal tone. It is also shown that CRF can vary based on the cancer type [14]. The CRF is defined as a distressing, persistent, and subjective sense of physical, emotional, and/or cognitive tiredness or exhaustion related to cancer or cancer treatment that is not proportional to recent activity and interferes with usual functioning [15]. Moreover, it can lead to a decrease in the participation of activities of daily living and impairment of the patient mood; moreover, it is an important predictor of reduced overall QoL [16,17]. The CRF has been estimated to affect between 25% and 99% of cancer patients and depends on several factors, including patient population, type of treatment received, and assessment method, which can persist for five or more years after cancer diagnosis [18].

Several interventions, such as exercise, heat, cryotherapy, or manual therapy, can be followed to ameliorate some of the above-mentioned side effects and improve QoL [19]. Different exercise programs offer benefits and are safe in cancer patients during and after cancer treatment [20], improving health and functional outcomes in these patients [21]. National guidelines recommend the prescription of exercise to cancer patients; however, it should be tailored to their needs and capabilities [22]. This physical activity has to be done 3–5 times/week and for at least 20 min to be effective and should involve aerobic, resistance exercises, or a combination of both [23].

Martial arts present several benefits to those who practice them. The benefits include physical and psychological aspects, including lessening negative emotional reactions, enhancing balance, and improving cardiovascular and musculoskeletal fitness [24]. Although there is limited evidence of studies with limited number of participants assessing the effects of practicing martial arts in cancer patients [25–27], there is a need to clarify their effects on CRF and QoL. This systematic review and meta-analysis aimed to comprehensively review the use of martial arts among cancer survivors and its impact on QoL and CRF. Furthermore, it was attempted to determine the benefits of these types of programs, identify the strengths and gaps in the evidence, and suggest directions to overcome the highlighted limitations.

2. Materials and Methods

Cochrane's handbook of systematic reviews of interventions and the Preferred Reporting Items for Systematic Reviews and Meta-Analyses (PRISMA) statement were utilized in this study to develop and perform this systematic review and meta-analysis [28].

2.1. Literature Search

Online databases, including PubMed (Medline), Cochrane Web, Web of Science, and Scopus, were searched from 1 January 2000 to 5 November 2020 using the keywords: (Martial Arts OR Hap Ki Do OR Judo OR Karate OR Jujitsu OR Tae Kwon Do OR Aikido OR Wushu OR Kung Fu OR Gong Fu OR Gongfu) AND (Cancer* OR Neoplasm* OR Tumor* OR Malignancy*). Furthermore, the search was continued for PubMed (Medline), which was then formatted to perform the search in other databases.

2.2. Eligibility Criteria

Following the PICO principles (patient, intervention, control, and outcomes) [29], the inclusion criteria were: (a) randomized controlled trials (RCTs) that investigated cancer patients with the primary intervention of martial arts and compared with any comparator for QoL and fatigue; (b) original articles in peer reviewed journals; and (c) eligible studies in English. Non-randomized or any other trials rather than RCTs, non-English RCTs, trials that did not assess the QoL or CRF, non-human studies, studies with no full text, single arm studies, and reviews and secondary works were excluded from this study.

2.3. Screening of Results

Initially, two authors (D.S. and S.S.) screened all titles and abstracts using the inclusion criteria. Subsequently, they coded the abstracts as "yes" for inclusion in full text-review and "no" for excluding the abstract. If both authors coded an abstract as "yes", they were considered for full text review. If both were coded as no, they were excluded. For abstracts where there were discrepancies, the decision was made through either mutual discussion or with the help of a third reviewer (S.A). In the next stage, a full text review of all articles was performed against the inclusion criteria. Following that, the full text was read carefully for eligibility criteria.

2.4. Data Extraction

The extracted data were divided into three categories. The first one was baseline characteristics, including author name, country, sample size, age, gender, marital status, and cancer treatment (surgery, chemotherapy, and radiation, as well as author name). The second contained the key characteristics of the included studies, such as country, cancer type, the timing of intervention, duration of the intervention (sessions, frequency, and period), and outcomes. The last one was outcome measures, including: (I) quality of life by European Organization for Research and Treatment of Cancer Quality of Life Questionnaire (EORTC QLQ-C30) [30], Functional Assessment of Cancer Therapy—General (FACT-G) [31], and The Short-Form 36 (SF-36) [32]; and (II) fatigue by The Brief Fatigue Inventory (BFI) [33], Functional Assessment of Chronic Illness Therapy—Fatigue (FACIT-F) [34], and the Multidimensional Fatigue Symptom Inventory—Short Form (MFSI-SF) [35,36].

2.5. Quality Assessment

The quality of this meta-analysis was judged based on the Grading of Recommendations, Assessment, Development, and Evaluations (GRADE) guideline [37]. GRADE is a transparent and reproducible system that allows the researcher to grade the quality and certainty of the evidence. Based on the quality of the evidence, the level of confidence was assessed that an estimate of the effect could be correct. Following that, two researchers (D.S. and S.S.) evaluated each study. An overall quality score was assigned to each study, ranging from high, moderate, low, to very low grade of evidence. These grades mean the grade certainty/quality of the evidence of the studies. If there was any uncertainty between the two independent researchers, a third researcher (S.A.) evaluated the evidence to obtain the conclusion. The risk of bias of the included studies was also evaluated using the Cochrane's risk of bias tool [38]. This tool was used to evaluate the RCTs regarding randomization tools; concealment of allocation; blinding of assessors, participants, and personnel; and selective reporting, attrition, and other biases. No paper evaluated was excluded from the results because of low quality or high risk of bias.

2.6. Statistical Analysis

The data were analyzed as a standardized mean difference (SMD) and 95% confidence interval (CI) under a random-effects model using the inverse-variance method in the Review Manager Software (version 5.3, The Nordic Cochrane Centre, Copenhagen, Denmark) package. The heterogeneity was considered when I-square test (I^2) and Chi-Square P were more and less than 50% and 0.1, respectively [38–40].

3. Results

3.1. Search Results and Summary of Included Studies

Our electronic search retrieved 801 records, 744 of which underwent title and abstract screening after removal of duplicates. Out of these, 38 records progressed for full-text screening, and 21 of them were excluded from the study. Finally, 17 RCTs were included for further analysis [41–57]. Figure 1 illustrates the study selection process. These studies included a total of 1103 cancer patients who were divided into control groups (n = 546) and treatment groups with martial arts (n = 557). The mean age of the included cancer patients was 58 ± 3.1 years. The baseline characteristics and summary of the included studies are shown in Tables 1 and 2.

3.2. Description of Intervention

Most of the studies analyzed martial arts, such as Tai Chi and Qigong, in one of the comparator arms. They compared the effect of martial arts with standard care, control, psychosocial support, strength training, and even dance. Tai Chi is a traditional Chinese martial art used for defense as well as for its health benefits [58]. Tai Chi and its derivates (Tai Chi Chih, Tai Chi Chuan, Tai Chi Qi Qong, and Tai Chi Easy) are efficient complementary approaches used in improving wellbeing and fatigue [59]. Qigong is considered a form of Chinese martial arts with benefits in immune regulation, balancing the "qi", and strengthening muscles and tendons [60]. These traditional martial arts forms involved meditation, breathing techniques, coordinating the movements, and relaxation exercises [61]. Another martial art used in the clinical trials was Kyoshu Jitsu. This martial art focuses on pressure points for self-defense as well as its benefits for healing [53]. The majority of the studies analyzed for this meta-analysis focused on breast cancer. Only a small number of studies considered other tumor types, such as lymphoma, ovary, colon, lung, prostate, and nasopharyngeal cancer (Tables 1 and 2).

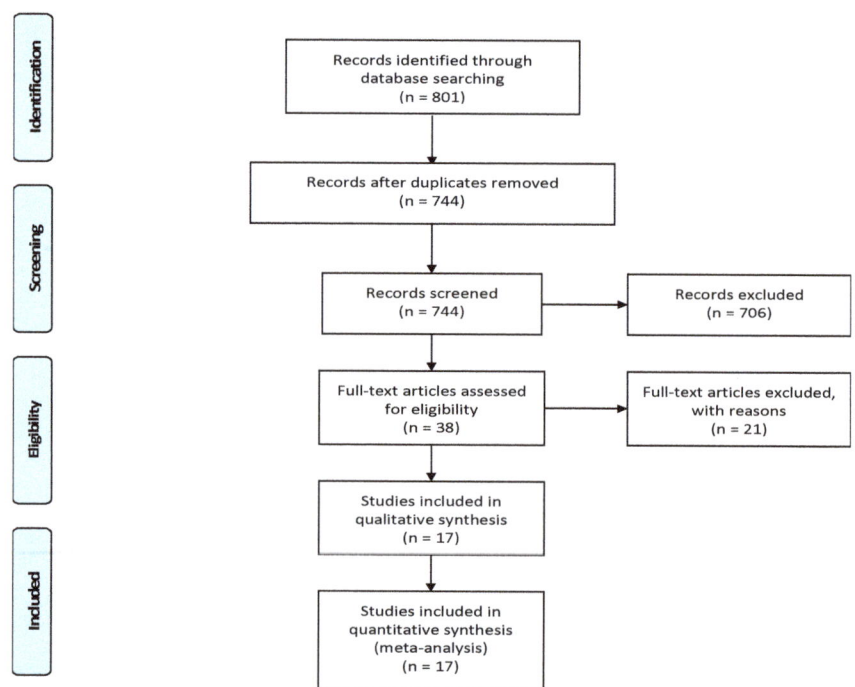

Figure 1. PRISMA flow diagram.

Table 1. Baseline characteristics of the included studies.

ID	Arms	Number	Age (Years)	Female n (% of Total)	Cancer Treatment		
					Surgery	Chemotherapy	Radiation
Campo 2013	Tai Chi Chih	32	66.54 (55–89) [1]	32 (100)	27	19	21
	Health Education Class	31	65.64 (57–84) [1]	31 (100)	28	19	20
Chen 2013	Qigong	49	45.3 (6.3)	49 (100)	49	-	49
	Usual care	47	44.7 (9.7)	47 (100)	46	-	45
Chuang 2017	Qigong	48	55.85 (16.78)	22 (45)	-	48	-
	Usual care	48	64.54 (15.51)	19 (40)	-	48	-
Irwin 2017	Tai Chi Chih	45	59.6 (7.9)	45 (100)	6	18	22
	Cognitive behavioral therapy for insomnia	45	60.0 (9.3)	45 (100)	4	21	34
Larkey 2016	Sham Qigong	45	59.8 (8.93)	45 (100)	-	-	-
	Qigong and Tai Chi Easy	42	57.7 (8.94)	42 (100)	-	-	-
Loh 2014	Qigong	32	18–65	32 (100)	32	23	18
	Line dance	31		31 (100)	31	23	18
McQuade 2017	Qigong/tai chi	21	62.2 (7.4)	21 (100)	-	-	21
	Waitlist control	24	66.0 (8.4)	24 (100)	-	-	24
Mustian 2004	Tai Chi Chuan	11	52 (9)	11 (100)	21	18	13
	Psychosocial support	10		10 (100)			
Mustian 2008	Tai Chi Chuan	11	52 (9)	11 (100)	21	18	13
	Psychosocial support	10		10			
Oh 2008	Qigong	15	54 (9)	12 (80)	-	-	-
	Usual care	15		12 (80)	-	-	-
Oh 2009	Qigong	79	60.1 (11.7)	48 (61)	-	-	-
	Usual care	83	59.9 (11.3)	45 (54)	-	-	-
Sprod 2011	Tai Chi Chuan	9	54.33 (3.55) [2]	9 (100)	9	6	8
	Standard support therapy	10	52.70 (2.11) [2]	10 (100)	10	3	9
Strunk 2018	Kyusho Jitsu	30	54.2 (7.8)	30 (100)	29	14	23
	Control	21	51.5 (8.4)	21 (100)	21	15	17
Thongteratham 2015	Tai Chi Qi Qong	15	-	15 (100)	15	15	15
	Usual care	15	-	15 (100)	15	15	15
Vanderbyl 2017	Qigong	11	66.1 (11.7)	4 (37)	-	-	-
	standard endurance and strength training	13	63.7 (7.7)	6 (46)	-	-	-
Zhang 2016	Tai Chi Chih	47	62.8	10 (21)	47	-	-
	Control	44		13 (30)	44	-	-
Zhou 2017	Tai Chi Chih	57	18–70	19 (33)	-	57	57
	Control	57		12 (21)	-	57	57

Values reflect number or mean (standard deviation); [1] median (range); [2] standard error of the mean.

Table 2. Summary of the included studies.

ID.	Country	Cancer Type	Timing of Intervention	Type of Treatment	Session, Minutes	Frequency, Times/Week	Period, Week	Outcomes	Time Questionnaires
Campo 2013	USA	Breast, colorectal, ovarian, cervical/uterine, thyroid, bladder, nasopharyngeal	≥3 months after TTT [3]	Surgery, radiation, chemotherapy, hormone, other	60	3	12	SF-36 [6]	Baseline and 1 week after
Chen 2013	China	Breast	During TTT	Radiation	60	5	5–6	FACT-G, BFI [7]	Baseline, during and at the end of treatment, and 1 and 3 months later.
Chuang 2017	Taiwan	Lymphoma	During TTT	Chemotherapy	60	2	10	EORTC QLQ-C30, BFI [4]	Baseline and 21 days after
Irwin 2017	USA	Breast	≥6 months after TTT	Surgery, radiation and/or chemotherapy	120 min weekly		12	MFSI-SF [9]	Baseline and 2, 3, 6, and 15 months
Larkey 2016	USA	Breast	6 months to 5 years after TTT	Surgery, radiation, or chemotherapy	30	5	12	SF-36	Baseline and 12 and 24 weeks
Loh 2014	Malaysia	Breast	TTT completed	NM	30	2	8	FACT-G [5]	Baseline and 8 weeks
McQuade 2017	USA	Prostate	During TTT	Radiation	60	3	6–8	BFI	Baseline, midway, during the last week of TTT, and 3 months after TTT.
Mustian 2004	USA	Breast	1 week to 30 months after TTT	NM	60	3	12	FACIT-F [8]	Baseline and 12 weeks after
Mustian 2008	USA	Breast	1 week to 30 months after TTT	NM	60	3	12	FACIT-F	Baseline and 12 weeks after intervention
Oh 2008	Australia	Breast, ovary, lung, lymphoma, colon	During or completed TTT	Cancer treatment, chemotherapy	60	1 or 2	8	EORTC QLQ-C30	Baseline and 8 weeks
Oh 2009	Australia	Breast, lung, prostate, colorectal, bowel	During or completed TTT	NM	90 min weekly		10	FACIT-F, FACT-G	Baseline and 10 weeks after intervention
Sprod 2011	USA	Breast	1 month to 30 months after TTT	NM	60	3	12	SF-36	Baseline and 6 and 12 weeks
Strunk 2018	German	Breast	≥6 months after TTT	Not hormone treatment	90	2	24	EORTC QLQ-C30	Baseline and 12 and 24 weeks
Thongteratham 2015	Thailand	Breast	TTT completed	NM	60	3	12	FACT-G	Baseline and 12 and 24 weeks
Vanderbyl 2017	Canada	NSCLC [1] or GI [2]	During TTT	Chemotherapy	45	2	6	FACT-G	Baseline and 6 weeks
Zhang 2016	China	Lung	During TTT	Chemotherapy	60	3	12	MFSI-SF	Baseline and 43 and 85 days
Zhou 2017	China	Nasopharyngeal carcinoma	During TTT	Chemotherapy	60	5	6	MFSI-SF	Baseline and after treatment

NM, not mentioned; [1] NSCLC, non-small cell lung cancer; [2] GI, gastrointestinal cancer; [3] TTT, treatment; [4] EORTC QLQ-C30, European Organization for Research and Treatment of Cancer Quality of Life Questionnaire; [5] FACT-G, Functional Assessment of Cancer Therapy—General; [6] SF-36, the Short-Form 36; [7] BFI, the Brief Fatigue Inventory; [8] FACIT-F, Functional Assessment of Chronic Illness Therapy—Fatigue; [9] MFSI-SF, the Multidimensional Fatigue Symptom Inventory—Short Form.

3.3. Outcomes

In total, three studies [43,50,53] assessed QoL using the European Organization for Research and Treatment of Cancer Quality of Life Questionnaire (EORTC QLQ-C30). A pooled analysis compared the impact of martial arts vs. no intervention among cancer patients and showed no significant improvement in global health, (SMD = 1.30, 95% CI: −1.18, 3.78; p = 0.30, I^2 > 95%), physical function (SMD = 0.84, 95% CI: −1.42–3.10; p = 0.47, I^2 > 95%), role function (SMD = 1.03, 95% CI: −1.01–3.08]; p = 0.32, I^2 > 95%), emotional function (SMD = 1.37, 95% CI: −1.12–3.85; p = 0.28, I^2 > 95%), cognitive function (SMD = 1.37, 95% CI: −0.82–3.55]; p = 0.22, I^2 > 95%), and social function (SMD = 1.17, 95% CI: −0.99–3.34; p = 0.29, I^2 > 95%) (Figure 2). It should be noted that the heterogeneity was solved after excluding the study by Chuang (2017) [43] (p > 0.1), and the results remained non-significant (Figure A1).

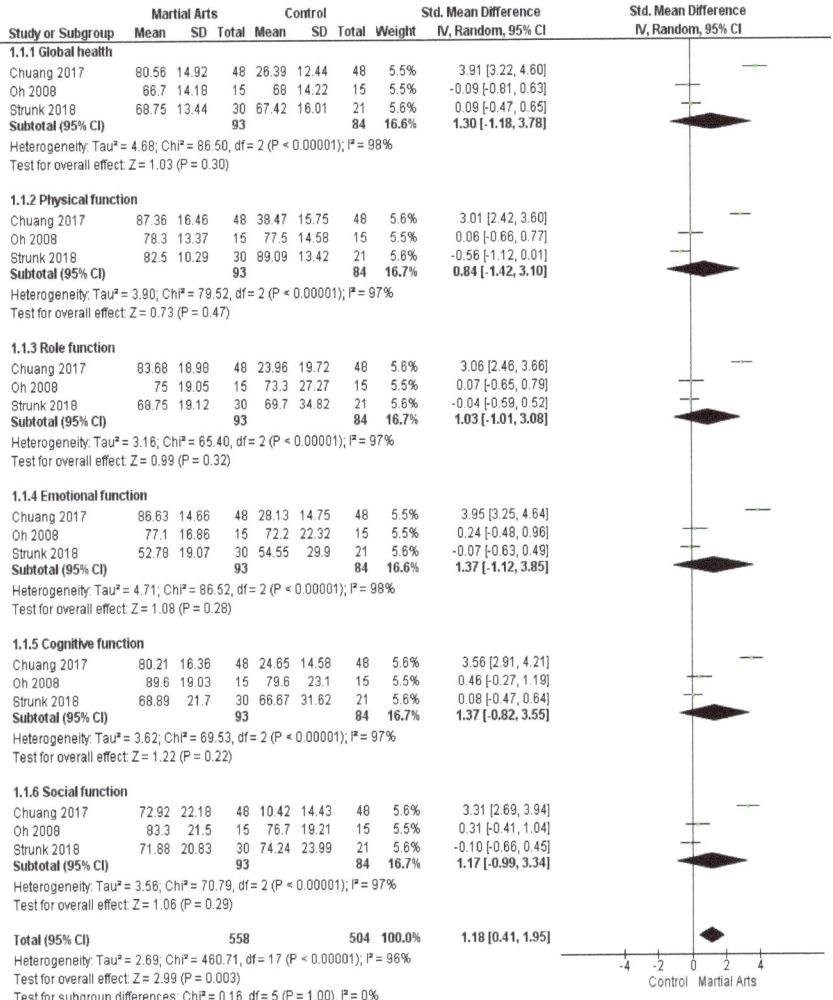

Figure 2. Analysis of European Organization for Research and Treatment of Cancer Quality of Life Questionnaire (QLQ-C30).

3.4. Functional Assessment of Cancer Therapy-General

In total, five studies [42,46,51,54,55] reported the effect of martial arts on QoL by FACT-G. Pooled data show non-significant improvement between the groups in terms of the Functional Assessment of Cancer Therapy—General (SMD = 0.34, 95% CI: −0.02–0.70]; p = 0.06) (Figure 3). The analysis was heterogeneous (p = 0.04, I2 = 61%), and the heterogeneity was solved when removing the study by Oh (2009) [51] (p = 0.70, I2 = 0%). The results remained non-significant (SMD = 0.16, 95% CI: −0.11–0.43; p = 0.25) (Figure A2).

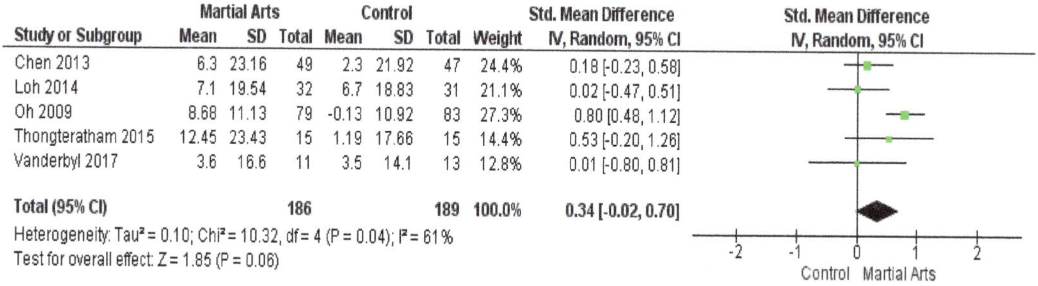

Study or Subgroup	Martial Arts Mean	SD	Total	Control Mean	SD	Total	Weight	Std. Mean Difference IV, Random, 95% CI
Chen 2013	6.3	23.16	49	2.3	21.92	47	24.4%	0.18 [−0.23, 0.58]
Loh 2014	7.1	19.54	32	6.7	18.83	31	21.1%	0.02 [−0.47, 0.51]
Oh 2009	8.68	11.13	79	−0.13	10.92	83	27.3%	0.80 [0.48, 1.12]
Thongteratham 2015	12.45	23.43	15	1.19	17.66	15	14.4%	0.53 [−0.20, 1.26]
Vanderbyl 2017	3.6	16.6	11	3.5	14.1	13	12.8%	0.01 [−0.80, 0.81]
Total (95% CI)			**186**			**189**	**100.0%**	**0.34 [−0.02, 0.70]**

Heterogeneity: Tau² = 0.10; Chi² = 10.32, df = 4 (P = 0.04); I² = 61%
Test for overall effect: Z = 1.85 (P = 0.06)

Figure 3. Analysis of Functional Assessment of Cancer Therapy—General.

3.5. The Short-Form 36 (SF-36)

The Short-Form 36 (SF-36) was reported in three studies [41,45,52]. The combined SMD between martial art and control groups showed non-significant results regarding physical function (SMD = 0.16, 95% CI: −0.18–0.50; p = 0.36), mental health (SMD = 0.05, 95% CI: −0.27–0.36; p = 0.77), and social function (SMD = 0.07, 95% CI: −1.87–2.01; p = 0.94). It is worth noting that the results of physical function and mental health were homogeneous (p = 0.33, I2 = 10% and p = 0.95, I2 = 0%, respectively) (Figure 4). However, the social function was heterogeneous (p < 0.00001, I2 = 97%), and the heterogeneity was solved by excluding the study by Larkey (2016) [45] (p = 0.47, I2 = 0%). The results after sensitivity analysis show that martial arts significantly reduced social function compared to the control group (SMD = −0.88, 95% CI: −1.36, −0.39]; p = 0.0004) (Figure A3).

3.6. The Brief Fatigue Inventory

Pooled data of three studies [42,43,47] report that the BFI showed no significant reduction of fatigue between the two groups (SMD = −1.04, 95% CI: −2.96–0.87; p = 0.29). According to the results, the analysis was heterogeneous (p < 0.00001, I2 = 98%) (Figure 5). Furthermore, the heterogeneity was solved after removing the study by Chuang (2017) [43] (p = 0.24, I2 = 26%), and the results remained non-significant (SMD = 0.01, 95% CI: −0.39–0.41; p = 0.96) (Figure A4).

3.7. Functional Assessment of Chronic Illness Therapy-Fatigue

Totally, three studies [48,49,51] reported the use of Functional Assessment of Chronic Illness Therapy—Fatigue (FACIT-F). The results show martial arts significantly improved fatigue, compared to the control group (SMD = 0.68, 95% CI: 0.39–0.96; p < 0.00001). According to the results, the data are homogeneous (p = 0.73, I2 = 0%) (Figure 6).

3.8. The Multidimensional Fatigue Symptom Inventory-Short Form

The multidimensional Fatigue Symptom Inventory—Short Form was used in three studies [44,56,57]. The results reveal that the SMD between martial art and control groups was non-significant (SMD = −0.31, 95% CI: −0.71–0.10; p = 0.14), and the data are heterogeneous (p = 0.06, I2 = 64%) (Figure 7). Furthermore, the heterogeneity was solved after excluding the study by Irwin (2017) [44] (p = 0.92, I2 = 0%), and the results show that martial arts significantly reduced fatigue, compared to the control group (SMD = −0.51, 95% CI: −0.80, −0.22]; *p* = 0.0005) (Figure A5).

	Martial Arts			Control				Std. Mean Difference
Study or Subgroup	**Mean**	**SD**	**Total**	**Mean**	**SD**	**Total**	**Weight**	**IV, Random, 95% CI**
1.3.1 Physical Function								
Campo 2013	70	12.5	29	65	8.75	25	11.6%	0.45 [-0.09, 0.99]
Larkey 2016	47.7	7.28	39	48.2	7.84	45	12.2%	-0.07 [-0.49, 0.36]
Sprod 2011	26.89	1.37	9	26.5	1.31	10	9.7%	0.28 [-0.63, 1.18]
Subtotal (95% CI)			**77**			**80**	**33.4%**	**0.16 [-0.18, 0.50]**
Heterogeneity: Tau² = 0.01; Chi² = 2.23, df = 2 (P = 0.33); I² = 10%								
Test for overall effect: Z = 0.92 (P = 0.36)								
1.3.2 Mental Health								
Campo 2013	80	4	29	80	5	25	11.7%	0.00 [-0.53, 0.53]
Larkey 2016	51.5	8.7	39	50.7	8.52	45	12.2%	0.09 [-0.34, 0.52]
Sprod 2011	24.78	0.68	9	24.8	1.01	10	9.7%	-0.02 [-0.92, 0.88]
Subtotal (95% CI)			**77**			**80**	**33.5%**	**0.05 [-0.27, 0.36]**
Heterogeneity: Tau² = 0.00; Chi² = 0.09, df = 2 (P = 0.95); I² = 0%								
Test for overall effect: Z = 0.29 (P = 0.77)								
1.3.3 Social Function								
Campo 2013	87.5	12.5	29	100	12.5	25	11.5%	-0.99 [-1.55, -0.42]
Larkey 2016	95.75	7.87	50	82.44	7.26	49	12.0%	1.74 [1.28, 2.21]
Sprod 2011	8.63	0.63	9	9	0.58	10	9.6%	-0.59 [-1.51, 0.34]
Subtotal (95% CI)			**88**			**84**	**33.0%**	**0.07 [-1.87, 2.01]**
Heterogeneity: Tau² = 2.82; Chi² = 58.92, df = 2 (P < 0.00001); I² = 97%								
Test for overall effect: Z = 0.07 (P = 0.94)								
Total (95% CI)			**242**			**244**	**100.0%**	**0.12 [-0.43, 0.67]**
Heterogeneity: Tau² = 0.59; Chi² = 65.02, df = 8 (P < 0.00001); I² = 88%								
Test for overall effect: Z = 0.43 (P = 0.67)								
Test for subgroup differences: Chi² = 0.23, df = 2 (P = 0.89), I² = 0%								

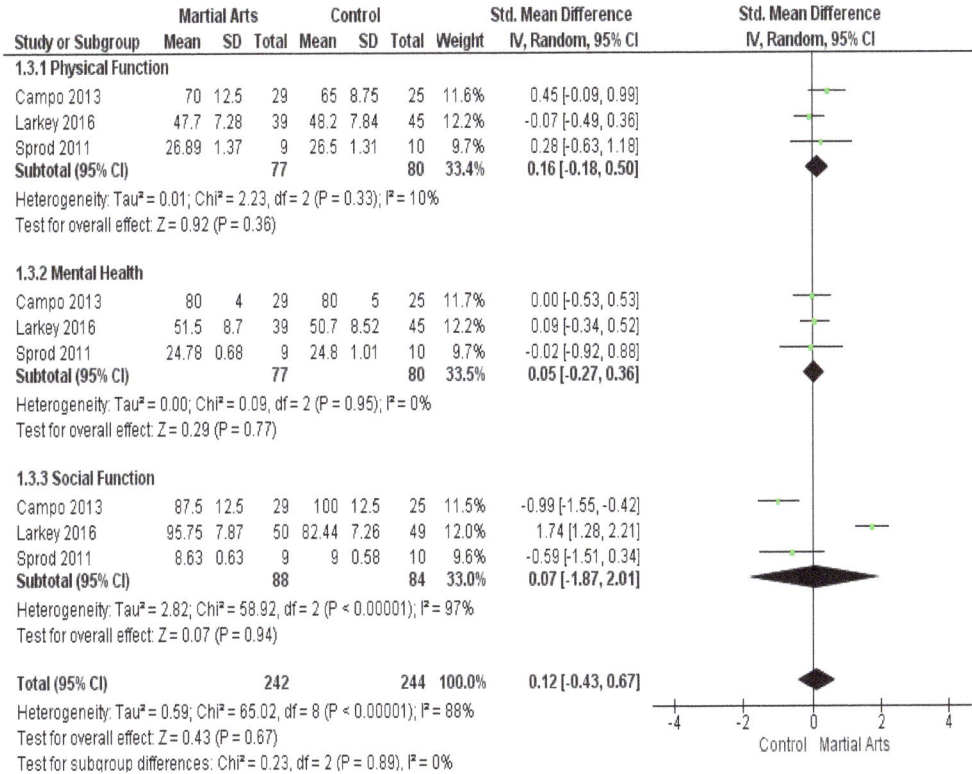

Figure 4. Analysis of the Short-Form 36.

	Martial Arts			Control				Std. Mean Difference
Study or Subgroup	**Mean**	**SD**	**Total**	**Mean**	**SD**	**Total**	**Weight**	**IV, Random, 95% CI**
McQuade 2017	1.45	1.6	21	1.87	1.61	24	33.2%	-0.26 [-0.85, 0.33]
Chuang 2017	0.37	1.39	48	4.95	1.57	48	33.1%	-3.06 [-3.66, -2.47]
Chen 2013	2.6	1.8	49	2.3	1.8	47	33.7%	0.17 [-0.24, 0.57]
Total (95% CI)			**118**			**119**	**100.0%**	**-1.04 [-2.96, 0.87]**
Heterogeneity: Tau² = 2.79; Chi² = 80.40, df = 2 (P < 0.00001); I² = 98%								
Test for overall effect: Z = 1.07 (P = 0.29)								

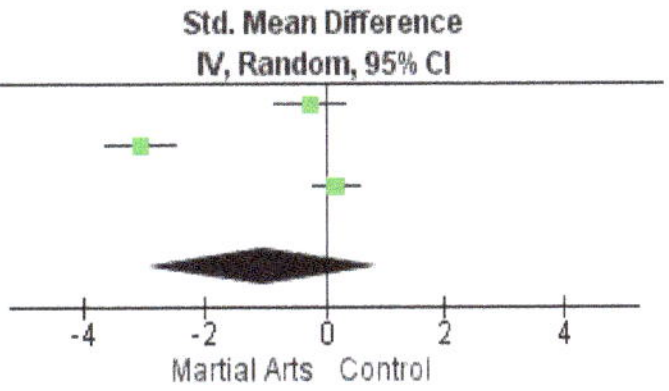

Figure 5. Analysis of the Brief Fatigue Inventory.

	Control			Control				Std. Mean Difference
Study or Subgroup	**Mean**	**SD**	**Total**	**Mean**	**SD**	**Total**	**Weight**	**IV, Random, 95% CI**
Mustian 2004	14.22	6.1	11	-0.11	44.7	10	10.6%	0.44 [-0.43, 1.31]
Mustian 2008	14.2	27.27	11	-0.4	32.37	10	10.6%	0.47 [-0.40, 1.34]
Oh 2009	6.34	8.88	79	0.64	6.41	83	78.9%	0.74 [0.42, 1.05]
Total (95% CI)			**101**			**103**	**100.0%**	**0.68 [0.39, 0.96]**
Heterogeneity: Tau² = 0.00; Chi² = 0.63, df = 2 (P = 0.73); I² = 0%								
Test for overall effect: Z = 4.69 (P < 0.00001)								

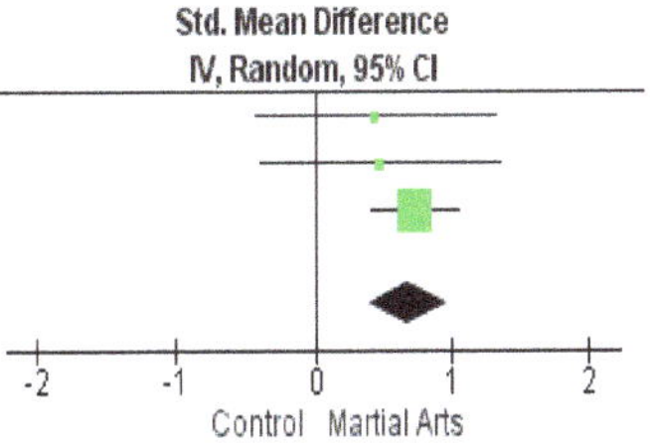

Figure 6. Analysis of Functional Assessment of Chronic Illness Therapy—Fatigue.

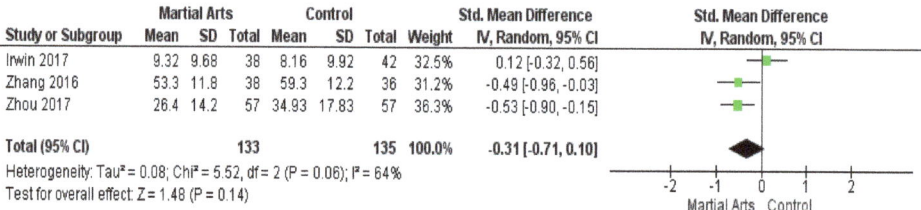

Figure 7. Analysis of the multidimensional fatigue symptom inventory-short form.

3.9. Quality Assessment of the Included Studies

An overall moderate risk of bias was found in selection, reporting, and other bias. Furthermore, performance, detection, and attribution biases were judged as having a high risk of bias. Detailed risk of bias summary and graph are shown in Figures 8 and 9.

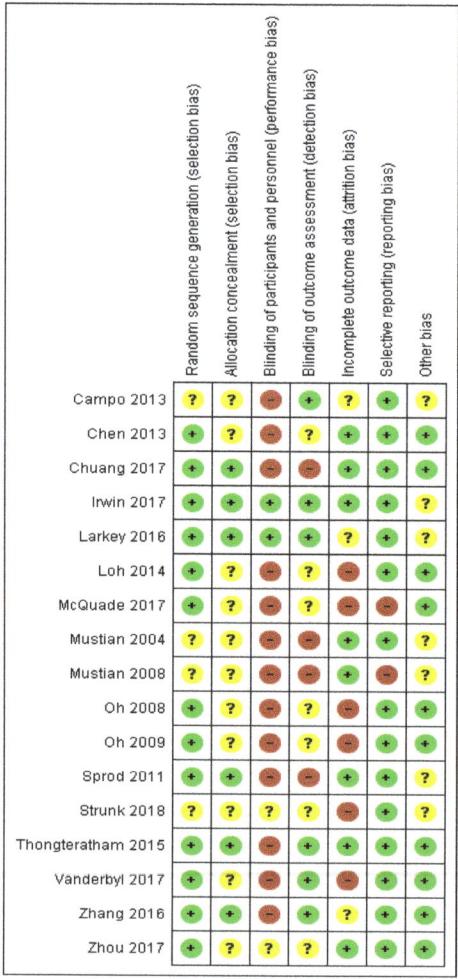

Figure 8. Risk of bias summary.

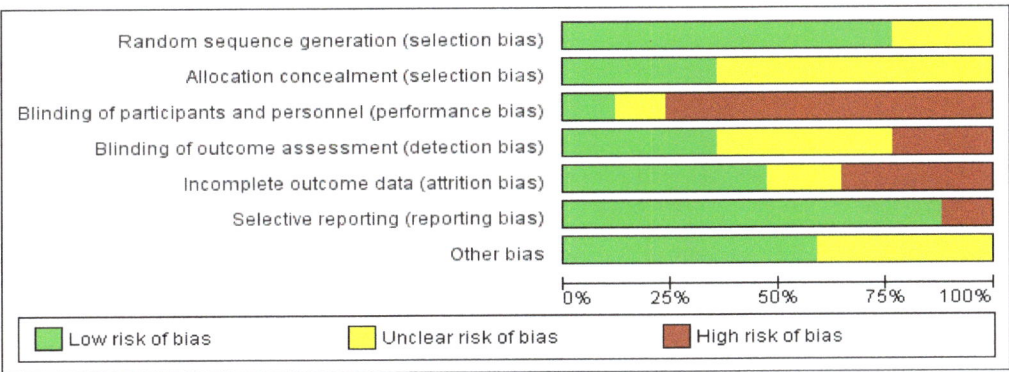

Figure 9. Risk of bias graph.

4. Discussion

Cancer patients are encouraged to participate in an exercise program during and following treatment [15]; however, there are still gaps related to regimes and forms of exercise appropriate for each individual. Improvement of QoL in cancer patients and management of their CRF have gained importance in recent years to enhance the general wellbeing of cancer patients and ameliorate the side effects of cancer therapies [62]. Multiple studies have covered the role of physical activity and exercise studying their effects on QoL and CRF of cancer patients during and after standard cancer treatment [63]. In this regard, martial arts have gained popularity in western countries as a new form of physical activity. In addition, martial arts combine musculoskeletal conditioning and training in cognitive skills, together with breathing exercises, which are typically delivered in group training sessions that also provide social support for cancer patients [24]. The results of the benefits of martial arts on QoL and CRF have been reported in several studies with a limited number of participants covering limited martial arts disciplines and cancer types [41–57].

This is the first systematic review and meta-analysis grouping martial arts and their effects on QoL and CRF as a primary intervention in cancer patients during and after treatment, regardless of the cancer type and treatment received. The data extracted from different studies of cancer patients practicing martial arts show a significant improvement of social function measured through SF-36 and a significant reduction of CRF measured using FACIT-F and MFSI-SF. The effects reported on social function by Campo et al. [41] and Sprod et al. [52] were positive but modest in their studied population. Social function is an important dimension for cancer patients since the disease and its treatment can affect diverse aspects, such as marital relationships, parental responsibilities, work environment, and social activities [64]. Regarding the significant reduction of CRF using the FACIT-F assessment scale, Oh et al. found a significant difference in their study of breast cancer survivors practicing Tai Chi Chuan for 60 min, 3 times per week, for 12 weeks [51]. Mustian et al. found a non-significant positive effect on fatigue measured by the same tool in breast cancer survivors practicing Tai Chi, possibly due to the small number of participants in their studies [48,49]. Considering the CRF measured through the MFSI-SF scale, Zhou et al. found a significant reduction of CRF in nasopharyngeal patients undergoing radiotherapy after practicing Tai chi for 60 min, 5 times per week, for 8 months [57]. In line with these results, another study found that lung cancer patients who followed a Tai Chi program of 60 min every other day for 12 weeks and underwent chemotherapy had a significant reduction of CRF, compared to those who were in a low-impact exercise program. This reduction was observed after 6 and 12 weeks of the program initiation [56]. Other outcomes analyzed in this meta-analysis did not reach a significant difference, even after heterogeneity was solved.

In the articles analyzed by our team, most of the patients in the trials were breast cancer patients who finished their treatment and started a program for physical activity or are undergoing chemotherapy or radiotherapy. The trials analyzed had small batches of patients enrolled and the population was too heterogeneous for us to be able to conclude about the optimal load and specifics of exercises. Furthermore, most of the martial arts sessions presented ranged from a period of 3 weeks to 24 weeks of practice, with a normal session being 40–60 min. The schedule of the sessions was from 2 weekly classes to 12 weekly classes depending on the type of martial arts. Taking into account the results of the analyzed trials, we consider that practicing martial arts is safe and recommended for patients undergoing treatment as well as for cancer survivors at the completion of their oncological therapy

Other meta-analyses have reviewed the effects of martial arts in QoL and/or CRF [64,65]. Tao et al. in a study analyzed the effects of acupuncture, Tuina, Tai Chi, Qigong, and traditional Chinese music therapy on symptom management and QoL in cancer patients. According to the results, Tai Chi and Qigong had no effect on QoL or CRF in breast cancer survivors [65]. Wayne et al. also analyzed the effects of Tai Chi and Qigong in cancer survivors, finding a significant improvement in CRF, sleep difficulty, depression, and overall QoL, as well as a non-significant trend in pain control [66].

Albeit all the evidence points to the benefits of physical activity in cancer patients, these changes to increase their physical activity seem harder to implement by cancer patients [67]. Martial arts have been demonstrated in several studies to be a feasible option for cancer patients [41,53]. Moreover, they may reduce some of the negative effects of cancer and improve physical as well as psychological health [68]. This study may help healthcare professionals involved in cancer management and patients decide to choose an activity to improve QoL and reduce CRF. Martial arts offer a wide variety of disciplines with different levels of intensity that would allow cancer patients the possibility of deciding the activity that fits better with their needs.

Different guidelines covering CRF, such as NCCN (National Comprehensive Cancer Network) guidelines, focused on CRF [15], and the guidelines from the Oncology Nursing Society "Putting Evidence into Practice" [69] proposed exercise and physical activity as a first-line intervention for CRF. Other interventions, in addition to erythropoiesis-stimulating agents and low-dose dexamethasone, do not offer effectiveness reducing CRF in patients with cancer [69]. The beneficial effects of martial arts in QoL of cancer patients can be due to the relaxation response and the immunomodulatory [50,70] and hormonal effects [71]. A recent meta-analysis has shown that Tai Chi has an impact on reducing cortisol levels in breast cancer survivors. The same study showed an impact on physical and mental health, improving limb-muscular function and promoted sleep [72].

There is some evidence showing that CRF and QoL are not improved only by physical exercises [73,74], supporting the concept that a more holistic approach should be considered in order to benefit these outcomes in cancer patients. Adverse effects due to martial arts practice did not exist in several studies [42,49,51].

Meta-analyses allow overcoming several limitations. First, pooling the data from different studies allows correcting the statistical limitation of the small sample data of some of the analyzed studies. Another strength is that meta-analyses allow detecting the heterogeneity existing in different studies that used martial arts as a primary intervention in cancer patients. It also helps settle the effect from conflicting results coming from different studies.

Regarding the limitations of this study, one can refer to the analysis of only studies that were published in English. This fact excludes the articles written in other languages that could represent the evidence better and make more general conclusions. Second, the diversity of the outcomes measured in the studies analyzed in this meta-analysis made the task of comparison arduous. Future studies should report outcomes in a more homogeneous way in order to be able to pool all available data. Another limitation is that the majority of the studies analyzed were performed on breast cancer survivors, limiting the conclusions drawn in this study to this group of patients. Accordingly, future studies involving the investigation of the effects on QoL and CRF of martial arts in cancer patients should cover other cancer types. In that way, it would be possible to stratify the results by cancer types and other variables, such as age or other interesting conditions, including gender or grade of disability, which could help tailor the interventions to the patients' needs. In addition, the control groups analyzed were very heterogeneous, and this could be a source of heterogeneity of this study. Another limitation comes from the fact that the analyzed studies covered broad inclusion criteria related to how fatigue was evaluated in those patients enrolled. Finally, some limitations are due to the sample size of the studies and the fact that the patients in some cases were not homogenously under cancer treatment, limitations that are intrinsic to the scarce available data in this regard.

Future studies should address the limitations existing in previous trials. Sample size was an issue in several trials, not providing enough statistical power to draw significant observations. Furthermore, martial arts should be studied in more cancer types, and patients should be stratified in order to be able to extract cancer- and population-specific conclusions. Moreover, trials should try to overcome a common issue where neither the participants nor the instructors or investigators were blinded to the condition against drug trial recommendations. Another limitation was related to the selection bias found in several of the analyzed studies. Longer intervention periods should be followed in order to see if the interventions have effects on cancer survivors.

5. Conclusions

The results of this systematic review and meta-analysis reveal that the effects of practicing martial arts on CRF and QoL in cancer patients and survivors are inconclusive. Although some potential effects were seen for social function and CRF, the results are inconsistent across different measurement methods. Therefore, larger and more homogeneous clinical trials encompassing different cancer types and specific martial arts disciplines are needed before definitive cancer- and symptom-specific recommendations can be made.

Author Contributions: Formal analysis, S.S.; Investigation, D.S., S.S. and S.A.; Resources, S.A.; Data curation, D.S., S.S. and S.A.; writing—original draft preparation, D.S.; and writing—review and editing, D.S., S.S. and S.A. All authors have read and agreed to the published version of the manuscript.

Funding: There is no financial support for this study.

Institutional Review Board Statement: Not applicable.

Informed Consent Statement: Not applicable.

Data Availability Statement: The data that support the findings of this study are available on request from the corresponding author.

Acknowledgments: The authors would like to thank all people who participated in this study and Antoni Torres for professional medical writing and editing services.

Conflicts of Interest: The authors have no conflict of interests regarding the publication of this study.

Appendix A

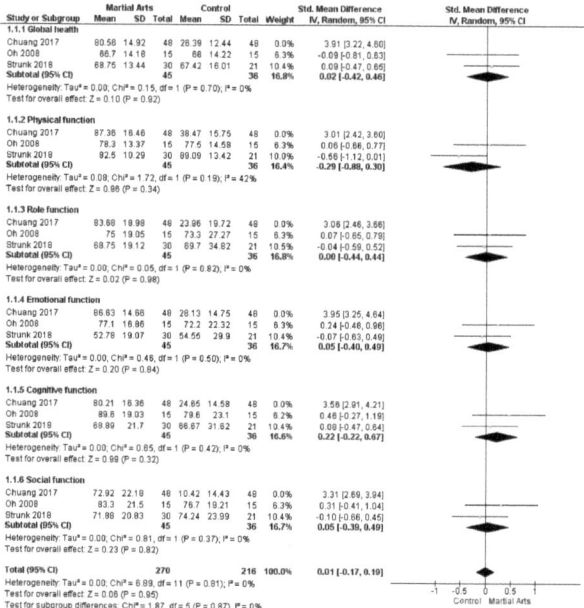

Figure A1. Results of EORTC QLQ-C30 after sensitivity analysis.

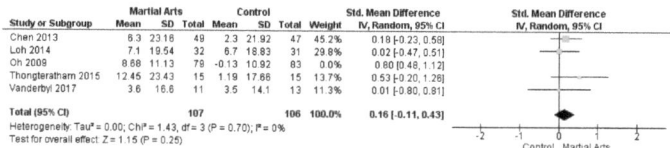

Figure A2. Results of FACT-G change after sensitivity analysis.

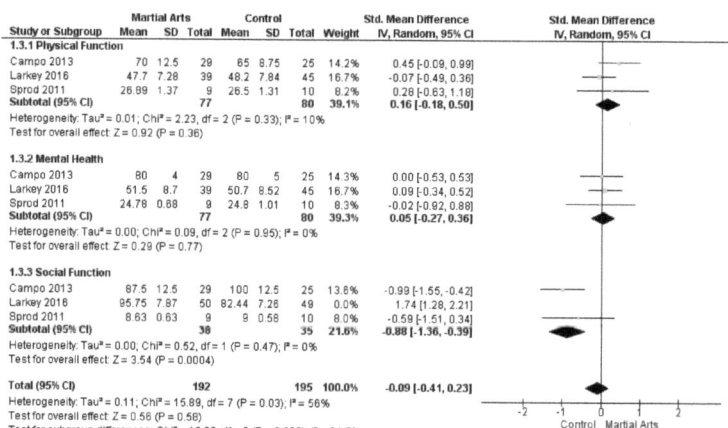

Figure A3. Results of SF-36 after sensitivity analysis.

Study or Subgroup	Martial Arts Mean	Martial Arts SD	Martial Arts Total	Control Mean	Control SD	Control Total	Weight	Std. Mean Difference IV, Random, 95% CI
McQuade 2017	1.45	1.6	21	1.87	1.61	24	36.5%	-0.26 [-0.85, 0.33]
Chuang 2017	0.37	1.39	48	4.95	1.57	48	0.0%	-3.06 [-3.66, -2.47]
Chen 2013	2.6	1.8	49	2.3	1.8	47	63.5%	0.17 [-0.24, 0.57]
Total (95% CI)			**70**			**71**	**100.0%**	**0.01 [-0.39, 0.41]**

Heterogeneity: Tau² = 0.02; Chi² = 1.35, df = 1 (P = 0.24); I² = 26%
Test for overall effect: Z = 0.06 (P = 0.96)

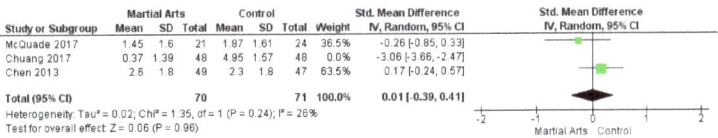

Figure A4. Results of BFI after sensitivity analysis.

Study or Subgroup	Martial Arts Mean	Martial Arts SD	Martial Arts Total	Control Mean	Control SD	Control Total	Weight	Std. Mean Difference IV, Random, 95% CI
Irwin 2017	9.32	9.68	38	8.16	9.92	42	0.0%	0.12 [-0.32, 0.56]
Zhang 2016	53.3	11.8	38	59.3	12.2	36	39.4%	-0.49 [-0.96, -0.03]
Zhou 2017	26.4	14.2	57	34.93	17.83	57	60.6%	-0.53 [-0.90, -0.15]
Total (95% CI)			**95**			**93**	**100.0%**	**-0.51 [-0.80, -0.22]**

Heterogeneity: Tau² = 0.00; Chi² = 0.01, df = 1 (P = 0.92); I² = 0%
Test for overall effect: Z = 3.46 (P = 0.0005)

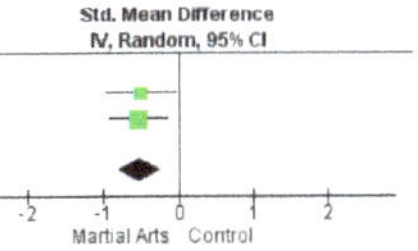

Figure A5. Results of MFSI-SF after sensitivity analysis.

References

1. Sung, H.; Ferlay, J.; Siegel, R.L.; Laversanne, M.; Soerjomataram, I.; Jemal, A.; Bray, F. Global cancer statistics 2020: GLOBOCAN estimates of incidence and mortality worldwide for 36 cancers in 185 countries. *CA Cancer J. Clin.* **2018**, *68*, 394–424. [CrossRef]
2. Mattiuzzi, C.; Lippi, G. Current cancer epidemiology. *J. Epidemiol. Glob. Health* **2019**, *9*, 217–222. [CrossRef]
3. Allemani, C.; Matsuda, T.; Di Carlo, V.; Harewood, R.; Matz, M.; Niksic, M.; Bonaventure, A.; Valkov, M.; Johnson, C.J.; Estève, J.; et al. Global surveillance of trends in cancer survival: Analysis of individual records for 37,513,025 patients diagnosed with one of 18 cancers during 2000–2014 from 322 population-based registries in 71 countries (CONCORD-3). *Lancet* **2018**, *391*, 1023–1075. [CrossRef]
4. Siegel, R.L.; Miller, K.D.; Jemal, A. Cancer statistics, 2020. *CA Cancer J. Clin.* **2020**, *70*, 7–30. [CrossRef]
5. Shah, S.C.; Kayamba, V.; Peek, R.M., Jr.; Heimburger, D. Cancer control in low- and middle-income countries: Is it time to consider screening? *J. Glob. Oncol.* **2019**, *5*, 1–8. [CrossRef]
6. Pearman, T. Quality of life and psychosocial adjustment in gynecologic cancer survivors. *Health Qual. Life Outcomes* **2003**, *1*, 1–6. [CrossRef]
7. Trask, P.C. Quality of life and emotional distress in advanced prostate cancer survivors undergoing chemotherapy. *Health Qual. Life Outcomes* **2004**, *2*, 1–5. [CrossRef]
8. WHO WHOQOL: Measuring Quality of Life 2020. Available online: https://www.who.int/toolkits/whoqol (accessed on 14 December 2020).
9. Hornquist, J.O. Quality of life: Concept and assessment. *Scand. J. Public Health* **1990**, *18*, 69–79. [CrossRef]
10. Schirrmacher, V. From chemotherapy to biological therapy: A review of novel concepts to reduce the side effects of systemic cancer treatment (review). *Int. J. Oncol.* **2019**, *54*, 407–419. [CrossRef]
11. Byar, K.L.; Berger, A.M.; Bakken, S.L.; Cetak, M.A. Impact of adjuvant breast cancer chemotherapy on fatigue, other symptoms, and quality of life. *Oncol. Nurs. Forum* **2006**, *33*, 18–26. [CrossRef]
12. Hickok, J.T.; Roscoe, J.A.; Morrow, G.R.; Mustian, K.; Okunieff, P.; Bole, C.W. Frequency, severity, clinical course, and correlates of fatigue in 372 patients during 5 weeks of radiotherapy for cancer. *Cancer* **2005**, *104*, 1772–1778. [CrossRef]
13. Meneses, K.; Benz, R. Quality of life in cancer survivorship: 20 years later. *Semin. Oncol. Nurs.* **2010**, *26*, 36–46. [CrossRef]
14. Berger, A.M.; Mitchell, S.A.; Jacobsen, P.B.; Pirl, W.F. Screening, evaluation, and management of cancer-related fatigue: Ready for implementation to practice? *CA Cancer J. Clin.* **2015**, *65*, 190–211. [CrossRef]
15. Berger, A.M.; Mooney, K.; Alvarez-Perez, A.; Breitbart, W.S.; Carpenter, K.M.; Cella, D.; Cleeland, C.; Dotan, E.; Eisenberger, M.A.; Escalante, C.P.; et al. Cancer-related fatigue, version 2. 2015. *J. Natl. Compr. Cancer Netw.* **2015**, *13*, 1012–1039. [CrossRef]
16. Siefert, M.L. Fatigue, pain, and functional status during outpatient chemotherapy. *Oncol. Nurs. Forum* **2010**, *37*, E114–E123. [CrossRef]
17. Lis, C.G.; Rodeghier, M.; Gupta, D. Distribution and determinants of patient satisfaction in oncology: A review of the literature. *Patient Prefer. Adherence* **2009**, *3*, 287–304. [CrossRef] [PubMed]
18. Bower, J.E. Cancer-related fatigue–mechanisms, risk factors, and treatments. *Nat. Rev. Clin. Oncol.* **2014**, *11*, 597–609. [CrossRef] [PubMed]
19. Maltser, S.; Cristian, A.; Silver, J.K.; Morris, G.S.; Stout, N.L. A focused review of safety considerations in cancer rehabilitation. *PM R* **2017**, *9*, S415–S428. [CrossRef] [PubMed]
20. Campbell, K.L.; Winters-Stone, K.M.; Wiskemann, J.; May, A.M.; Schwartz, A.L.; Courneya, K.S.; Zucker, D.S.; Matthews, C.E.; Ligibel, J.A.; Gerber, L.H.; et al. Exercise guidelines for cancer survivors: Consensus statement from international multidisciplinary roundtable. *Med. Sci. Sports Exerc.* **2019**, *51*, 2375–2390. [CrossRef] [PubMed]
21. Silver, J.K.; Gilchrist, L.S. Cancer rehabilitation with a focus on evidence-based outpatient physical and occupational therapy interventions. *Am. J. Phys. Med. Rehabil.* **2011**, *90*, 5–15. [CrossRef] [PubMed]

22. Demark-Wahnefried, W.; Rogers, L.Q.; Alfano, C.M.; Thomson, C.A.; Courneya, K.S.; Meyerhardt, J.A.; Stout, N.L.; Kvale, E.; Ganzer, H.; Ligibel, J.A. Practical clinical interventions for diet, physical activity, and weight control in cancer survivors. *CA Cancer J. Clin.* **2015**, *65*, 167–189. [CrossRef] [PubMed]
23. Hayes, S.C.; Newton, R.U.; Spence, R.R.; Galvão, D.A. The exercise and sports science australia position statement: Exercise medicine in cancer management. *J. Sci. Med. Sport* **2019**, *22*, 1175–1199. [CrossRef]
24. Burke, D.T.; Al-Adawi, S.; Lee, Y.T.; Audette, J. Martial arts as sport and therapy. *J. Sports Med. Phys. Fit.* **2007**, *47*, 96–102.
25. Pons van Dijk, G.; Leffers, P.; Lodder, J. The effectiveness of hard martial arts in people over forty: An attempted systematic review. *Societies* **2014**, *4*, 161–179. [CrossRef]
26. Lomas-Vega, R.; Obrero-Gaitán, E.; Molina-Ortega, F.J.; Del-Pino-Casado, R. Tai chi for risk of falls. A meta-analysis. *J. Am. Geriatr. Soc.* **2017**, *65*, 2037–2043. [CrossRef]
27. Witte, K.; Kropf, S.; Darius, S.; Emmermacher, P.; Böckelmann, I. Comparing the effectiveness of karate and fitness training on cognitive functioning in older adults—A randomized controlled trial. *J. Sport Health Sci.* **2016**, *5*, 484–490. [CrossRef]
28. Shamseer, L.; Moher, D.; Clarke, M.; Ghersi, D.; Liberati, A.; Petticrew, M.; Shekelle, P.; Stewart, L.A.; Altman, D.G.; Booth, A.; et al. Preferred reporting items for systematic review and meta-analysis protocols (prisma-p) 2015: Elaboration and explanation. *BMJ* **2015**, *349*, 1–25. [CrossRef]
29. Aslam, S.; Emmanuel, P. Formulating a researchable question: A critical step for facilitating good clinical research. *Indian J. Sex. Transm. Dis. AIDS* **2010**, *31*, 47–50. [CrossRef]
30. Fayers, P.; Aaronson, N.; Bjordal, K.; Groenvold, M. *EORTC QLQ-C30 Scoring Manual*, 3rd ed.; European Organisation for Research and Treatment of Cancer: Brussels, Beigium, 2001.
31. Cella, D.F.; Tulsky, D.S.; Gray, G.; Sarafian, B.; Linn, E.; Bonomi, A.; Silberman, M.; Yellen, S.B.; Winicour, P.; Brannon, J.; et al. The functional assessment of cancer therapy scale: Development and validation of the general measure. *J. Clin. Oncol.* **1993**, *11*, 570–579. [CrossRef]
32. Ware, J.E.; Kosinski, M.A.; Keller, S.D. *SF-36 Physical and Mental Health Summary Scales—A User's Manual*; Health Assessment Lab.: Boston, MA, USA, 1994; pp. 1–147.
33. Mendoza, T.R.; Wang, X.S.; Cleeland, C.S.; Morrissey, M.; Johnson, B.A.; Wendt, J.K.; Huber, S.L. The rapid assessment of fatigue severity in cancer patients. *Cancer* **1999**, *85*, 1186–1196. [CrossRef]
34. Cella, D.; Nowinski, C.J. Measuring quality of life in chronic illness: The functional assessment of chronic illness therapy measurement system. *Arch. Phys. Med. Rehabil.* **2002**, *83*, 10–17. [CrossRef]
35. Donovan, K.A.; Stein, K.D.; Lee, M.; Leach, C.R.; Ilozumba, O.; Jacobsen, P.B. Systematic review of the multidimensional fatigue symptom inventory-short form. *Support. Care Cancer* **2015**, *23*, 191–212. [CrossRef] [PubMed]
36. Pien, L.C.; Chu, H.; Chen, W.C.; Chang, Y.S.; Liao, Y.M.; Chen, C.H.; Chou, K.R. Reliability and validity of a Chinese version of the multidimensional fatigue symptom inventory-short form (MFSI-SF-C). *J. Clin. Nurs.* **2011**, *20*, 2224–2232. [CrossRef]
37. The Grading of Recommendations Assessment, Development and Evaluation (Grade) Guidelines 2020. Available online: https://www.gradeworkinggroup.org/ (accessed on 10 December 2020).
38. Higgins, J.P.T.; Thomas, J.; Chandler, J.; Cumpston, M.; Li, T.; Page, M.J.; Welch, V.A. *Cochrane Handbook for Systematic Reviews of Interventions, version 6.1 (updated September 2020)*; John Wiley & Sons: Hoboken, NJ, USA, 2020; Available online: www.training.cochrane.org/handbook (accessed on 10 December 2020).
39. Matthews, J.N.S.; Altman, D.G. Statistics notes: Interaction 3: How to examine heterogeneity. *BMJ* **1996**, *313*, 862. [CrossRef] [PubMed]
40. Terrin, N.; Schmid, C.H.; Lau, J.; Olkin, I. Adjusting for publication bias in the presence of heterogeneity. *Stat. Med.* **2003**, *22*, 2113–2126. [CrossRef]
41. Campo, R.A.; O'Connor, K.; Light, K.C.; Nakamura, Y.; Lipschitz, D.L.; Lastayo, P.C.; Pappas, L.; Boucher, K.; Irwin, M.R.; Agarwal, N.; et al. Feasibility and acceptability of a Tai Chi Chih randomized controlled trial in senior female cancer survivors. *Integr. Cancer Ther.* **2013**, *12*, 464–474. [CrossRef]
42. Chen, Z.; Meng, Z.; Milbury, K.; Bei, W.; Zhang, Y.; Thornton, B.; Liao, Z.; Wei, Q.; Chen, J.; Guo, X.; et al. Qigong improves quality of life in women undergoing radiotherapy for breast cancer: Results of a randomized controlled trial. *Cancer* **2013**, *119*, 1690–1698. [CrossRef] [PubMed]
43. Chuang, T.Y.; Yeh, M.L.; Chung, Y.C. A nurse facilitated mind-body interactive exercise (Chan-Chuang Qigong) improves the health status of non-Hodgkin lymphoma patients receiving chemotherapy: Randomised controlled trial. *Int. J. Nurs. Stud.* **2017**, *69*, 25–33. [CrossRef] [PubMed]
44. Irwin, M.R.; Olmstead, R.; Carrillo, C.; Sadeghi, N.; Nicassio, P.; Ganz, P.A.; Bower, J.E. Tai Chi Chih compared with cognitive behavioral therapy for the treatment of insomnia in survivors of breast cancer: A randomized, partially blinded, noninferiority trial. *J. Clin. Oncol.* **2017**, *35*, 2656–2665. [CrossRef] [PubMed]
45. Larkey, L.K.; Roe, D.J.; Smith, L.; Millstine, D. Exploratory outcome assessment of Qigong/Tai Chi easy on breast cancer survivors. *Complement. Ther. Med.* **2016**, *29*, 196–203. [CrossRef]
46. Loh, S.Y.; Lee, S.Y.; Murray, L. The Kuala Lumpur Qigong trial for women in the cancer survivorship phase-efficacy of a three-arm RCT to improve QOL. *Asian Pac. J. Cancer Prev.* **2014**, *15*, 8127–8134. [CrossRef]

47. McQuade, J.L.; Prinsloo, S.; Chang, D.Z.; Spelman, A.; Wei, Q.; Basen-Engquist, K.; Harrison, C.; Zhang, Z.; Kuban, D.; Lee, A.; et al. Qigong/Tai Chi for sleep and fatigue in prostate cancer patients undergoing radiotherapy: A randomized controlled trial. *Psychooncology.* **2017**, *26*, 1936–1943. [CrossRef] [PubMed]
48. Mustian, K.M.; Katula, J.A.; Gill, D.L.; Roscoe, J.A.; Lang, D.; Murphy, K. Tai Chi Chuan, health-related quality of life and self-esteem: A randomized trial with breast cancer survivors. *Support. Care Cancer* **2004**, *12*, 871–876. [CrossRef] [PubMed]
49. Mustian, K.; Palesh, O.; Flecksteiner, S. Tai Chi Chuan for breast cancer survivors. *Med. Sport Sci.* **2008**, *52*, 209–217. [CrossRef]
50. Oh, B.; Butow, P.; Mullan, B.; Clarke, S. Medical qigong for cancer patients: Pilot study of impact on quality of life, side effects of treatment and inflammation. *Am. J. Chin. Med.* **2008**, *36*, 459–472. [CrossRef]
51. Oh, B.; Butow, P.; Mullan, B.; Clarke, S.; Beale, P.; Pavlakis, N.; Kothe, E.; Lam, L.; Rosenthal, D. Impact of medical qigong on quality of life, fatigue, mood and inflammation in cancer patients: A randomized controlled trial. *Ann. Oncol.* **2009**, *21*, 608–614. [CrossRef]
52. Sprod, L.K.; Janelsins, M.C.; Palesh, O.G.; Carroll, J.K.; Heckler, C.E.; Peppone, L.J.; Mohile, S.G.; Morrow, G.R.; Mustian, K.M. Health-related quality of life and biomarkers in breast cancer survivors participating in Tai Chi Chuan. *J. Cancer Surviv.* **2012**, *6*, 146–154. [CrossRef] [PubMed]
53. Strunk, M.A.; Zopf, E.M.; Steck, J.; Hamacher, S.; Hallek, M.; Baumann, F.T. Effects of kyusho jitsu on physical activity-levels and quality of life in breast cancer patients. *In Vivo* **2018**, *32*, 819–824. [CrossRef]
54. Thongteratham, N.; Pongthavornkamol, K.; Olson, K.; Ratanawichitrasin, A.; Nityasuddhi, D.; Wattanakitkrilert, D. Effectiveness of Tai Chi Qi Qong program for Thai women with breast cancer: A randomized control trial. *Pac. Rim Int. J. Nurs. Res.* **2015**, *19*, 280–294.
55. Vanderbyl, B.L.; Mayer, M.J.; Nash, C.; Tran, A.T.; Windholz, T.; Swanson, T.; Kasymjanova, G.; Jagoe, R.T. A comparison of the effects of medical Qigong and standard exercise therapy on symptoms and quality of life in patients with advanced cancer. *Support. Care Cancer* **2017**, *25*, 1749–1758. [CrossRef] [PubMed]
56. Zhang, L.L.; Wang, S.Z.; Chen, H.L.; Yuan, A.Z. Tai Chi exercise for cancer-related fatigue in patients with lung cancer undergoing chemotherapy: A randomized controlled trial. *J. Pain Symptom Manag.* **2016**, *51*, 504–511. [CrossRef]
57. Zhou, W.; Wan, Y.H.; Chen, Q.; Qiu, Y.R.; Luo, X.M. Effects of Tai Chi exercise on cancer-related fatigue in patients with nasopharyngeal carcinoma undergoing chemoradiotherapy: A randomized controlled trial. *J. Pain Symptom Manag.* **2018**, *55*, 737–744. [CrossRef]
58. Huston, P.; McFarlane, B. Health benefits of Tai Chi. *Can. Fam. Physician* **2016**, *62*, 881–890.
59. Chang, P.S.; Knobf, T. Qigong exercise and Tai Chi in cancer care. *Asia Pac. J. Oncol. Nurs.* **2019**, *6*, 315–317. [CrossRef] [PubMed]
60. Klein, P. Qigong in cancer care: Theory, evidence-base, and practice. *Medicines* **2017**, *4*, 2. [CrossRef]
61. Jahnke, R.; Larkey, L.; Rogers, C.; Etnier, J.; Lin, F. A comprehensive review of health benefits of qigong and tai chi. *Am. J. Health Promot.* **2010**, *24*, e1–e25. [CrossRef]
62. Charalambous, A.; Kouta, C. Cancer related fatigue and quality of life in patients with advanced prostate cancer undergoing chemotherapy. *Biomed. Res. Int.* **2016**, *2016*. [CrossRef]
63. Velthuis, M.J.; Agasi-Idenburg, S.C.; Aufdemkampe, G.; Wittink, H.M. The effect of physical exercise on cancer-related fatigue during cancer treatment: A meta-analysis of randomised controlled trials. *Clin. Oncol.* **2010**, *22*, 208–221. [CrossRef]
64. Hahn, E.A.; Kallen, M.A.; Jensen, R.E.; Potosky, A.L.; Carol, M.; Ramirez, M.; Cella, D.; Teresi, J.A. Measuring social function in diverse cancer populations: Evaluation of measurement equivalence of the Patient Reported Outcomes Measurement Information System® (PROMIS®) ability to participate in social roles and activities short form. *Psychol. Test. Assess. Model.* **2016**, *58*, 403–421. [PubMed]
65. Tao, W.W.; Jiang, H.; Tao, X.M.; Jiang, P.; Sha, L.Y.; Sun, X.C. Effects of acupuncture, tuina, tai chi, qigong, and traditional chinese medicine five-element music therapy on symptom management and quality of life for cancer patients: A meta-analysis. *J. Pain Symptom Manag.* **2016**, *51*, 728–747. [CrossRef] [PubMed]
66. Wayne, P.; Lee, M.; Novakowski, J.; Osypiuk, K.; Ligibel, J.; Carlson, L.; Rong, S. Tai Chi and Qigong for cancer-related symptoms and quality of life: A systematic review and meta-analysis. *J. Cancer Surviv.* **2018**, *12*, 256–267. [CrossRef]
67. Yaw, Y.H.; Shariff, Z.M.; Kandiah, M.; Weay, Y.H.; Saibul, N.; Sariman, S.; Hashim, Z. Diet and physical activity in relation to weight change among breast cancer patients. *Asian Pac. J. Cancer Prev.* **2014**, *15*, 39–44. [CrossRef]
68. Abbott, R.; Lavretsky, H. Tai Chi and Qigong for the treatment and prevention of mental disorders. *Psychiatr. Clin. North. Am.* **2013**, *36*, 109–119. [CrossRef]
69. Mitchell, S.A.; Hoffman, A.J.; Clark, J.C.; Degennaro, R.M.; Poirier, P.; Robinson, C.B.; Weisbrod, B.L. Putting evidence into practice: An update of evidence-based interventions for cancer-related fatigue during and following treatment. *Clin. J. Oncol. Nurs.* **2015**, *18*, 38–58. [CrossRef] [PubMed]
70. Bower, J.E.; Irwin, M.R. Mind-body therapies and control of inflammatory biology: A descriptive review. *Brain Behav. Immun.* **2016**, *51*, 1–11. [CrossRef]
71. Rassovsky, Y.; Harwood, A.; Zagoory-Sharon, O.; Feldman, R. Martial arts increase oxytocin production. *Sci. Rep.* **2019**, *9*, 1–8. [CrossRef]
72. Ni, X.; Chan, R.J.; Yates, P.; Hu, W.; Huang, X.; Lou, Y. The effects of Tai Chi on quality of life of cancer survivors: A systematic review and meta-analysis. *Support. Care Cancer* **2019**, *27*, 3701–3716. [CrossRef] [PubMed]

73. Mutrie, N.; Campbell, A.M.; Whyte, F.; McConnachie, A.; Emslie, C.; Lee, L.; Kearney, N.; Walker, A.; Ritchie, D. Benefits of supervised group exercise programme for women being treated for early stage breast cancer: Pragmatic randomised controlled trial. *Br. Med. J.* **2007**, *334*, 517–520. [CrossRef]
74. Courneya, K.S.; Segal, R.J.; Mackey, J.R.; Gelmon, K.; Reid, R.D.; Friedenreich, C.M.; Ladha, A.B.; Proulx, C.; Vallance, J.K.H.; Lane, K.; et al. Effects of aerobic and resistance exercise in breast cancer patients receiving adjuvant chemotherapy: A multicenter randomized controlled trial. *J. Clin. Oncol.* **2007**, *25*, 4396–4404. [CrossRef] [PubMed]

MDPI
St. Alban-Anlage 66
4052 Basel
Switzerland
Tel. +41 61 683 77 34
Fax +41 61 302 89 18
www.mdpi.com

International Journal of Environmental Research and Public Health Editorial Office
E-mail: ijerph@mdpi.com
www.mdpi.com/journal/ijerph

www.ingramcontent.com/pod-product-compliance
Lightning Source LLC
LaVergne TN
LVHW070641100526
838202LV00013B/851